Digital Transformation in Healthcare

Digital Transformation in Healthcare

Editor

Marco P. Soares dos Santos

MDPI • Basel • Beijing • Wuhan • Barcelona • Belgrade • Manchester • Tokyo • Cluj • Tianjin

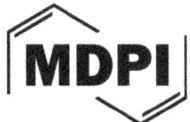

Editor
Marco P. Soares dos Santos
Departamento de Engenharia
Mecânica
Universidade de Aveiro
Aveiro
Portugal

Editorial Office
MDPI
St. Alban-Anlage 66
4052 Basel, Switzerland

This is a reprint of articles from the Special Issue published online in the open access journal *Healthcare* (ISSN 2227-9032) (available at: www.mdpi.com/journal/healthcare/special_issues/digital_transformation_healthcare).

For citation purposes, cite each article independently as indicated on the article page online and as indicated below:

LastName, A.A.; LastName, B.B.; LastName, C.C. Article Title. *Journal Name* **Year**, *Volume Number*, Page Range.

ISBN 978-3-0365-4870-8 (Hbk)
ISBN 978-3-0365-4869-2 (PDF)

© 2022 by the authors. Articles in this book are Open Access and distributed under the Creative Commons Attribution (CC BY) license, which allows users to download, copy and build upon published articles, as long as the author and publisher are properly credited, which ensures maximum dissemination and a wider impact of our publications.

The book as a whole is distributed by MDPI under the terms and conditions of the Creative Commons license CC BY-NC-ND.

Contents

About the Editor vii

Gaute Terning, Eric Christian Brun and Idriss El-Thalji
Modeling Patient Flow in an Emergency Department under COVID-19 Pandemic Conditions: A Hybrid Modeling Approach
Reprinted from: *Healthcare* **2022**, *10*, 840, doi:10.3390/healthcare10050840 1

Lersi D. Durán, Ana Margarida Almeida, Ana Cristina Lopes and Margarida Figueiredo-Braga
Impact of a Digital Intervention for Literacy in Depression among Portuguese University Students: A Randomized Controlled Trial
Reprinted from: *Healthcare* **2022**, *10*, 165, doi:10.3390/healthcare10010165 29

Andrej Thurzo, Veronika Kurilová and Ivan Varga
Artificial Intelligence in Orthodontic Smart Application for Treatment Coaching and Its Impact on Clinical Performance of Patients Monitored with AI-TeleHealth System
Reprinted from: *Healthcare* **2021**, *9*, 1695, doi:10.3390/healthcare9121695 41

Ibrahim El rube', David Heatley and Mohamed Abdel-Maguid
Detecting a Stroke-Affected Region in the Brain by Scanning with Low-Intensity Electromagnetic Waves in the Radio Frequency/Microwave Band
Reprinted from: *Healthcare* **2021**, *9*, 1170, doi:10.3390/healthcare9091170 65

Mohamed Yaseen Jabarulla and Heung-No Lee
A Blockchain and Artificial Intelligence-Based, Patient-Centric Healthcare System for Combating the COVID-19 Pandemic: Opportunities and Applications
Reprinted from: *Healthcare* **2021**, *9*, 1019, doi:10.3390/healthcare9081019 85

Tania Pereira, Joana Morgado, Francisco Silva, Michele M. Pelter, Vasco Rosa Dias and Rita Barros et al.
Sharing Biomedical Data: Strengthening AI Development in Healthcare
Reprinted from: *Healthcare* **2021**, *9*, 827, doi:10.3390/healthcare9070827 107

Gianluca Tornese, Riccardo Schiaffini, Enza Mozzillo, Roberto Franceschi, Anna Paola Frongia and Andrea Scaramuzza et al.
Telemedicine in the Time of the COVID-19 Pandemic: Results from the First Survey among Italian Pediatric Diabetes Centers
Reprinted from: *Healthcare* **2021**, *9*, 815, doi:10.3390/healthcare9070815 119

Na-Eun Cho
The Impact of Health Information Sharing on Hospital Costs
Reprinted from: *Healthcare* **2021**, *9*, 806, doi:10.3390/healthcare9070806 129

Chung-Feng Liu, Chien-Cheng Huang, Jhi-Joung Wang, Kuang-Ming Kuo and Chia-Jung Chen
The Critical Factors Affecting the Deployment and Scaling of Healthcare AI: Viewpoint from an Experienced Medical Center
Reprinted from: *Healthcare* **2021**, *9*, 685, doi:10.3390/healthcare9060685 139

Norbert Hosten, Britta Rosenberg and Andrzej Kram
Project Report on Telemedicine: What We Learned about the Administration and Development of a Binational Digital Infrastructure Project
Reprinted from: *Healthcare* **2021**, *9*, 400, doi:10.3390/healthcare9040400 151

Svea Storjohann, Michael Kirsch, Britta Rosenberg, Christian Rosenberg, Sandra Lange and Annika Syperek et al.
The Accuracy of On-Call CT Reporting in Teleradiology Networks in Comparison to In-House Reporting
Reprinted from: *Healthcare* **2021**, *9*, 405, doi:10.3390/healthcare9040405 173

Juan Uribe-Toril, José Luis Ruiz-Real and Bruno José Nievas-Soriano
A Study of eHealth from the Perspective of Social Sciences
Reprinted from: *Healthcare* **2021**, *9*, 108, doi:10.3390/healthcare9020108 183

Keunbada Son, Jung-Ho Lee and Kyu-Bok Lee
Comparison of Intaglio Surface Trueness of Interim Dental Crowns Fabricated with SLA 3D Printing, DLP 3D Printing, and Milling Technologies
Reprinted from: *Healthcare* **2021**, *9*, 983, doi:10.3390/healthcare9080983 201

Moon-Il Joo, Satyabrata Aich and Hee-Cheol Kim
Development of a System for Storing and Executing Bio-Signal Analysis Algorithms Developed in Different Languages
Reprinted from: *Healthcare* **2021**, *9*, 1016, doi:10.3390/healthcare9081016 211

Mateusz Świtała, Wojciech Zakrzewski, Zbigniew Rybak, Maria Szymonowicz and Maciej Dobrzyński
The Use of Modern Technologies by Dentists in Poland: Questionnaire among Polish Dentists
Reprinted from: *Healthcare* **2022**, *10*, 225, doi:10.3390/healthcare10020225 227

Xiao Wen Kok, Anisha Singh and Bahijja Tolulope Raimi-Abraham
A Design Approach to Optimise Secure Remote Three-Dimensional (3D) Printing: A Proof-of-Concept Study towards Advancement in Telemedicine
Reprinted from: *Healthcare* **2022**, *10*, 1114, doi:10.3390/healthcare10061114 241

About the Editor

Marco P. Soares dos Santos

Since 2020, Marco P. Soares dos Santos has held the tenured position of Assistant Professor in the Department of Mechanical Engineering, University of Aveiro, Portugal. He was also the Principal Investigator of the research project "SelfMED - The next-generation of biomechanical self-powering systems for multifunctional implantable medical devices" (POCI-01-0145-FEDER-031132). He has authored >30 publications in international peer-reviewed journals, including in journals with the highest impact in the areas of mechanical engineering, energy, applied physics, applied mathematics, and materials science. His scientific education was multidisciplinary, as is his scientific research path. He attained a 5-year graduation in Electrical and Computers Engineering, and later postgraduation in Industrial Automation Engineering (MSc degree) and Mechanical Engineering (PhD Degree). His research activity has been to explore the frontiers of automation engineering.

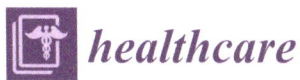

Article

Modeling Patient Flow in an Emergency Department under COVID-19 Pandemic Conditions: A Hybrid Modeling Approach

Gaute Terning [1,*], Eric Christian Brun [1] and Idriss El-Thalji [2]

[1] Department of Safety, Economics, and Planning, University of Stavanger, 4036 Stavanger, Norway; eric.brun@uis.no

[2] Department of Mechanical and Structural Engineering and Materials Science, University of Stavanger, 4036 Stavanger, Norway; idriss.el-thalji@uis.no

* Correspondence: gaute.terning@uis.no

Abstract: Emergency departments (EDs) had to considerably change their patient flow policies in the wake of the COVID-19 pandemic. Such changes affect patient crowding, waiting time, and other qualities related to patient care and experience. Field experiments, surveys, and simulation models can generally offer insights into patient flow under pandemic conditions. This paper provides a thorough and transparent account of the development of a multi-method simulation model that emulates actual patient flow in the emergency department under COVID-19 pandemic conditions. Additionally, a number of performance measures useful to practitioners are introduced. A conceptual model was extracted from the main stakeholders at the case hospital through incremental elaboration and turned into a computational model. Two agent types were mainly modeled: patient and rooms. The simulated behavior of patient flow was validated with real-world data (Smart Crowding) and was able to replicate actual behavior in terms of patient occupancy. In order to further the validity, the study recommends several phenomena to be studied and included in future simulation models such as more agents (medical doctors, nurses, beds), delays due to interactions with other departments in the hospital and treatment time changes at higher occupancies.

Keywords: healthcare; emergency department; patient flow; simulation modeling; agent-based modeling; pandemic decision support

1. Introduction

Emergency departments (EDs) are complex and crucial systems for accommodating patients in urgent and responsive need of health care [1]. Lately, there has been a particular focus on the ED under COVID-19 pandemic conditions [2], forcing us to rethink its organization [3]. Due to the pandemic conditions, EDs have had to adjust their operations according to regulations while cost-effectively managing their resources.

In order to comply with restrictions and guidelines, several management policies have been imposed simultaneously, e.g., changes in patient arrival handling, priorities of patients with suspected virus contamination, structural changes in patient flow, and the use of available space. Although such measures have put unprecedented strain on the department and its vital resources, they aim to ensure less overcrowding and treatment time while keeping the risk of contamination as low as possible.

In the past, ED crowding has been shown to have adverse effects on patient response time [4–8]. Overcrowding and treatment time can be regarded as systemic effects of several agent behaviors and multiple operating scenarios, which might be hard to explain by medical staff or revealed by field experiments or surveys. Computer modeling and simulation, in particular agent-based modeling, can thus be useful, as it allows to model organizational participants with their collective behavior [1,9–12]. It can further be used for decision support and to evaluate interventions, scenarios, operational risks, and cost-effectiveness of policies.

Overall, there is an increasing body of literature on modeling and simulation of ED patient flow [13,14]. There are several simulation models where the discrete event or system dynamics approaches mimic ED patient flow during normal conditions [13]. Such modeling and simulation approaches have also been used to model COVID-19 spread and transmission [4] and mass-vaccination facilities [15]. However, there is an unmet need for simulation models that mimic, explain, and predict ED patient flow under pandemic conditions while considering multiple agent behaviors [11], a feature not available in the discrete event or system dynamics approaches. Moreover, there is a lack of studies demonstrating rigorous and transparent construction of a conceptual model of an ED, which leads to difficulties for readers to understand, assess and build trust in such models. Furthermore, from a practitioner's point of view, there are several performance measures that ED managers use (such as time to treatment, the average length of stay, % full of triage room, etc.) that are not yet considered in existing simulation models.

This paper thus aims to answer the following research question:

How can we build a simulation model of the emergency department patient flow during COVID-19 pandemic conditions while considering multiple agent behaviors?

In this paper, we present a thorough description of how we developed such a simulation model. We first detail how we developed a conceptual model building on system knowledge and expertise from a case organization. Following that, we show how this conceptual model was incorporated into a hybrid computational model, where agent-based modeling was used to model patient behavior, and discrete event modeling was used to model resources (e.g., treatment rooms, triage beds, extra treatment rooms, pre-triage). The modeling approach we used consisted of (1) case study and systems analysis, (2) conceptual modeling, (3) computational modeling, and (4) verification and validation. Moreover, the main key performance indicators (KPIs) for patient flow used by practitioners were integrated and visualized.

The remainder of this article is organized as follows: the following Materials and Methods section will briefly illustrate the applied four-step simulation modeling process, fundamentals of the main methods used, description of the case study (process, facility), and input data (patient arrival data). Next, the Results section will provide rigorous documentation of the conceptual model, including the purpose, KPIs, interfaces, process flows, and sequential interactions between agents. Additionally, the computational model and a comparison between the simulated and real-world data will be presented. Finally, the Discussion section will go through the implications and possibilities drawn from the results, and the Conclusions section will state the final, conclusive remarks of the research findings.

2. Materials and Methods

This section will present the modeling methodology and empirical case. First, the simulation modeling methodology and methods to collect and analyze the model inputs and structure will be presented for both conceptual and computational models. Next, we will present our case organization—the ED of the Stavanger University Hospital in Norway—and the case data that were used to build, validate, and verify the models.

2.1. Simulation Modeling Methodology: Randers' Model

In the original literature on modeling and simulation, there are several formalized ways of carrying out simulation studies [16]. In this study, we followed the process defined by Randers' [17], which divides the process of modeling into four main phases: (1) conceptualization, (2) formulation, (3) testing, and (4) implementation (see Figure 1).

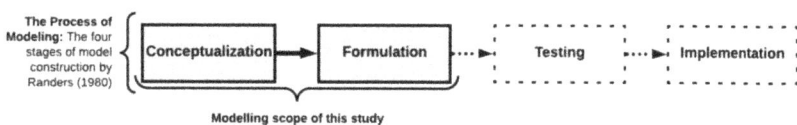

Figure 1. Randers' modeling methodology.

Randers' structure was chosen because it focuses on model purpose rather than a singular and finite problem as a starting predicate for the model. More importantly, Randers' approach is perhaps the most paradigm-independent among the available modeling protocols from the research literature. Therefore, in the context of a hybrid model which combines two or more paradigms (discrete-event and agent-based modeling) into one simulation study, Randers' protocol was considered the most appropriate. The methodological aspects that will be given primary focus hereunder are those of the "conceptualization" and "formulation" steps. The last two steps were out of scope for this paper but will be pursued by the authors in a subsequent paper.

2.1.1. Conceptual Modeling

In a previous paper [18], we developed and presented a general model for an ED, mimicking the patient flow process before the pandemic situation. In this study, the model has been expanded and presented in further detail to cover patient regimens during a pandemic situation. Like the general model, this model expansion was carried out in collaboration with the case organization through several meetings. As recommended in the literature, this stage was started before any computational modeling was made [19].

The conceptual modeling followed the four steps of Albin's [20] process for constructing rigid conceptual models, shown in Figure 2. The four steps are: "Step 1–Define the purpose of the model", "Step 2–Define the boundary and key variables", "Step 3–Describe the system behavior", and "Step 4–Describe the basic mechanisms of the system". Although the steps here are numbered from 1 to 4, it does not imply a necessity for a strict chronological enactment. The overall simulation modeling process is a recursive and iterative process that will be developed in a back-and-forth manner, an issue we will revert to in Section 2.3.4.

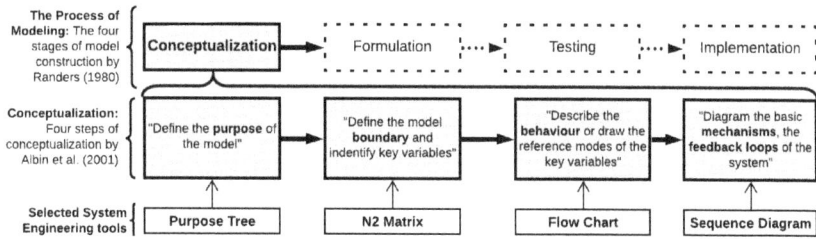

Figure 2. Model conceptualization process defined by Albin [20] and the associated systems engineering tools.

For each step we used a system engineering tool to aid communication with the case organization and to help analyze and understand the processes together with the stakeholders. The steps and their corresponding tools are shown in Figure 2.

The following subsections describe these four systems engineering tools.

2.1.2. Purpose Tree

A purpose tree, shown in Figure 3, is an illustrative tool representing the purpose behind the simulation model of interest and its measurable key performance indicators (KPIs). Different versions of tree structures are commonly used in management disciplines, e.g., work breakdown structure in the project management discipline, and organization charts. The purpose tree is used similarly to elaborate the fundamental aim of the model and decompose it to achieve an overview of the model purpose and what system elements the model purpose builds upon.

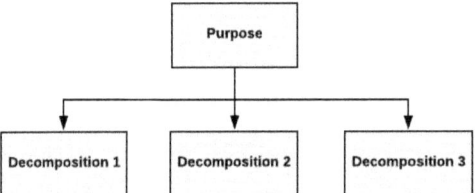

Figure 3. A generic purpose tree and its KPIs decomposition.

2.1.3. Interface Diagram

The interface diagram, shown in Figure 4, also known under the name "N^2-matrix", visually illustrates the interfaces between involved entities or agents, as well as external inputs. The principal diagonal (Principal diagonal: the diagonal going from the uppermost left corner, "Subssytem 1" in Figure 4, to the lowermost right corner, "Subssystem 3" in Figure 4.) in the matrix constitutes different subsystems. The remaining squares in the matrix constitute interfaces between the various subsystems. The blocks above the principal diagonal constitute downstream interfaces, and the blocks below the principal diagonal constitute interface feedback upstream in the system. The top row of the matrix contains descriptions of subsystem input from external parts. The rightmost column of the matrix illustrates the output from the subsystems.

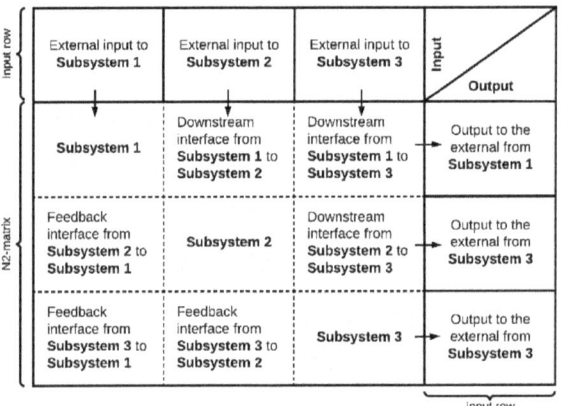

Figure 4. Generic interface diagram.

The principal diagonal of the N^2-matrix may be procedural steps of a process, or a distinct group of assets used by system agents. Figure 4 shows a generic interface diagram where subsystems 1–3 are considered. Like the purpose tree, this tool is flexible as it can be used at several different units (e.g., health, patient, medicine, information) and levels (e.g., health trust, hospital, department, ward, treatment room) of analysis. For multi-purpose models, one can construct one diagram for each purpose and analyze them separately.

2.1.4. Flow Chart

A flow chart, shown in Figure 5, is a high-level description of the system's behavior. It describes the process in terms of connected steps necessary to accomplish a task. In our study, the flow chart representation was divided into states that coincide with the most important and distinct processes the patient goes through in the ED.

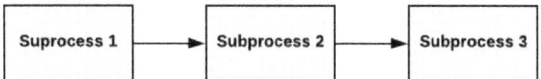

Figure 5. A generic flow chart of a process containing three linearly connected subprocesses.

2.1.5. Sequence Diagram

The sequence diagram, shown in Figure 6, is a detailed-level description that shows the entity/agent interactions arranged in a time sequence. Complex social systems, e.g., EDs, rarely have a linear progression through the system's different subprocesses. The system may have several feedback loops, resulting in a plethora of different system realizations, depending on specific details of the agent traveling through the system.

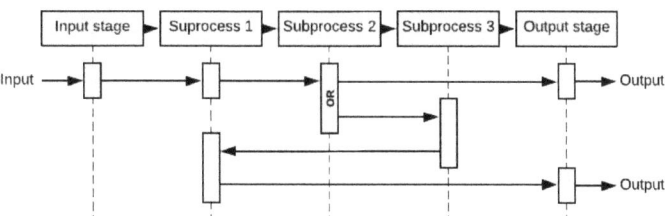

Figure 6. Simple illustration of a sequence diagram progressing through three subprocesses.

The sequence diagram provides a systemic way to capture, analyze, and discuss how different system agents progress throughout the various subprocesses of the system. A fully detailed sequence diagram thus visualizes all the unique passages an agent can take through the system in a more detailed manner than a flow chart can illustrate.

2.2. Computational Modeling–Hybrid Simulation Modeling

Following the conceptualization step, the next step in the overall modeling was to perform the Formulation step, as shown in Figure 7. The formulation is about structuring the conceptual model into software by using a computer programming language. A computational model will thus be another layer of codification on the conceptual model and be significantly contingent on the software's codification abilities (i.e., a meta-model).

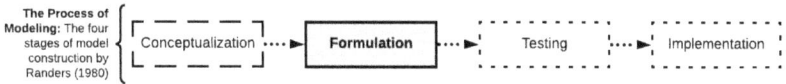

Figure 7. In the process of modeling, the next step after the conceptual modeling is formulation.

In order to carry out the modeling, it was found necessary to use an agent-based simulation in order to be able to adequately implement the complex patient flow logic of the case organization. However, a pure agent-based modeling approach was found to be insufficient when we were to model the resources and their use by the patient agents. Some agents would behave dominantly in a discrete-event manner, e.g., room seizing and releasing.

This required us to expand from strictly agent-based modeling (ABM) to a hybrid combination by including discrete event simulation (DES) model elements. To implement this type of hybrid model that allowed for the utilization of both ABM and DES, we used AnyLogic 8 Personal Learning Edition 8.7.2.

Agent behavior was defined using the statechart, which is an integrated feature in AnyLogic describing agent behavior. A statechart is a blueprint for the behavior of each agent. The statechart is common for every agent (of the same type) that becomes initiated into the model. However, every patient will each have their individual realization of the statechart. The resource allocation logic, which included elements of discrete-event modeling, was codified by using the "process modeling" flow chart in AnyLogic.

In making the model, we collected data about how the emergency department in our case study normally works in a pre-pandemic situation. This model served as a basis for the model development. We then added the complexities introduced by the pandemic restrictions, e.g., a waiting zone, extra treatment rooms, and the associated procedures.

We then validated the model in two manners: Firstly, we set the patient contamination rate (PCR) to 0% to simulate a pre-pandemic situation, ran the model with real-life pre-pandemic patient arrival data and compared the output of the run with real-life pre-pandemic patient crowding data.

Secondly, we ran the model with peri-pandemic patient arrival data, using a PCR set to 30%, since this was the actual patient contamination rate in the real peri-pandemic data, and again compared to the real-life peri-pandemic patient crowding data.

2.3. Case Study: ED of Stavanger University Hospital

In order to obtain a good understanding of the studied ED, three aspects will be presented in this section:
(1). The facility and layout to understand the capacity, routes, and waiting zones.
(2). The data management systems that store and visualize the patient arrival and crowding rates, (in this case, two systems called Meona and Smart Crowding, respectively).
(3). The involved experts who provided descriptions of operations, policies, and expected performance measures.

2.3.1. Facility and Layout

The case subject of this study is the ED of the public hospital Stavanger University Hospital, located in the city of Stavanger in the south-western part of Norway. The hospital is a large hospital with more than 500 beds, over 7800 employees, and 33 wards serving 369,000 city inhabitants. The case ED serves approximately 35,000 patients each year, averaging around a hundred patients daily. During normal circumstances, the case ED is equipped with 13 treatment rooms, 11 triage beds, and seven medical doctors (1 foundation house officer, three surgeons, two neurologists, and one orthopedist) [21–24].

2.3.2. Case Data

Three categories of data were utilized in this study, displayed in Figure 8; (1) data used as inputs to run the simulation model, (2) data used to construct the simulation model, and (3) data used to validate the simulation output. Figure 8 shows a schematic overview of the case data categories.

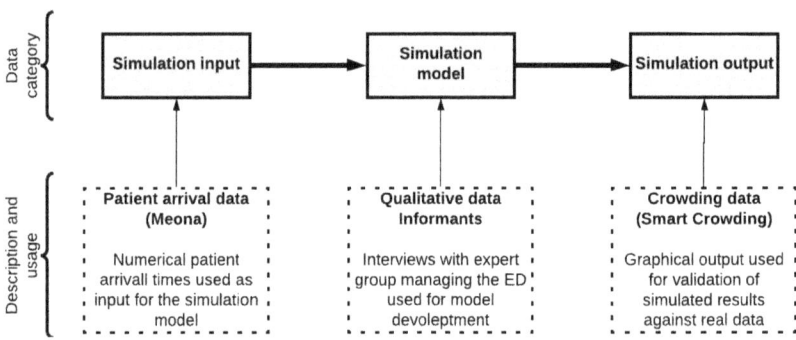

Figure 8. The data categories used in constructing, running, and validating the simulation model.

The first category—data used for simulation input—consisted of anonymized patient arrival time registrations for patients in the ED. These data were pre-existing data recorded independently of this study and were thus secondary data. The dataset we utilized was collected from a local database in an information and communication technology (ICT) system called Meona at the case hospital. Each record of data in Meona represented the time of arrival to the ED of one new patient. The number of data entries on a particular day in Meona thus represented the number of patients arriving at the ED that day.

The second category—data used for simulation model developments—was mainly obtained through interviews with knowledgeable stakeholders from the case organization. This category of data represented information about the patent flow process in the ED. These data were thus primary qualitative data. The steps in the patient flow process, and the criteria for the choice of alternative routes through the system, were explained to us by a group of key stakeholders at the case hospital.

Furthermore, we were given a blueprint of the layout of the ED, shown in Figure 9, which served as an outset for the construction of the computational model.

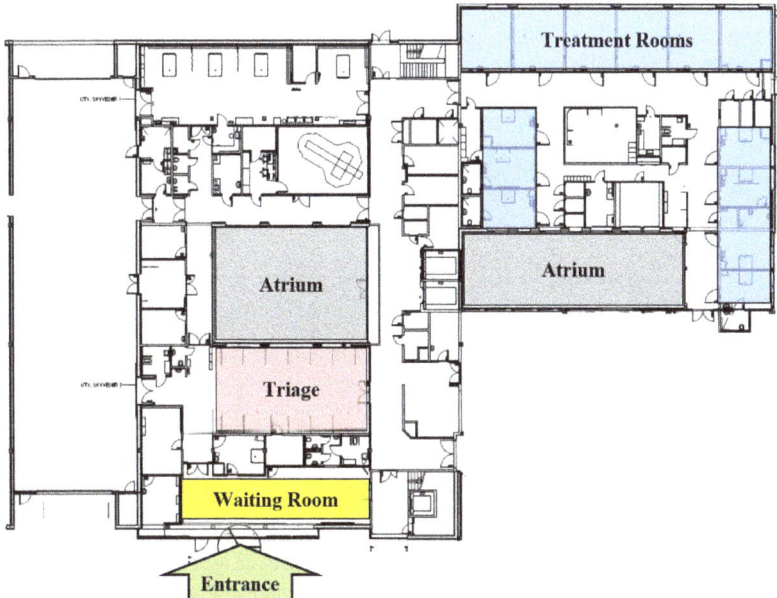

Figure 9. Blueprint of the studied ED before the pandemic measures was put in place.

Using the blueprint eased the process of mapping out the patient movement path and laying out the resources. In addition to being informative in the model layout, this was also an important part of data collection to understand how the ED operates. For example, knowing the spatial positioning of the resources was necessary for ensuring that the model represented the actual system. Additionally, it directly revealed how many resources there were, e.g., number of treatment rooms which were limited to 13, and amount of triage beds limited to 11.

Additionally, we were given a walkthrough inside the case ED to observe the daily operation and obtain an understanding the workings of the real system.

For the final category—data used for the simulation output—we used secondary data retrieved from an ICT system at the hospital called SmartCrowding for verification and validation. These data consisted of graphs showing the patient flow development throughout the time of the days. Patient flow development was represented through a number of measures, such as time of day when crowing reached a certain percentage of room capacity, peak crowding level, etc. Thus, while the data from Meona represented the actual arrival of patients to the ED on a particular day, the data from SmartCrowding showed the actual resulting patient flow development on the same day.

2.3.3. Arrival and Crowding

The set of real-life numerical data we were given, gathered from Meona, consisted of registration times for each patient's arrival at the ED. The record of the data spanned over two full days, altogether 48 h. Our informants selected these two days as two representative days. These two days of data collection were two regular separate working days at the hospital (i.e., *not in sequence*) in the *pre-pandemic* situation, i.e., *prior* to the COVID-19 pandemic onset. The crowding data for the same two days, gathered from SmartCrowding, are shown in Table 1a.

Table 1. a. Patient crowding in the ED gathered from Smart Crowding for two regular days in a pre-pandemic situation. **b.** Patient crowding in the ED gathered from Smart Crowding for two separate days in a peri-pandemic situation.

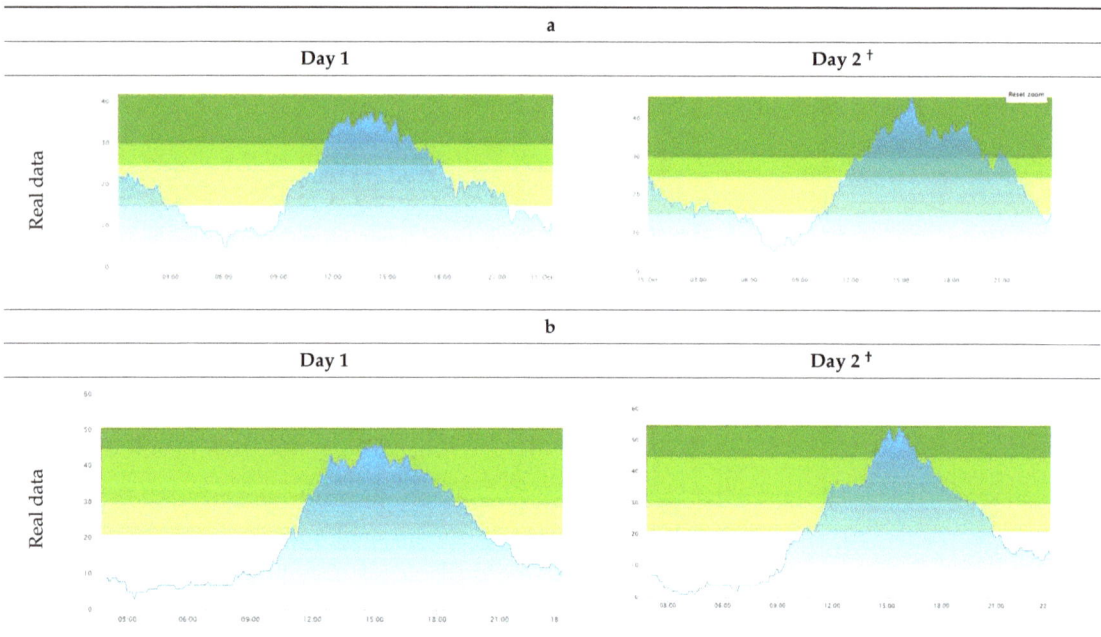

† Graph "Day 2" is not immediately the following day after "Day 1" as the naming may suggest.

We were also given a similar set of real-life numerical data gathered from Meona during the pandemic, i.e., in a peri-pandemic situation, which consisted of registration times for patients arriving at the ED in the case hospital. Data spanning over two separate full days were selected also from this dataset. The real-life crowding data for the same two days, gathered from SmartCrowding, are shown in Table 1b.

2.3.4. Operations and Experts' Descriptions

Dialog with a case organization is essential for a modeling process to succeed and benefit the system stakeholders. Accordingly, a significant portion of the data for this study was the qualitative data gathered through talking with the organization's stakeholders. These individuals are personnel that work closely with the ED on a day-to-day basis.

The communication occurred as a mix of meetings on both a scheduled basis and an on-need basis for clarification in the model development. Development of both the conceptual and the computational model required intensive gathering of qualitative data by direct communication with the case organization. Testing of the computational model would quickly reveal misunderstandings in the conceptual modeling, resulting in an iterative development process in dialog with the stakeholders, as we indicated in Section 2.1.1. The development process, shown in the overall modeling methodology in Figure 2, was, thus, in practice, a nonlinear process, where the steps had to be revisited continually and iteratively throughout the lifetime of the model's development process.

3. Results

Applying Randers' model of simulation modeling [17] allowed us to obtain three main results:

(1) The conceptual model that represents the real-world structure and context of the ED during both pre-pandemic and peri-pandemic status.
(2) The computational model that mimics the patient flow behavior in the ED during both the pre-pandemic and peri-pandemic situations.
(3) The output (the simulated behaviors) of the computational model, where both real (from the patient crowding data) and simulated behavior are compared.

3.1. Result from Conceptual Modeling of the Case

Performing the conceptual modeling process described in Section 2.1.1 and Figure 2, resulted in a model including the following elements:

(1) Definition of the model purpose and twelve performance measures that the simulation model should be able to perform.
(2) Definition of model boundary and key variables, including critical interfaces between the *layout agents* of the ED (pre-treatment, triage, treatment rooms, waiting-zones, discharge).
(3) Description of the system behavior, including interactions between *patient agents* (ordinary and contaminated patient) and *layout agents* to describe the room seizing/releasing process, and
(4) Description of the basic mechanisms of the system.

3.1.1. Step 1 – Definition of the Purpose of the Model

The model's primary purpose was to model the patient flow behavior in the ED to test several policies and interventions in a virtual and low-cost environment. From an operational perspective, the patient flow could be divided into three main segments, as illustrated in Figure 10: patient inflow, patient throughput within the department, and patient output.

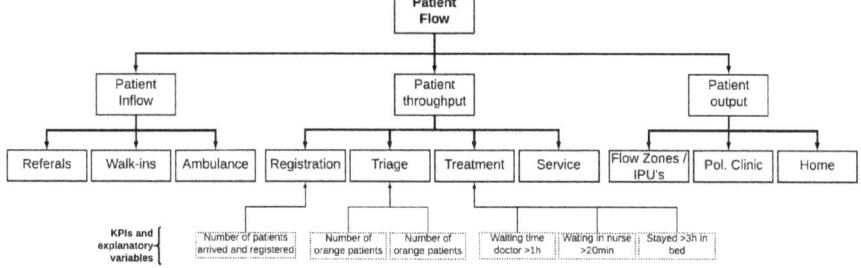

Figure 10. Purpose tree breakdown structure and KPIs for ED operations.

Implementation of the Patient Flow Key Performance Indicators

Performance indicators were selected and constructed within the simulation software to measure relevant aspects of patient flow within the ED. The following comprises a brief description of the KPI implementation as well as their mathematical equations (main contributor of this paper is the author of these equations), illustrating the calculations programmed into the simulation model.

1. Time to treatment (TTT) [h/pt]: This KPI tracks the time spent on all the activities prior to the treatment. Then, it is calculated as an average. TTT is calculated for all the patients (Tot.), the patients that are suspected to be pathogen contagious (Cont.), and the patients that are found likely not to be pathogen carrying (Ord.).

$$\text{TTT}(t) = \frac{1}{N_{out}(t)} \cdot \sum_{n=0}^{N_{out}(t)} \left(P_{\text{Time entering TR}}(n) - P_{\text{Time entering ED}}(n) \right)$$
$$\forall\ P \in [P(0), \ldots, P(N_{out}(t))]$$

$P(n)$–nth patient agent, $P_x(n)$–parameter x of the nth patient agent, $N_{in}(t)$–Number of patients who entered the ED at time t, $N_{out}(t)$–Number of patients left the ED at time t, t–time; acting as the independent discrete-time variable going from 00:00:00 to 23:59:59, running in increments of seconds.

2. The average length of stay (ALOS) [h/pt]: This calculates the average time the patients spend in the ED. This measure can also be calculated individually for the different patient populations.

$$\text{ALOS}(t) = \frac{1}{N_{out}(t)} \cdot \sum_{n=0}^{N_{out}(t)} \left(P_{\text{Time leaving ED}}(n) - P_{\text{Time entering ED}}(n) \right)$$
$$\forall\ P \in [P(0), \ldots, P(N_{out}(t))]$$

$P(n)$–nth patient agent, $P_x(n)$–parameter x of the nth patient agent, $N_{in}(t)$–Number of patients who entered the ED at time t, $N_{out}(t)$–Number of patients left the ED at time t, t–time; acting as the independent discrete-time variable going from 00:00:00 to 23:59:59, running in increments of seconds.

3. Crowding [%]: Crowding is defined as the number of patients simultaneously staying within the ED facility, i.e., prevalence. This measure tracks how long the crowding in the ED is above certain predefined levels and divides it by the total amount of time passed. The crowding levels are selected according to the case organization's plan for high activity, 15, 20, and 30.

$$\text{Crowding}_{>15}(t) = \frac{\sum_{n=0}^{t} u(t)}{t} \cdot 100\%, \quad u(t) = \begin{cases} 1 \text{ if } (N_{out}(t) - N_{in}(t)) > 15 \\ 0 \text{ otherwise} \end{cases}$$

$P(n)$–nth patient agent, $P_x(n)$–parameter x of the nth patient agent, $N_{in}(t)$–Number of patients who entered the ED at time t, $N_{out}(t)$–Number of patients left the ED at time t, t–time; acting as the independent discrete-time variable going from 00:00:00 to 23:59:59, running in increments of seconds.

4. Peak crowding: This measure is intended to present information on how many patients are present at the peak of the day.

$$\text{Peak crowding}(t) = max[N_{out}(t) - N_{in}(t)]$$
$$\forall\ t \in [0, t]$$

$P(n)$–nth patient agent, $P_x(n)$–parameter x of the nth patient agent, $N_{in}(t)$–Number of patients who entered the ED at time t, $N_{out}(t)$–Number of patients left the ED at time t, t–time; acting as the independent discrete-time variable going from 00:00:00 to 23:59:59, running in increments of seconds.

5. Time of peak [time]: This measure states records at which the previously mentioned peak of crowding occurs.
6. Time start use [time]: This measure keeps track of when the different resources start being used within the ED. Measures were chosen to be tracking the use of the extra treatment rooms (E.Tr.), triage (Tri.), and the waiting zone (WZ).

7. Time in use [%]. This estimates the amount of time the resources are used as a proportion of the total time simulated. Equation (5) shows the calculation for the extra treatment rooms (*E.Tr.*).

$$\text{Time in use}_{E.Tr.}(t) = \frac{\sum_{n=0}^{t} u(t)}{t} \cdot 100\%, \quad u(t) = \begin{cases} 1 \text{ if } N_{@E.Tr.}(t) > 0 \\ 0 \text{ otherwise} \end{cases}$$

$P(n)$–nth patient agent, $P_x(n)$–parameter x of the nth patient agent, $N_{in}(t)$–Number of patients who entered the ED at time t, $N_{out}(t)$–Number of patients left the ED at time t, t–time; acting as the independent discrete-time variable going from 00:00:00 to 23:59:59, running in increments of seconds.

8. Time full [time]: Similar to the "time start use", this measure keeps track of when the resource first reached its full capacity (i.e., there was no more left of the resource for a new patient for the first time).
9. Waiting time pr pts [h/pt]: This measure calculates the average waiting time in WR across the different patient agent groups.
10. Times TR blocked for contaminated patients [#]: This measure keeps track of the number of times a patient with virus suspicion is blocked from going directly to a treatment room after undergoing the pre-triage screening. Such a blockage occurs under the following conditions: (1) all the ordinary and all the extra treatment rooms are fully utilized, and (2) no ordinary patients can leave their treatment room, either due to the lack of a waiting zone available or because none of the patients currently in the treatment rooms have stayed their minimum amount of time in their treatment rooms. Therefore, this measure is critical, because if this condition occurs, it means that a potentially contaminated patient has to wait, which poses an increased risk of contamination.
11. Times TR (WZ) seized [#]: Similar to the previous, this one is a pure counter. This measure counts the number of times a treatment room (or waiting zone) is seized by a patient agent. The main reason for keeping track of this is that seizing rooms is work intensive. Rooms need to be set up and sanitized and thus constitute an economic and resource burden both directly and indirectly. Additionally, besides the pure labor aspect, the management of seizing and releasing may cause an error and be costly. In addition, having patients leave their rooms might be a high cost for the individual patients, as this might yield stress and other discomforts for the patient.

3.1.2. Step 2—Definition of Model Boundary and Key Variables

The organizational structures of EDs may vary across hospitals. In the case organization, the ED was organized as its own independent department, not as a subdivision of another department, which is typical in smaller Norwegian hospitals.

In this step, the overall purpose was to convey patient flow elements in the simulation model. Figure 11 illustrates the inputs and outputs of each process step, identified by applying to our case the Interface (N2) diagram tool presented in Section 2.1.3.

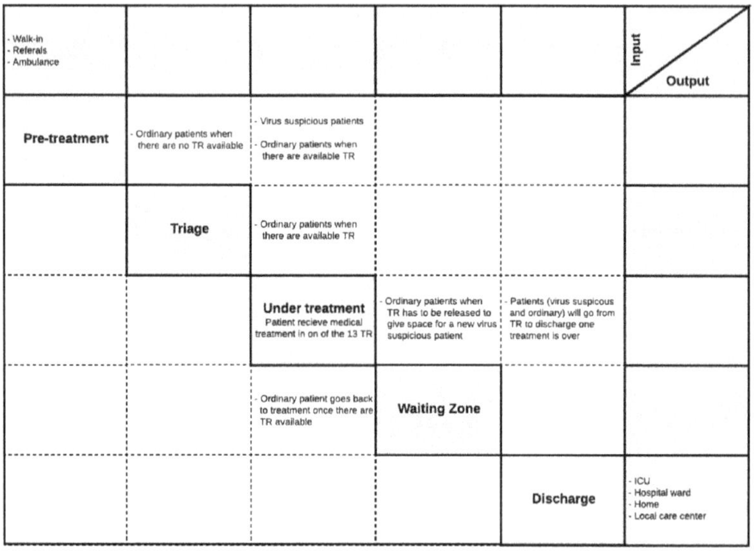

[Figure 11 diagram – N2 diagram content]

Figure 11. N2 diagram for ED facilities under pre- and peri-pandemic conditions.

3.1.3. Step 3—Description of the System Behavior

In this step, a simple flowchart depiction of the patient flow process was developed. The result is shown in Figure 12. The following descriptions explain each element in the flowchart:

Pre-pandemic operation

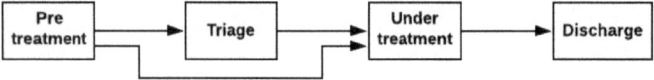

Peri-pandemic operation

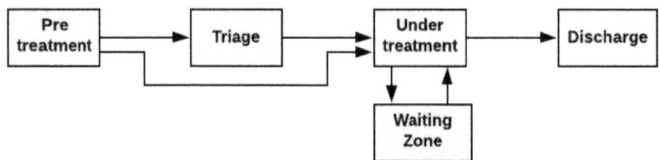

Figure 12. Flow chart for patient flow under the pre-and peri-pandemic situation.

"Pre-Treatment"

The first stage in the flow chart was pre-treatment. This stage included everything from when the patient arrived at the ED until the patient left registration to be admitted into either the triage or treatment room. Imposed by the pandemic situation, the ED had decided to install a pre-triage area outside the entrance of the ED, where all patients arriving at the ED needed to be pre-screened. From here, if it was found likely that the patient was infected by the COVID-19 virus, the patient would immediately be directed to a prepared treatment room (TR) to ensure a reduction in intra-departmental contamination.

This implied that a treatment room was de-sanitized whenever it had been used to treat a patient who was suspected to have COVID-19.

"Triage"

Triage here refers to the physical location where admitted patients wait for treatment. It is used in situations where no treatment rooms are vacant. We will later address the distinction between action and physical location, as triage can refer to both the action of triaging a patient according to a specific triage system and the physical location within the ED where the triaging of patients is primarily taking place.

"Under Treatment"

This stage of the patient pathway is where the actual treatment takes place. Then, according to the prescribed medical protocol, the patient receives medical treatment from doctors and nurses. The standard treatment rooms in use before the pandemic amounted to 13. Extra treatment rooms were introduced for expanded capacity to cope with the pandemic situation. Once the standard treatment rooms were filled, the extra treatment rooms would be used to accommodate more patients.

To cope with the risk of transmission between the patients, patients suspected of being contaminated would be expedited to a treatment room. After treatment, the treatment room would be de-sanitized before accepting a new patient. If the regular treatment rooms were full and a new patient with suspected contamination arrived, then a patient that had stayed in the room for at least 1 h would have to leave their treatment room and move over to a waiting zone.

"Waiting Zone"

As said in the previous stage, the waiting zone was for patients evaluated not to be incumbents of the virus. Here, patients would wait until there was an available treatment room that they could return to for their treatment to continue.

"Discharge"

The last stage in the flow chart was the discharge. This step is where the patient finally has undergone the treatment and is ready to be discharged from the ED.

3.1.4. Step 4—Description of the Basic Mechanisms of the System

The fourth step in the development procedure was to capture the basic mechanisms of the system at a more detailed level than the simple flowchart. Discussions with the stakeholders in the case organization revealed a variety of possible pathways through the ED. These are illustrated in the sequence diagram in Figure 13, where the conditions for each route are indicated. These will be further elaborated in Table 2 in our computational model.

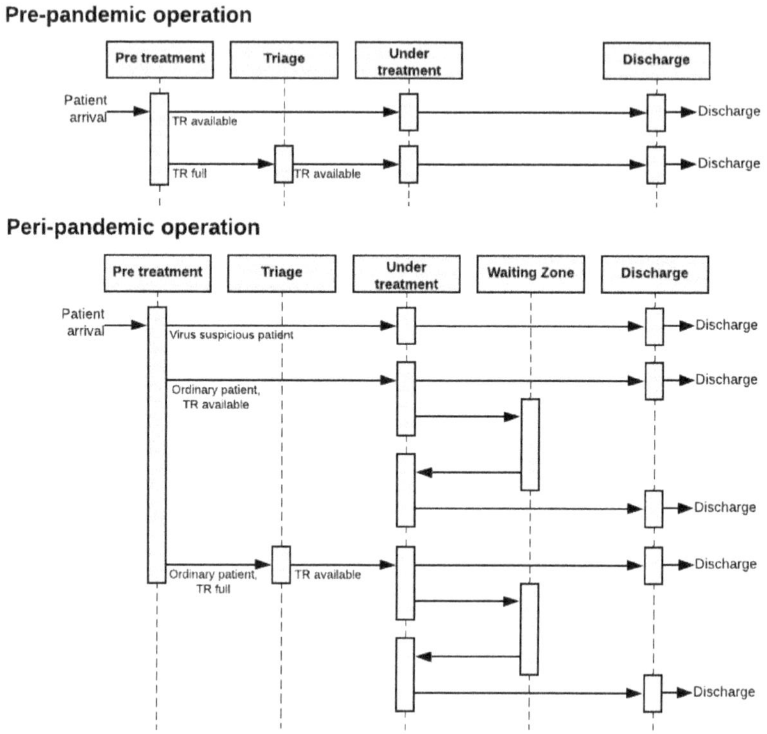

Figure 13. Effect on patient flow operation illustrated in sequence diagram pre- and peri-pandemic situation.

Table 2. Description of the elements (states, transitions and initial conditions) of the patient agent statechart.

Name	Description	Logic	Code
	Patient arrival will be arriving according to the numerical data attained from the case organization. Arrivals can be programmed based on a probability distribution that will make for a stochastical model. Alternatively, arrivals can be programmed according to recorded arrival times; the model will then be deterministic.		
'Stay'	State-Stay: The sole purpose of this state-block is to calculate the length of stay of patients throughout their lifetime, i.e., the entire statechart. Timer3 here does the counting. No other logic is contained within this state block.	Timeout for each second in simulation in order to increment the timer value within Timer3 according to criteria in the code. Variables: (integer) v_LOS	Action: v_LOS += inState(Stay) ? 1: 0;
'S1'	State-Pre-treatment: First compound state in the overall patient flow. This state contains all the states for the pre-treatment activities a patient is undergoing. Like the previous state, counting is performed. It is worth noting counter is placed here instead of the 'Stay' state block to reduce the calculation power needed for each discrete increment.	Timeout for each second in simulation in order to increment the timer value within Timer1 according to code. Variables: v_time_in_PreTriage, v_time_in_WR	Action: v_time_in_PreTriage += inState(PreTriage)? 1: 0; v_time_in_WR += inState(WaitingInWR) ? 1: 0;

Table 2. Cont.

Name	Description	Logic	Code
's1-1'	State-Incidence: Patient agent takes place into the statechart after being transferred from the 'Exit' block in DES (Figure 14). The sole purpose of this state block is that t serves the programmatic purpose of letting the patient agent enter the statechart. Once the patient agent is instantiated into this state, it is immediately passed onto the transition.	-	-
't1-1'	Transition: Patient agent arrives from the DES. Transition is triggered on the string message "occurrence," which is sent from the 'Exit'-block in the DES model.	-	-
's1-2'	State–PreTriage: Patient agent is getting moved from the entry node to the Pre-triage node, i.e., light green field in Figure 14.	The patient agent initiates movement from the Entry node to the te pre triage node.	Action: moveTo(main.PreTriageNode);
't1-2'	Transition: Transition from the state PreTriage to branch B1.	Transition is executed periodically for every fixed time interval in order to ensure. Parameter used:main.p_RegistrationCheckInterval	
'B1'	Branch: This branch carries out the selection for what path the patient agent should proceed in.	Three different outgoing transitions: (1) If there is a suspicion that the patient is contaminated, the patient will go to S2. (2) If the patient agent is found not to be contaminated, the patient will go to the waiting room after a specified waiting time, i.e., state s1-3. (3) T3: If the patient agent has virus suspicion and there are no more treatment rooms, the patient must wait in the Pre-triage.	(1) Condition: p_contaminated && !f_is_TR_full() (1) Action: main.enter_SeizeTR.take(this); (2) Condition: !p_contaminated && (v_time_in_PreTriage > main.p_minTimeInPreTriage) (3) Action: if (p_contaminated && f_is_TR_full() && v_BlockFlag == false) { main.v_Virus_Patient_TR_Decline ++; v_BlockFlag = true;}
's1-3'	State–WalkingToWR: Patient agent walking to the waiting room from the pre triage.	The patient agent walks along the path between the pre-triage and waiting room shown in Figure 14.	Action: moveTo (main.waitingRoomNode);
't1-3'	Transition: The patient agent is simply transitioning between walking to the waiting room and waiting in the waiting room.	This transition is triggered once the patient agent stops walking and arrives at its place in the waiting room.	-
's1-4'	State–WaitingInWR: This state for the patient agents when waiting in the waiting room (WR); see the node in Figure 14.	-	-
't1-4'	Transition: Here, the patient agent will attempt to see if it is ready to proceed.	This transition will trigger periodically. It will check if it can fulfill any of the transitions branch B4 for each periodic interval.	-

Table 2. Cont.

Name	Description	Logic	Code
'B4'	Branch: This is the pathway forward after the PreTreatment state. Patient agents from here either have to go to the treatment room, triage or wait further if the above-mentioned is full.	Three outgoing transitions: (1) T1–Going to triage if there are no more treatment rooms left, (2) T2–Going to a treatment room, and (3) Stay in the waiting room if the above-mentioned transitions do not fulfill their execution conditions. None of the transitions have dependencies on the patient virus suspicious status, as these are already sorted in the previous branch B1.	(1) Conditions: f_is_TR_full() && !f_is_Triage_full() && (v_time_in_WR > main.p_minTimeInWR) (1) Action: main.enter_seize_Triage.take(this); (2) Action: main.enter_SeizeTR.take(this); (3) Conditions: !f_is_TR_full() && f_is_WZ_empty() && f_is_Triage_empty() && (v_time_in_WR >main.p_minTimeInWR)
'S2'	State–IntraTreatment: This is the second major compound state of the overall patient flow. As the name suggests, this is where the patient finally undergoes treatment. The patient agent is released from the treatment room seizing pathway shown in the DES block diagram (Figure 14)	The treatment is simulated by the patient agent waiting inside the treatment room. The treatment time differs according to whether the patient has suspicion of virus contamination. (1) Timer variable: v_time_in_TR. (2) Counter variable: main.p_number_room_exit	v_time_in_TR += inState(Treatment) ? 1: 0; main.p_number_room_exit++
's2-1'	State–WalkingToAndSeizingTR: This is the state the patient agent is contained within until it has been transferred from the seize-path, as mentioned earlier.	-	-
't2-1'	Transition–The patient agent is transitioned to the next state once the message is received from the	The patient agent is transitioned to the next state once the message is received from the	-
's2-2'	State–Treatment: This is the state in which the patient agent is under treatment.	The patient agent stays in this state while the counter is increasing.	-
't2-2'	Transition–Transition out of treatment leads to a branch where there are three options possible.	This transition is cyclical and repeats every second during model runtime for patients' agents that stay within the treatment state.	-
'B2'	Branch: This branch leads the patient agent to go to the waiting zone, leave the ED, or stay to continue the treatment.	The branch is leading to three outgoing transitions (1) T6: Patient agents pause the treatment and makes the patient go to the waiting zone. (2) T7: Patient agent has completed treatment and will head to exit the ED. (3) Treatment is not carried out, and it will proceed until it is either completed or has to pause because the treatment room needs to be seized by a patient suspicious of contamination.	(1) Action: main.enter_seize_WZ.take(this); (1) Condition: !p_contaminated && f_is_TR_full() && !f_is_WZ_full() && v_time_in_TR > main.p_minTimeTR && f_is_this_longest_in_TR(this) && f_is_any_contaminated_in_WR() && main.b_is_WZ_in_use (2) Action: main.enter.take(this); (2) Condition: p_contaminated ? v_time_in_TR > main.p_TreatmentTime_VirusSuspicion: v_time_in_TR > main.p_TreatmentTime_OrdinaryPatient

Table 2. Cont.

Name	Description	Logic	Code
'S3'	State–Triage: Compound state element emulating the patient standing by in the triage until there is room for the patient in the treatment rooms.	Time is tracked. Variable: v_time_in_Triage	v_time_in_Triage += inState(Triage) ? 1: 0;
's3-1'	State-WalkingToTriage: The patient agent walks from the waiting room node to the triage node. The patient agent is retrieved from the DES path shown in Figure 14, distributing the triage bed to the patient agent.	-	-
't3-1'	Transition–Transition is executed once the patient agent is transferred from the DES flow chart.	-	-
's3-2'	State–WaitingInTriage:	This state emulates the waiting time in the triage.	-
't3-2'	Transition: Transition for checking if it is time to leave the triage. Decision-making through the branch (B5) in the next row.	Transition executed periodically; every second patient stays state 'WaitingInTriage.'	-
'B5'	Branch: Checking if the patient agent can leave the triage to go to a treatment room.	The branch is leading to two outgoing transitions. (1) Transition for when there is a treatment room ready. (2) No treatment room is available for the patient agent, returning to the previous state.	(1) Condition: !f_is_TR_full() && f_is_WZ_empty() && !f_is_any_contaminated_in_WR() && (v_time_in_Triage > main.p_minTimeInTriage) (1) Action: main.enter_SeizeTR.take(this);
'S4'	State-WaitingZone: This is the compound state encompassing the states that emulate the waiting zone for the patient agents.	This compound statement has no time counters as the time is directly relevant for when a patient agent will leave this state. However, as seen in the outgoing transition (T5), the patient agent can leave once there is room again for the patient agent to return to the treatment room.	-
's4-1'	State–GoingToWZ: The patient is retrieved from the DES chart, it has been allocated to a waiting zone, and walking to the spot it has been granted.	-	main.enter_seize_WZ.take(this);
't4-1'	Transition: Patient agent is finished walking to the waiting zone and will proceed by waiting in the waiting zone.	This transition is carried out once the patient agent has arrived at the granted waiting zone spot. This transition is executed by receiving a message from the DES-chart	-
's4-2'	State-WaitingInWZ: The patient agent is waiting in the waiting zone.	-	-
't4-2'	Transition: Transition going out from waiting in the waiting zone.	This transition is periodically executed every second of runtime.	-

Table 2. *Cont.*

Name	Description	Logic	Code
'B3'	Branch: Branch for going further to the treatment room or keep on waiting.	This branch does have two outgoing transitions for the patient agents staying in the triage (1) T4–Going to the IntraTreatment state. (2) Keep on waiting in the triage.	(1) Condition: !f_is_TR_full() && f_is_WZ_empty() && !f_is_any_contaminated_in_WR() && (v_time_in_Triage > main.p_minTimeInTriage) (1) Action: main.enter_SeizeTR.take(this);
'S5'	State–Discharge: Patient agent is here on its way out of the model. The state does not do anything besides being a mediator between the two states.	-	-

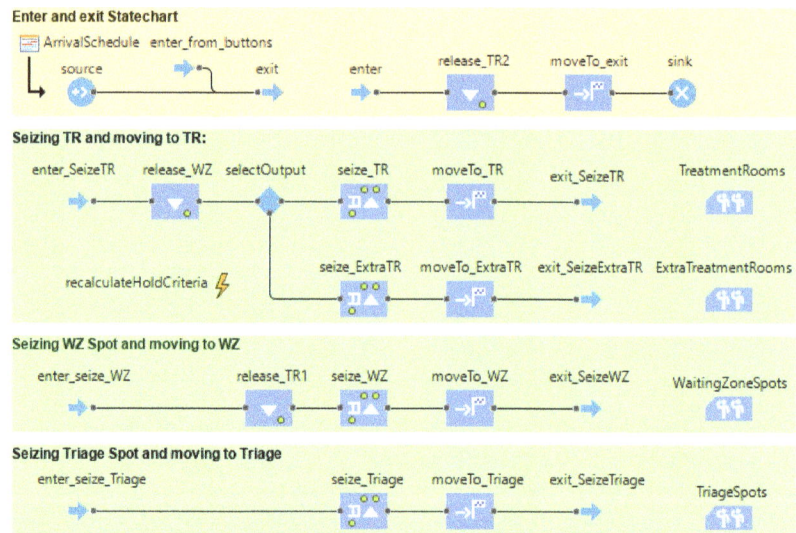

Figure 14. Process diagram programmatically carrying out the resource allocation. Patients are input in the source and output in the sink; resources will be seized and released depending on the individual patient agent's situation.

3.2. Computational Model

The following documentation of the computational model will be segmented into the following subjects: Environment, Resources, Agents, and Interaction topology, which are some of the elements STRESS guidelines suggested for documenting DES and ABS models [25].

The computational modeling process resulted in:

(1) Animated layout to visualize the patient flow behavior in a virtual ED environment.
(2) A discrete-event model for facility resources (treatment rooms, waiting zones, triage) and patient arrival rate.
(3) An agent-based model for patient flow (for ordinary and COVID-19 contaminated patients), where the sequence (state and transitions), policies (conditions, triggers), and service time (treatment time, waiting time) are modeled.

These will be presented in the following, and the modeling assumptions will be listed.

3.2.1. Virtual ED Model

The computational model was modeled using AnyLogic 8.0 Learning Edition, and the present study was limited to considering the spatial resources of the ED. These resources were overlaid on top of the case organization's blueprints for convenience and accuracy.

3.2.2. Resource Allocation Model

The resource allocation of this model was programmed through a process flow chart using the discrete-event modeling approach.

3.2.3. Patient Flow Behavior Model

The agents, depending on variable characteristics, will progress through the following main groups of activities:

- Pre-treatment;
- Triage;
- Intra treatment;
- Waiting Zone;
- Discharge.

In Figure 15, the patient flow sequence is described in a statechart, where the main states (physical locations, e.g., triage, treatment room, waiting zones) and the triggers to move from one state to another are illustrated. The statechart is the programmatic entity that orchestrates the behavior of the individual agents in the model [26].

In our current model, the only agents acting are patients. Whether the patients are ordinary, or COVID-19 contaminated, patients have a clear flow throughout several facilities (triage, treatment rooms, waiting zones). Specific conditions trigger the flow or patient movement, e.g., if a treatment room is empty, a patient moves from triage into that treatment room. Thus, there are several states and transitions that each patient has to undergo within the ED. As there are specific transitions that are time-dependent and executed depending on how much time the patient agents have spent in different states, it was necessary to implement timers to keep track of the duration patients stay in different parts of the patient flow process.

As seen in the statechart (Figure 15), there is a correlation between the flowchart in the conceptual model developed in the previous subsections (Figure 12) and the resulting statechart. The main blocks in the flowchart and statechart are the same. However, the statechart has one more level of granularity as some of the main blocks ("PreTreatment", "Triage", "IntraTreatment", "WaitingZone") have a flow chart of activities within them.

In Figure 15, there is a unique transition (T3) for COVID-19 contaminated patients to move from the pre-triage room (S1-2) at B1 to treatment rooms (S2). This particular transition represents the mentioned priority rule that our case organization implemented in the ED during the pandemic for channeling the patients directly to treatment rooms.

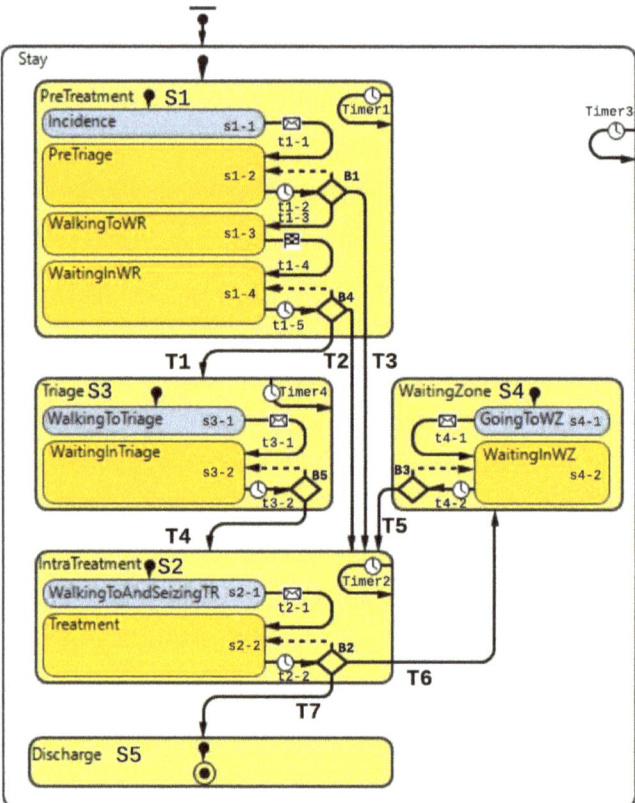

Figure 15. Statechart of patient flow behavior at the studied ED.

In Table 2, the first three columns describe each state and transition and their logic in the following table. These were all discussed and verified by our stakeholders in the case organization. The rightmost column shows the code of each element implemented in the computational model.

3.3. Model Outcome and Output Validation

There are two primary outcomes from the computational model:
(1) Patient crowding timeline in the ED;
(2) Key performance indicators of patient flow, e.g., waiting time and time to treatment.

Table 3 show comparisons between simulation output and actual patient crowding data in a pre-pandemic and peri-pandemic setting, respectively. Figures 16 and 17 show snapshots of simulated key performance indicators during the same pre-pandemic and peri-pandemic settings, respectively.

Table 3. a. Model output validation comparing graphs of patient crowding in the ED in a pre-pandemic situation. (**a**) Actual patient crowding data gathered from SmartCrowding, (**b**) Simulated patient crowding. **b.** Model output validation comparing graphs of patient crowding in the ED in a peri-pandemic situation. (**a**) Actual patient crowding data gathered from SmartCrowding, (**b**) Simulated patient crowding.

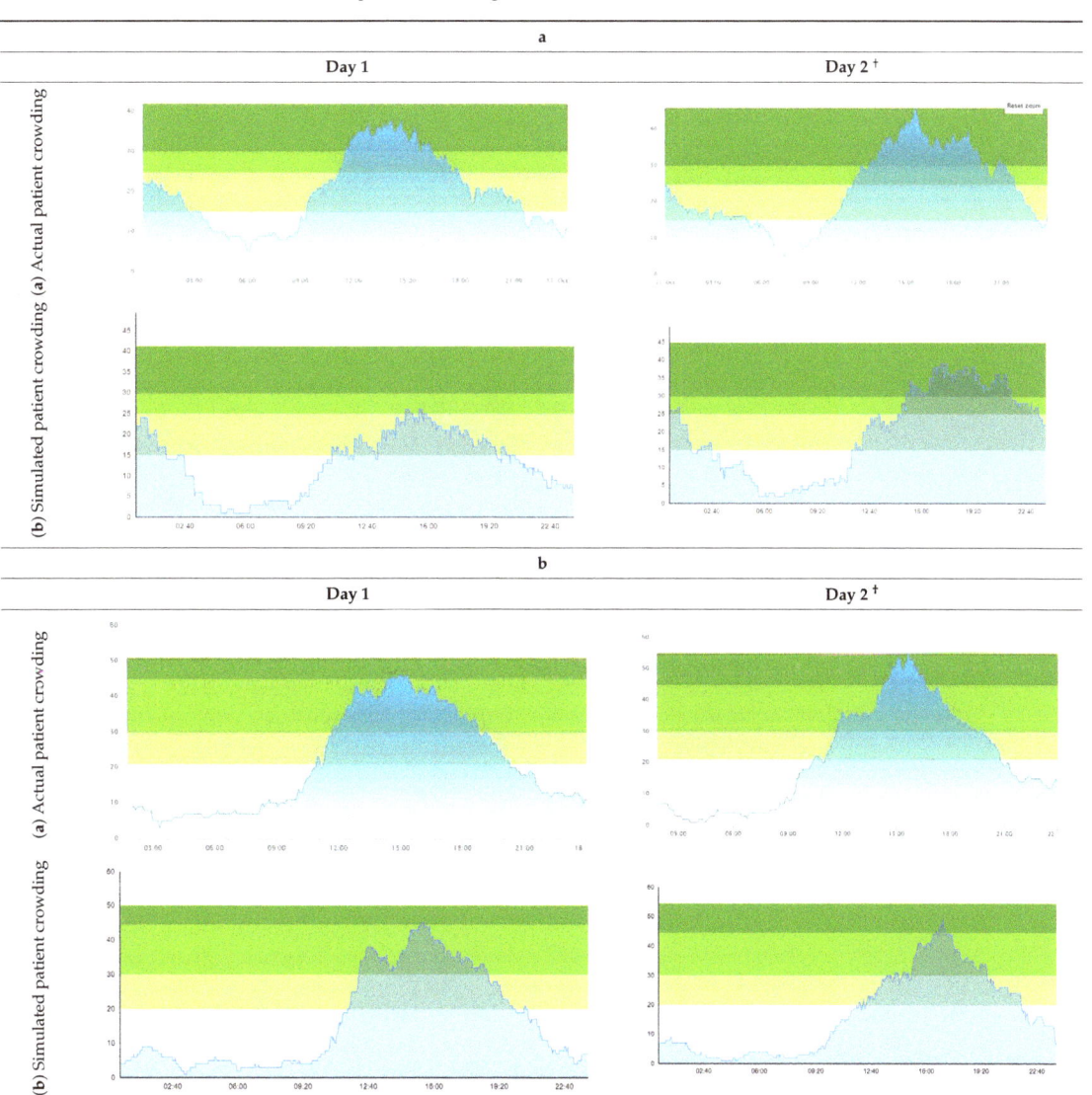

† Graph "Day 2" is not the immediately following day after "Day 1" as the naming may suggest.

	Total	Ordinary pts	Contaminated pts
Waiting time pr pts (h/pt)	--	0.066	--
Time to treatment pr pt (h/pt)	0.481	0.587	0.037
ALOS (h)	2.606	2.616	2.567
	>15 pts	>20 pts	>30 pts
Crowding - Day 1 (%)	23.793 (10:45)	6.859 (12:00)	0 (null)
Crowding - Day 2 (%)	43.6 (11:30)	36.533 (12:15)	8.953 (15:15)
	Extra TR	Triage	WZ
Time start use - Day 1 [time] ([%])	10:33 (36.599)	11:18 (15.116)	12:15 (3.873)
" - Day 2 [time] ([%])	11:33 (51.443)	12:18 (39.885)	12:45 (13.207)
Time full - Day 1 [time] ([%])	10:48 (21.631)	null (0.0)	null (0.0)
" - Day 2 [time] ([%])	11:48 (42.499)	15:35 (11.918)	null (0.0)
Times TR blocked for cont. pts (#)	7		
Times TR (WZ) seized (#)	249 (20)		
Peak crowding - Day 1 (#, time)	24 (14:45)		
" - Day 2 (#, time)	36 (17:30)		

Figure 16. Snapshot of simulated KPI of patient flow in a pre-pandemic setting.

	Total	Ordinary pts	Contaminated pts
Waiting time pr pts (h/pt)	--	0.478	--
Time to treatment pr pt (h/pt)	1.208	1.625	0.028
ALOS (h)	3.369	3.655	2.558
	>15 pts	>20 pts	>30 pts
Crowding - Day 2 (%)	46.177 (11:20)	31.499 (13:21)	20.695 (14:03)
	Extra TR	Triage	WZ
Time start use- Day 2 [time] ([%])	11:00 (54.778)	11:30 (41.012)	11:48 (21.851)
Time full - Day 2 [time] ([%])	11:29 (41.489)	14:06 (22.115)	null (0.0)
Times TR blocked for cont. pts (#)	0		
Times TR (WZ) seized (#)	145 (23)		
Peak crowding - Day 2 (#, time)	44 (16:58)		

Figure 17. Snapshot of simulated KPIs of patient flow in a peri-pandemic setting.

As can be seen in Table 3, the curve shapes from the actual patient crowding data in the case organization system (SmartCrowding) in row (a) and our simulated patient crowding in row (b) show a reasonably close resemblance. There are, however, discrepancies of the primary two main types. Firstly, the curves from the actual data (row a) are more elevated than the simulation output curves (row b) and secondly, a slight time lag seems present between the actual curves and the simulated output curves. These discrepancies will be further discussed in Section 4.2.1 of this paper's Discussion chapter.

In the conceptualization stage, we presented the key performance indicators of patient flow to be implemented and estimated by the simulation model. Figure 16 shows how these measures were represented in a table within the simulation software. The values will change dynamically throughout the simulation runtime.

As shown in Table 3, the curve shapes from the actual patient crowding data in row (a) and simulated patient crowding in row (b) also show reasonably close resemblance in a peri-pandemic setting. The same discrepancies between the curves for simulated and actual patient crowding (i.e., slight differences in elevation level and time lag) discussed above for Table 3 can also be observed here.

Figure 17 shows how key performance indicators were represented in the peri-pandemic setting. As in the pre-pandemic setting, the values will change dynamically throughout the simulation runtime.

4. Discussion

In this section, the conceptual and computational modeling process is discussed, followed by a discussion of the simulated results and their validity. Finally, some implications and future work will be highlighted.

4.1. Discussion of the Conceptual Modeling

The conceptual model in this present paper is documented in a paradigm-independent manner, providing freedom for modelers. Additionally, this approach provides transparency of the fundamental logic of the model. It makes it accessible for researchers determined to use a simulation paradigm or a mix of simulation paradigms different from the one used in this study. Furthermore, using systems engineering methods for conceptual modeling supports several purposes.

The purpose tree provided a direction for modeling by identifying and decomposing the over-arching purpose of the model. It also helped establish what key variables were essential to communicate in any output dashboard of the end product. The interface diagram aided us in mapping out both downstream and upstream patient flow interfaces between subcomponents of the system. Thereby one sets the model's boundary by determining the input and output, in addition to giving a systemic view of the process interactions between subcomponents.

The flow chart offers a simple overview of the whole patient flow process and provides valuable direct guidance on how to construct the statechart of the following computational model.

Lastly, in the conceptual modeling process, the sequence diagram captured and highlighted the feedback loops and the plethora of different realizations throughout the patient flow system that the ED entails. In particular, the sequence diagram highlighted how much the complexity of the patient flow increased when the ED had to perform the prioritization of regular and contamination suspected patients.

In their unique way, each of these tools helped arrive at the necessary understanding of the patient flow complexities to proceed to the computational modeling. We assert that this understanding goes beyond the understanding one can gain by solely using a flowchart as a conceptualizing tool, as commonly seen in many patient-flow simulation studies.

Utilizing the conceptual modeling approach as demonstrated in this study is useful as it demonstrates the use of a set of tools for data collection and communication with the stakeholders. It can also be used to verify and validate if the conceptual model represents a credible understanding of the real-world case and to validate if the computational model is traceable to the conceptual model. It is important to emphasize the benefit of the tools being software independent.

The synergic effect of the combination of the different tools is essential. The tools represent four abstractions of the same patient flow process. They serve as four different low-resolution lenses to perceive the actual process. We believe that the diversity within these "lenses" forces the simulation modeler and the participating stakeholders to perceive the system from different conceptual perspectives. This, in turn, helps extract as much relevant information as possible, in line with the stated purpose(s) of a conceptual model, thus increasing the chance of representing the actual system behavior. We believe the approach we have followed helps the stakeholders articulate important elements they otherwise might consider too obvious to mention or that they may have not reflected thoroughly upon.

4.2. Computational Model

The computational model, represented by a discrete event process diagram and statecharts, has been structured based on the conceptual model diagrams. It is clear that any computational model has a structure, behavior (formulas, rules, etc.) and inputs. The rules and conditions have been extracted from interviews with staff working and managing the ED at SUS. The input data such as 'time of arrival' was extracted from a real-time database, i.e., Meona. The service time for treatment and waiting time are assumed based on expert experience. Finally, the simulated results were validated in two manners: (1) compared with real-life patient flow data (2) dialogue with stakeholders in the ED to ensure that our understanding has mimicked real-world structure and relationships.

The comparison between the actual real-life data provided by SmartCrowding and the simulation results provided by our model, illustrated in Table 3, clearly shows similarities in the daily pattern (i.e., curve shape) of the patient prevalence in the ED. Producing a realistic output that reasonably replicates the system behavior, confirmed by the expert group in the meetings as being credible, gained confidence from the group. We experienced that this confirmation was a sign of trustworthiness of the model and yielded our acceptance with the system stakeholders as the model continued to develop.

One particular problem experienced during the model development, which had a practical solution, was the way to emulate the limited resources (i.e., emergency treatment rooms). This was solved by making these model elements use discrete-event modeling rather than agent-based modeling. There were, thus, interfaces between the DES portion of the model and the ABM part of the model. Agents would be programmed to temporarily exit their statechart, seize their supposed resources, and return to progress through the statechart.

The resulting model ended up fairly complex. Data will be gathered and calculated every second, and the agents will check conditions for several transitions. However, a regular modern laptop can run this model, simulating 24 h of operation in less than one minute.

The computational model provides reliable and consistent results in several runs. However, three assumptions have been taken regarding the model: (1) static patient infection rate, (2) no intra-hospital contamination, and (3) perfect sorting of the patients in the pre-screening. The patient rate is modeled as a variable that users of the model will have the ability to vary. However, intra-hospital contamination and imperfect sorting might require further development to model such complex phenomena. It is worth highlighting that the developed simulation model is generalizable in two terms. First, it can be utilized for other EDs in Norway or hospitals with similar operating procedures. The process of ED patient flow in our case organization widely coincides with the commonly used process described in the ED report from the Norwegian Directorate of Health [27]. Second, it has the potential to be utilized for other pandemics with different types of diseases.

The resulting computational model constitutes perhaps the biggest contribution of this paper. Being a hybrid model, including two major simulation paradigms: agent-based simulation and discrete event simulation, it is a result consistent with the recommendation of other studies to use more advanced simulation methods to incorporate more of the underlying complexities of the healthcare delivery system [10].

4.2.1. Simulation Model Validity

The conceptual model, represented by the purpose tree, N2-matrix flowchart, and sequence diagram, has been extracted from discussions with staff working at and managing the ED at SUS. Through continual and incremental verification from the system experts, the model was developed and tailored to mimic the patient flow system of the entire ED in the case hospital.

Confidence in the computational model was achieved by running the model and comparing the simulation output with actual data, both in a pre-pandemic and a peri-pandemic setting. There were sufficient overall similarities between real-world data and simulated data in both settings to gain confidence in the model's accuracy.

Our simulation model does not yet provide point prediction [28] in the sense that the simulation results yielded the same results at every time point as the empirical data from the same period. As mentioned, the simulation output from our computational model (Table 3, row b) showed some discrepancies in the empirical data (Table 3, row a) that covered the same periods (2 separate days) as our simulations. The discrepancies between (a) the real and (b) the simulation output data were subject to discussion with the case organization stakeholders and possible explanations were offered.

One explanation could be our simplified assumption of a 2,0-hour treatment time for every patient. Although our participating stakeholders at the case hospital suggested this simplification, they did indicate that treatment times would vary in practice. In particular, they stated that under periods of high patient crowding, most procedures tend to take longer than average, thereby extending the treatment time. Under these conditions, patients will stay in the system longer than the current simulation model assumes, thereby elevating the empirical curves higher than the simulation curves, as shown in Table 3. Our stakeholders based this perception (calling it the "syrup effect") on their experience rather than any available empirical data. We intend to develop our simulation model to address this issue in our future simulation studies. However, given the underlying assumptions and simplifications necessary in any simulation model, we assert that our model provides a reasonably good pattern prediction [28].

Another explanation offered by the stakeholder group was the subtle difference present in reporting between the two datasets. The real data gathered from the SmartCrowding system, plotted in row 'a' of Table 3, tracks the number of patients registered to the ED. This means that patients traveling to the hospital from their general practitioners or via an ambulance are registered as prevalent patients. However, the data used in the simulation model has a registration based upon actual arrival in the physical ED space. This difference results in a delay between the curves, as observed in Table 3, where the simulation output is slightly lagging behind the real data. This discrepancy will also be taken into consideration in future model development.

The differences between our simulation output and the actual patient flow data might also be explained by other phenomena that take an active role in the ED, such as the latency associated with higher crowding, staff shifts, or higher variation in the treatment times. The differences might also highlight the implication of the model delimitations that we have taken. For example, patients and rooms were the only two modeled agents; medical staff (doctors, nurses) and beds were excluded. Moreover, the interactions between the ED and other departments were excluded, such as blood test, and X-ray laboratories, where patients are usually sent to those departments between their stay at the ED.

The "syrup effect," potential delays in availability of doctors, nurses, and beds, and time spent at other departments all directly affect patient flow in the ED. In fact, such issues show the need and implication of using a multi-method simulation approach instead of only a discrete event or system dynamics approach. In future model development, more agents shall be considered in order to mimic the real-world behavior of the ED.

4.3. Assumptions and Simplifications

In addition to the above, there are other assumptions and simplifications that were taken at this stage of model development, as follows:

1. The percentage of COVID-19-contaminated patients out of total patients entering the ED, i.e., the patient contamination rate (PCR), was considered 30% in the peri-pandemic scenarios and 0% in the pre-pandemic scenarios. This percentage was constant throughout the entire day, while it may have varied throughout the day in real life.
2. Treatment time for each patient agent was assumed to be constant. However, realistically, the treatment time will most likely vary throughout the day according to what types of patients arrive to the emergency department. In this model, the treatment time was set static to a 2-hour average, based on an assessment by the case stakeholders.
3. No intra-hospital contamination was put into the model.
4. Therefore, the model implicitly assumes that there is a perfect sorting, i.e., a sorting error is not taken into consideration regarding the patients in the pre-triage.

4.4. Practical Implications

This work was carried out in the context of the COVID-19 pandemic. However, the model we have developed can be applied to other pandemic contexts, provided they require similar patient flow operation and intervention policies similar the ones used in this paper, i.e., that infected patients needs to go directly to their own treatment room and should avoid the waiting room and triage. On the other hand, the transparency of our account should facilitate other researchers to make necessary modifications to the model to suit their particular contexts.

Although the interventions (i.e., pre-triage, waiting zone) might be unique for this particular ED in our study's context, this paper shows how such interventions can be brought into a computational model.

The interventions shown here are a snapshot of one particular time in the case organization. Such policies will need to change in accordance with the best medical knowledge at the time in order to maintain the required quality of treatment. Detailed modeling can be quite time-consuming, and in the worst case, a model can be deemed obsolete by the time it is ready to be used. Additionally, it might be difficult for researchers to gain access to relevant stakeholders in such a high-paced and hands-on environment as an ED. There will likely be a need and demand from these to achieve fast-paced tangible outcomes to maintain stakeholder interest.

4.5. Further Work

As the scope of this paper was only to show the model building itself, a natural continuation from this is to carry out actual simulation tests. A natural expansion of the work presented in this paper is to progress further onto the next step in Randers' overall simulation modeling process, as illustrated in Figure 3. In subsequent work, we will demonstrate how our simulation model can be used to study the effects of pandemic-related policies on patient flow. For example, introducing a waiting zone and/or an extra treatment room in the ED are some of these policies.

Although the model resulting from the study presented in this paper is relatively advanced compared to previous studies, since multiple agents and multi-method simulation approaches are considered, we believe this study is merely scratching the surface of what truly is the potential of ABM in conveying patient flow problematics. The proposed model can be expanded in several different directions. In this regard, there are several avenues for further work in the modeling work presented in this study. Examples are:

- Replacing our assumption of a constant contamination rate with a dynamically changing rate as a pandemic develops through time throughout a population.
- Replacing our assumption of no intra-hospital contamination with a probability of such contamination.
- Replacing our assumption of perfect sorting of incoming patients with a probability of classification inaccuracies.

5. Conclusions

This study set out to model the patient flow behavior in the ED under pandemic conditions. We conclude, based on a comparison between actual and simulated behavior of patients, that patient flow behavior under pandemic conditions with multiple agents (patients, department resources) and operational complexities (transitions, conditions, priorities, processing time, resource limitations) can be modeled with an acceptable degree of accuracy. We found that the prioritization of COVID-19-contaminated patients has complicated the ED behavior and has significantly affected the studied key performance measures. Moreover, compared to the actual data, the simulated results highlight the need for further study, including other vital agents (doctors, nurses, beds, other departments) and behavioral phenomena related to the studied patient flow regiment.

The final simulation model could emulate the patient flow behavior, as this research set out to accomplish. This was confirmed with stakeholder informants who had extensive knowledge and familiarity with the system itself. By this, the model was confirmed to pose a valid re-representation of the patient flow process of the case organization.

We found and concluded that neither discrete-event nor agent-based modeling on their own was effectively able to encompass the resulting patient flow complexities stemming from the COVID-19 pandemic. However, combining the two in a hybrid simulation model capitalized on the strengths from both discrete-event and agent-based modeling.

The strength utilized from discrete-event modeling was the ability to model the resource allocation between patient agents. Similarly, the strength utilized from agent-based modeling was the ability to model the patient agent's complex journey through the system.

In line with our stated research goals, this paper has provided:

- A conceptual and a computational model that mimics, explains, and predicts ED behavior under pandemic conditions while considering multiple agent behaviors.
- An account demonstrating the rigorous and transparent implementation of conceptual modeling of patient flow in the ED, to a greater extent than shown in previous research literature. By documenting the entire thought process behind each step of the modeling process and showing the resulting model, we believe that we contribute to modeling practice by making these steps transparent and accessible to others. This will be helpful to other researchers to understand, assess and build trust in such models, and provides an example than can be emulated by others to build their own thoroughly validated models.
- The computational model we have provided includes several performance measures that will be useful for practitioners but have not been previously introduced in simulation studies of patient flow in the ED.
- Furthermore, we have discussed the broader applicability of our models and are currently undertaking further research using the presented model to study patient flow in the ED under pandemic conditions.

Author Contributions: Conceptualization, G.T., E.C.B. and I.E.-T.; data curation, G.T.; formal analysis, G.T.; investigation, G.T. and E.C.B.; methodology, G.T., E.C.B. and I.E.-T.; project administration, G.T. and E.C.B.; resources, G.T.; software, G.T.; supervision, G.T., E.C.B. and I.E.-T.; validation, G.T., E.C.B. and I.E.-T.; visualization, G.T., E.C.B. and I.E.-T.; Writing—Original draft, G.T., E.C.B. and I.E.-T.; Writing—Review and editing, G.T., E.C.B. and I.E.-T. All authors have read and agreed to the published version of the manuscript.

Funding: This research received no external funding.

Institutional Review Board Statement: Not applicable.

Informed Consent Statement: Not applicable.

Data Availability Statement: The numerical data used in this study is not publicly available and thus is not for distribution.

Acknowledgments: The development, including Even Frørenæs, Linda Halle Nordahl, and Maria Endresen team at SUS, has been instrumental in the progression of this research.

Conflicts of Interest: The authors declare no conflict of interest.

Abbreviations

ABM—Agent-based modeling, **ED**—Emergency departments, **PF**—Patient flow, **SUS**—Stavanger Universitetssykehus (The University Hospital of Stavanger), **WZ**—Waiting zone, **TR**—Treatment room.

References

1. Ahsan, K.B.; Alam, M.R.; Morel, D.G.; Karim, M.A. Emergency department resource optimisation for improved performance: A review. *J. Ind. Eng. Int.* **2019**, *15*, 253–266. [CrossRef]
2. Quah, L.J.J.; Tan, B.K.K.; Fua, T.-P.; Wee, C.P.J.; Lim, C.S.; Nadarajan, G.; Zakaria, N.D.; Chan, S.-E.J.; Wan, P.W.; Teo, L.T.; et al. Reorganising the emergency department to manage the COVID-19 outbreak. *Int. J. Emerg. Med.* **2020**, *13*, 32. [CrossRef] [PubMed]
3. Nadarajan, G.D.; Omar, E.; Abella, B.S.; Hoe, P.S.; Do Shin, S.; Ma, M.H.-M.; Ong, M.E.H. A conceptual framework for Emergency department design in a pandemic. *Scand. J. Trauma Resusc. Emerg. Med.* **2020**, *28*, 118. [CrossRef] [PubMed]
4. Ronen, B.; Pliskin, J.S.; Pass, S. *The Hospital and Clinic Improvement Handbook: Using Lean and the Theory of Constraints for Better Healthcare Delivery*; Oxford University Press: Oxford, UK; New York, NY, USA, 2018; ISBN 978-0-19-084345-8.
5. Hoot, N.R.; Aronsky, D. Systematic Review of Emergency Department Crowding: Causes, Effects, and Solutions. *Ann. Emerg. Med.* **2008**, *52*, 126–136.e1. [CrossRef] [PubMed]

6. Hwang, U.; McCarthy, M.L.; Aronsky, D.; Asplin, B.; Crane, P.W.; Craven, C.K.; Epstein, S.K.; Fee, C.; Handel, D.A.; Pines, J.M.; et al. Measures of Crowding in the Emergency Department: A Systematic Review: ED Crowding Measures. *Acad. Emerg. Med.* **2011**, *18*, 527–538. [CrossRef] [PubMed]
7. Moskop, J.C.; Sklar, D.P.; Geiderman, J.M.; Schears, R.M.; Bookman, K.J. Emergency Department Crowding, Part 1—Concept, Causes, and Moral Consequences. *Ann. Emerg. Med.* **2009**, *53*, 605–611. [CrossRef] [PubMed]
8. Pitts, S.R.; Pines, J.M.; Handrigan, M.T.; Kellermann, A.L. National Trends in Emergency Department Occupancy, 2001 to 2008: Effect of Inpatient Admissions Versus Emergency Department Practice Intensity. *Ann. Emerg. Med.* **2012**, *60*, 679–686.e3. [CrossRef] [PubMed]
9. Dooley, K. Simulation Research Methods. In *The Blackwell Companion to Organizations*; Baum, J.A.C., Ed.; Blackwell Publishing Ltd: Oxford, UK, 2017; pp. 829–848, ISBN 978-1-4051-6406-1.
10. Currie, C.S.M.; Fowler, J.W.; Kotiadis, K.; Monks, T.; Onggo, B.S.; Robertson, D.A.; Tako, A.A. How simulation modelling can help reduce the impact of COVID-19. *J. Simul.* **2020**, *14*, 83–97. [CrossRef]
11. Gul, M.; Guneri, A.F. A comprehensive review of emergency department simulation applications for normal and disaster conditions. *Comput. Ind. Eng.* **2015**, *83*, 327–344. [CrossRef]
12. Ostermann, T. Agent-based modelling for simulating patients flow in a community hospital. In Proceedings of the International Conference on Health Informatics (HEALTHINF-2015), Lisbon, Portugal, 12–15 January 2015; pp. 14–19.
13. Bhattacharjee, P.; Ray, P.K. Patient flow modelling and performance analysis of healthcare delivery processes in hospitals: A review and reflections. *Comput. Ind. Eng.* **2014**, *78*, 299–312. [CrossRef]
14. Roberts, S.D. Tutorial on the simulation of healthcare systems. In Proceedings of the 2011 Winter Simulation Conference (WSC), Phoenix, AZ, USA, 11–14 December 2011; pp. 1403–1414.
15. Asgary, A.; Najafabadi, M.M.; Karsseboom, R.; Wu, J. A Drive-through Simulation Tool for Mass Vaccination during COVID-19 Pandemic. *Healthcare* **2020**, *8*, 469. [CrossRef] [PubMed]
16. Luna, L.F.; Andersen, D.L. Using Qualitative Methods in the Conceptualization and Assessment of System Dynamics Models. In Proceedings of the 20th International System Dynamics Conference, System Dynamics Society, Palermo, Italy, 28 July–1 August 2002.
17. Randers, J. *Elements of the System Dynamics Method*; MIT Press: Cambridge, MA, USA, 1980.
18. Terning, G.; Brun, E. Systemic Conceptual Modeling of Patient Flow in a Hospital Emergency Department: A case example. In Proceedings of the System Dynamics Society Record of the 38th International Conference of the System Dynamics Society 2020, Bergen, Norway, 19–24 July 2020; Volume 38.
19. Gunal, M.M. A guide for building hospital simulation models. *Health Syst.* **2012**, *1*, 17–25. [CrossRef]
20. Albin, S.; Forrester, J.W.; Breierova, L. *Building a System Dynamics Model: Part 1: Conceptualization*; MIT: Cambridge, MA, USA, 2001.
21. Suh, H. Key Figures. 2018. Available online: https://helse-stavanger.no/om-oss/nokkeltall-2018 (accessed on 14 February 2019).
22. Suh, H. Om Oss. Available online: https://helse-stavanger.no/om-oss (accessed on 7 February 2019).
23. Gallagher Healthcare. What Are the Different Types of Hospitals? Available online: https://www.gallaghermalpractice.com/blog/post/what-are-the-different-types-of-hospitals (accessed on 14 February 2019).
24. Minge, A. Hun skal hele tiden være orakelet og ta raske og rette avgjørelse. Denne dagen varte pausen i 30 sekunder. *Stavanger Aftenblad* **2020**. Available online: https://www.aftenbladet.no/magasin/i/EWgGxa/hun-skal-hele-tiden-vaere-orakelet-og-ta-raske-og-rette-avgjoerelse-denne-dagen-varte-pausen-i-30-sekunder (accessed on 14 February 2019).
25. Monks, T.; Currie, C.S.M.; Onggo, B.S.; Robinson, S.; Kunc, M.; Taylor, S.J.E. Strengthening the reporting of empirical simulation studies: Introducing the STRESS guidelines. *J. Simul.* **2019**, *13*, 55–67. [CrossRef]
26. Borshchev, A. *The Big Book of Simulation Modeling: Multimethod Modeling with AnyLogic 6*; AnyLogic North America: Chicago, IL, USA, 2013; ISBN 978-0-9895731-7-7.
27. Helsedirektoratet—Avdeling sykehustjenester Faglige og organisatoriske kvalitetskrav for somatiske akuttmottak. *Nas. Faglige Retningslinjer-2236* **2014**. Available online: https://www.helsedirektoratet.no/retningslinjer/kvalitetskrav-for-somatiske-akuttmottak/Faglige%20og%20organisatoriske%20kvalitetskrav%20for%20somatiske%20akuttmottak%20%E2%80%93%20Nasjonal%20faglig%20retningslinje.pdf/_/attachment/inline/aea8baff-94d2-44f5-b525-f6c1f518aed5:029310dc7ad46980ba0fe85bdd9887148d4206b1/Faglige%20og%20organisatoriske%20kvalitetskrav%20for%20somatiske%20akuttmottak%20%E2%80%93%20Nasjonal%20faglig%20retningslinje.pdf (accessed on 14 February 2019).
28. Senge, P.M.; Forrester, J.W. Tests for building confidence in system dynamics models. *Syst. Dyn. TIMS Stud. Manag. Sci.* **1980**, *14*, 209228.

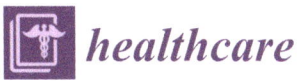

Article

Impact of a Digital Intervention for Literacy in Depression among Portuguese University Students: A Randomized Controlled Trial

Lersi D. Durán [1,*], Ana Margarida Almeida [1], Ana Cristina Lopes [2] and Margarida Figueiredo-Braga [3]

1 Department of Communication and Art, University of Aveiro/DigiMedia, 3810-193 Aveiro, Portugal; marga@ua.pt
2 Entre o Douro e Vouga Hospital Center, 4520-211 Santa Maria da Feira, Portugal; anacristinalopes.sp@gmail.com
3 Department of Clinical Neurosciences and Mental Health, School of Medicine, Porto University, 4200-450 Porto, Portugal; mmfb@med.up.pt
* Correspondence: ldquintero@ua.pt

Citation: Durán, L.D.; Almeida, A.M.; Lopes, A.C.; Figueiredo-Braga, M. Impact of a Digital Intervention for Literacy in Depression among Portuguese University Students: A Randomized Controlled Trial. *Healthcare* **2022**, *10*, 165. https://doi.org/10.3390/healthcare10010165

Academic Editor: Abraham Rudnick

Received: 15 December 2021
Accepted: 10 January 2022
Published: 15 January 2022

Publisher's Note: MDPI stays neutral with regard to jurisdictional claims in published maps and institutional affiliations.

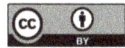

Copyright: © 2022 by the authors. Licensee MDPI, Basel, Switzerland. This article is an open access article distributed under the terms and conditions of the Creative Commons Attribution (CC BY) license (https://creativecommons.org/licenses/by/4.0/).

Abstract: Digital interventions are important tools to promote mental health literacy among university students. "Depression in Portuguese University Students" (Depressão em Estudantes Universitários Portugueses, DEEP) is an audiovisual intervention describing how symptoms can be identified and what possible treatments can be applied. The aim of this study was to evaluate the impact of this intervention. A random sample of 98 students, aged 20–38 years old, participated in a 12-week study. Participants were recruited through social media by the academic services and institutional emails of two Portuguese universities. Participants were contacted and distributed into four study groups (G1, G2, G3 and G4): G1 received the DEEP intervention in audiovisual format; G2 was given the DEEP in text format; G3 received four news articles on depression; G4 was the control group. A questionnaire was shared to collect socio-demographic and depression knowledge data as a pre-intervention method; content was then distributed to each group following a set schedule; the depression knowledge questionnaire was then administered to compare pre-intervention, post-intervention and follow-up literacy levels. Using the Scheffé and Least Significant Difference (LSD) multiple comparisons test, it was found that G1, which received the DEEP audiovisual intervention, differed significantly from the other groups, with higher depression knowledge scores in post-intervention stages. The DEEP audiovisual intervention, compared to the other formats used (narrative text format; news format), proved to be an effective tool for increasing depression knowledge in university students.

Keywords: digital interventions; mental health literacy; audiovisual

1. Introduction

There are many digital resources that provide mental health information and support. Digital technology has become an addictive element used by young university students as a privileged tool to access information [1]. It is not surprising that young people seek support and information about mental health on the Internet [2–4]. However, much of the digital content on the Internet does not have scientific validity [5,6], which can become a problem due to the use of unreliable information.

Providing mental health knowledge and promoting health literacy to young university students is a challenge for universities and the public health system [7,8]. Nowadays, an increasing number of cases of young people with depression are undetected, unrecognized and undertreated, leading to tragic episodes such as suicide and causing a great impact on the family and social environment [9–11]. According to the World Health Organization, depression is the leading cause of disability worldwide [12]. University students are exposed to specific challenges given their new responsibilities and are reported as a risk population for mental health problems, namely anxiety and/or depression [13], which can trigger other, more serious, disorders [11]. Young people are often reluctant to seek professional help for a mental/psychological disorder [7,14], due to preconceived ideas imposed by society, low mental health literacy and fear of being exposed [15,16].

Depression, according to Becken [17], is caused by a negative view of the world. A person with depressive symptoms has a negative cognition of the things around them. Depression is an illness in which feelings of deep sadness, emptiness, tiredness and lack of interest are present, which can lead to serious consequences such as suicide, causing great difficulties in family and social contexts [11].

Health literacy is of fundamental importance to guarantee a better quality of life on a personal and social level. This is a process that comprises three fundamental points, namely the capacity to analyze, understand and communicate [16,18], and depends on the skills that the individual or society develops in order to obtain the expected results. The significance of mental health literacy highlights the need to increase knowledge of mental-psychological disorders, so that help and information are sought and stigma is reduced [8,18].

In recent years, digital programs have been developed for the promotion, education and prevention of mental illnesses and/or disorders, with an emphasis on depression [18]. According to Frank, Pong, Asher and Soares [19], the use of digital programs may have positive effects on the understanding of depressive symptoms. The use of digital media to support interventions on depressive symptoms has been the subject of recent studies [20,21], which demonstrates the potential for using technology as a tool for the distribution of digital content in the area of depression [22]. Despite the wide variety of digital resources to treat and prevent depression, only a small number have been validated by specialists in the field [6,23]. For this reason, it is essential to develop further studies to validate the use of digital interventions on depression [24,25], and to better understand how the use of digital resources can provide well-being and mental health for university students.

Digital interventions can be used to provide a set of educational strategies with a cognitive orientation, allowing participants to learn about and/or face situations related to psychiatric disorders [26]. These interventions promote the integration of participants regardless of their geographical location [26,27] and can therefore bring together a large number of people. This makes the learning and/or treatment process more productive, easier and more enjoyable [28]. Digital interventions aimed at mental health promotion and education address specific needs and have a high success rate in overcoming stigma [29]. Importantly, digital resources have great potential for health information provision [30]. Social support, lack of geographic boundaries, free access and ease of access are some of the advantages of digital resources for health promotion and literacy [19,31,32]. However, there are several concerns, such as disparities in Internet access, the quality of online health information and the lack of real support to monitor how this information is processed [1,29,33].

For Michie et al. [34], Hollis et al. [35] and Alkhaldi et al. [36], digital interventions for mental health promotion and care must pay close attention to the content and information to be presented [33,37]. These are special interventions that, because they deal with sensitive issues, must be supported and monitored by specialists to prevent them from being non-beneficial resources for the participants [38]. Similarly, these digital resources for mental health promotion and literacy are based on pedagogical techniques, adapted to the needs of the participants. The information and content developed must have a technological, educational and explanatory context to ensure that the objective of a digital mental health literacy intervention is met [39].

The incorporation of an audiovisual format in the area of mental health literacy is considered an effective strategy to communicate, promote and support mental health literacy [40–42].

The evolution of technology and the digital world are part of the general population's life, especially among young people, thus allowing digital social media to be used as a tool to carry information in the area of mental health [43,44]. The concept of literacy that is associated with the ability to read and write thus expands and becomes the competence to promote or acquire information about, in this case within the scope of mental health [20,45]. The concept of literacy linked to technology is represented through images, sounds and videos, among other things [46]; therefore, the audiovisual format can be defined as a strategy to carry information in different forms of representation that generate interest in young audiences [47].

The digital audiovisual intervention DEEP consists of 23 short videos interspersed between a web series called "The Sara Wound" and informational videos about depression, divided into two stages. The first stage is "DEEP IN", which exposes the onset and acceptance of depressive symptoms, and the second stage "DEEP OUT", which presents the phase of seeking help and recovery.

This study aimed to evaluate the impact of the DEEP digital audiovisual intervention on Portuguese university students. The study considered their knowledge about the relevance they should give to symptoms and possible treatments, compared the audiovisual format of the intervention with the narrative text format and the news format and assessed the level of literacy before and after the intervention.

2. Materials and Methods

2.1. Study Context and Ethical Considerations

This study was conducted as part of the eMental project (evaluation of digital interventions for depression and suicide promotion and literacy), which aims to develop digital interventions for young university students and to understand the role they play in depression and suicide literacy. This research was developed as a randomized controlled trial, and the research protocol was approved by the Ethics Board of the University of Aveiro, Portugal (46-CED/2019).

2.2. Study Design and Sample

The evaluation of the impact of the intervention was conducted over a period of 14 weeks with an initial sample of 98 students, aged between 18 and 38 years old, of which 66% were female and 34% were male. The participants were students from two Portuguese universities and were randomly and equally divided into four groups, each group having access to information through different formats during the intervention. It should be noted that Group 1 received the DEEP intervention in audiovisual format and Group 4 was the control group. The purpose of having four groups was to allow comparison of the audiovisual format of DEEP intervention with the narrative text format of the same intervention, the narrative news format and to have a control group. It is important to note that only 71 students completed the first phase of the study.

Full access to the final version of this intervention cannot be presented in this paper as DEEP is still under analysis and development.

2.3. Recruitment of Participants

Students from two Portuguese universities were invited to participate in the study by means of an institutional email sent to all students, poster publications on the social networks of the universities' academic associations and printed posters placed in the common areas of the universities. The only criterion for participation was to be a university student, and the willingness to participate. No exclusion criteria were applied.

2.4. Instruments

After the recruitment campaign, those who were interested responded to the email quieroparticipar@ua.pt, sharing their intention to participate in the study. One week afterwards, participants were randomly divided into four groups. All groups were then sent a link via email to the initial questionnaire containing an introduction, an informed consent to participate form, a socio-demographic assessment (age and gender) and the pre-intervention knowledge literacy questionnaire. The literacy questionnaire was adapted from Griffiths et al. [15], Hart et al. [38] and Heickie et al. [48] and was tested in a pilot evaluation [25]. The questionnaire consists of true and false questions, divided into two parts: a first part of 25 questions on symptoms of depression, and a second part with 11 questions related to possible treatments. For the elaboration of the questionnaires and data collection, the software LimeSurvey was used on the platform https://forms.ua.pt/ (accessed in 10 January 2022), from the University of Aveiro, Portugal.

Subsequently, content was sent via email to each group, ranging from DEEP intervention in the digital format for G1, to DEEP intervention in narrative text for G2, to four news items on depression for G3, and it followed a distribution schedule (Appendix A) for a period of 23 working days between 3 p.m. and 8 p.m. At the end of the distribution of content for each group, the literacy questionnaire was sent as a post-intervention measurement instrument.

The purpose of the literacy questionnaire was to characterize participants' knowledge about depression at pre-intervention, post-intervention and follow-up. Finally, and after receiving the follow-up responses, DEEP intervention was sent in audiovisual format to all groups, including the control group (G4). Figure 1 represents the timeline of the assessment design.

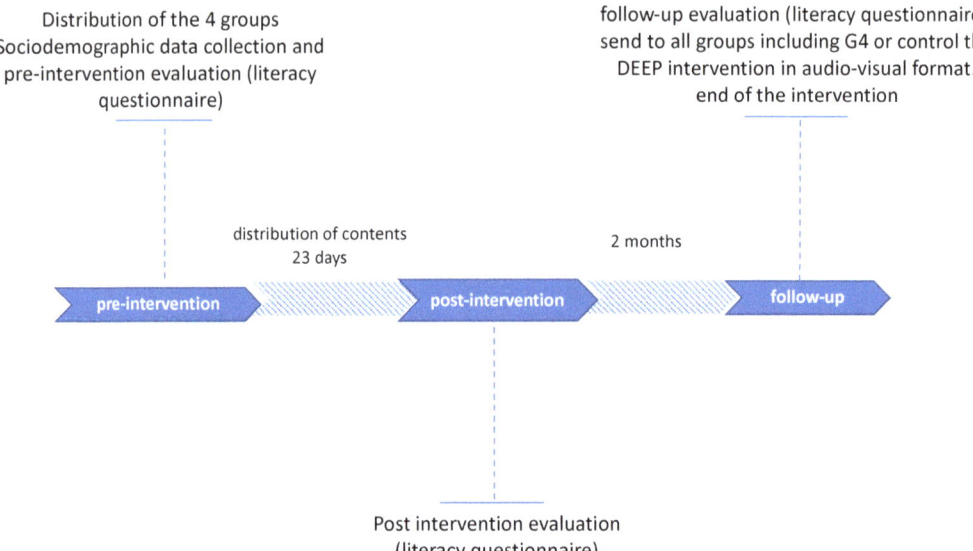

Figure 1. Timeline of the assessment design.

2.5. Statistical Analysis

For the quantitative data analysis, IBM® SPSS® software, version 24.0 for Windows®, was used to compare the total scores of the four groups in the three evaluation phases (pre-, post-intervention and follow-up), using one-factor ANOVA. When it was verified that there was no normality in the sample, the Kruskal–Wallis test was used as a non-parametric alternative. Since significant differences were found, multiple comparison tests were carried out using the Scheffé and Least Significant Difference (LSD) tests as they are adjusted when there is no normality and homogeneity of variances. For all cases, a level of 5% was used for the statistically significant value ($p < 0.05$).

3. Results

The results of the socio-demographic data are shown in Table 1. Considering the 71 university students who completed the entire literacy questionnaire and the socio-demographic data questionnaire in the pre-intervention phase, the age range was from 18 to 38 years old, the largest number of participants were female, and for the marital status of the participants, 60 out of the 71 were single. Regarding the place where they lived during the class period, 51 had to move from the family residence into a university residence due to the geographical distance between their home residences and the university.

Table 1. Socio-demographic characteristics of participants ($n = 71$).

$n = 71$	Gender		Marital Status			Place of Residence during the Period of University Classes	
Age Range	Male	Female	Single	Married	Partnership	Student Residence	At Home with Their Family
20 and 38 years old	24	47	60	9	2	51	20

It is important to note that the initial sample decreased when comparing each of the phases (pre-, post- and follow-up) of the intervention. Only 36 students reached the end of the study, a drop-out rate of 63.36%. Table 2 shows the number of students per group throughout the study and the results per group of the two literacy questionnaire sections.

Table 2. Results per literacy questionnaire group: number of participants, significant differences, and means in each phase of the study.

Study Group	Pre-Intervention ($n = 71$)				Post-Intervention ($n = 56$)				Follow-Up ($n = 36$)			
	Section 1		Section 2		Section 1		Section 2		Section 1		Section 2	
	Mean	p Value	Mean	p Value	Mean	p Value	Mean	p Value	Mean	p Value	Mean	p Value
G1	20.85	0.056	7.55	0.35	22.19	0.019 *	8.88	0.015 *	20.53	0.095	8.90	0.092
G2	20.82	0.107	6.71	0.451	21.36	0.175	7.14	0.118	20.11	0.264	7.00	0.242
G3	21.81	0.054	7.41	0.262	19.33	0.045	7.33	0.092	18.40	0.043	5.50	0.468
G4	20.41	0.118	7.71	0.094	20.42	0.091	7.50	0.059	20.80	0.191	7.60	0.445

* The mean difference is significant at the 0.05 level.

To measure the knowledge of respondents in the three phases of the intervention (pre-, post- and follow-up), the literacy questionnaire was used, divided into two sections: "Symptom identification" (Section 1) and "Possible treatments" (Section 2). For each section, the number of correct answers was added together, resulting in a final score. Therefore, the scores for Section 1 ranged from 0 to 25, and for Section 2, the scores ranged from 0 to 11.

It was necessary to test the normality of G1 data in the post-intervention phase, and no statistical significance was obtained. Hence, the assumption that G1 follows a normal distribution was rejected, and therefore, a non-parametric Kruskal–Wallis test was performed to measure if there were significant differences and to determine if the level of knowledge was equal or not in all phases.

In Table 3, the results of the Kruskal–Wallis test can be observed. For Sections 1 and 2 of G1, it can be seen that the significant group differences for each section are under 5%, thus rejecting the hypothesis that knowledge about depression is the same in all three phases.

After rejecting the hypothesis of equality, it was important to know which phase was responsible for this difference by creating a score-ordering variable for multiple comparisons between phases, using the Scheffé test for Section 1 and the LSD (least significant difference) test for Section 2.

Table 3. Kruskal–Wallis test results.

Teste	G1	
	Section 1	Section 2
Kruskal–Wallis H	12.367	7.126
p value	0.028 *	0.02 *

* The mean difference is significant at the 0.05 level.

The results of these multiple comparison statistical tests are in Table 4. The significant differences are marked with an asterisk, where it can be observed that G1 in the follow-up phase showed higher literacy levels compared to the pre-intervention phase. In Sections 1 and 2 in the pre-intervention phase, G1 had lower literacy levels than in the post-intervention and follow-up phases.

Table 4. Results of multiple comparison tests between phases of G1.

Group G1	Group G1	Sheffeé Test			LSD test		
		Section 1			Section 2		
Phase (I)	Phase (J)	Mean Difference (I–J)	Std. Error	Sig.	Mean Difference (I–J)	Std. Error	Sig.
Pre-intervention	Post-intervention	−9.506250	3.872342	0.060	−10.275000 *	4.140478	0.017
	Follow-up	−17.450000	4.471395	0.001	−10.700000 *	4.781013	0.030
Post-intervention	Pre-intervention	9.506250	3.872342	0.060	10.275000 *	4.140478	0.017
	Follow-up	−7.943750	4.653976	0.244	−0.425000	4.976236	0.932
Follow-up	Pre-intervention	17.450000 *	4.471395	0.001	10.700000 *	4.781013	0.030
	Post-intervention	7.943750	4.653976	0.244	0.425000	4.976236	0.932

* The mean difference is significant at the 0.05 level.

4. Discussion

This study evaluated the impact of the DEEP audiovisual intervention on university students. When comparing the results obtained in the pre- and post-intervention phases, it becomes clear that the mean number of correct answers in both sections only increased in groups G1 and G2. Significant differences ($p > 0.05$) were only obtained in G1. Therefore, depression literacy levels were significantly higher in this group, which demonstrates that digital content has a high potential to provide mental health literacy [25,26,33,39,40,49].

It is noteworthy that the knowledge of G3, who received information about depression in narrative notecard format, decreased, and that G4, or the control group, maintained the same knowledge in these phases. These results may suggest that young university students find it easier to obtain information through digital content because of the importance they place on the use of technology. At the same time, based on study findings, it may be inferred that the use of other formats may discourage young university students from acquiring new knowledge [2,8,9,13].

According to Carbonell et al. [1], Horgan and Sweeney [2], Griffiths et al. [15] and Uddin et al. [30], university students are immersed in the world of digital technology, so they are more interested in obtaining information and knowledge when the content is digital, which was corroborated by this study's findings, since it was shown that the format used for G3 and G4 was not as captivating as the digital format to generate interest in learning. However, for the follow-up phase, 2 months afterward, the scores did not increase. Despite this, the G1 and G2 groups maintained a level of knowledge very close to that of the pre-intervention phase. Although a decrease in knowledge of digital literacy interventions over time has been described in the literature [21,47,50], the DEEP intervention managed to maintain relatively unchanged knowledge levels of depression in the participants in the follow-up phase. It is important to further explore the impact of these results and the factors that influenced them by conducting an evaluation with more students and analyzing the different scenarios for each group.

The G4 or control group increased knowledge between the post-intervention and follow-up phases, but this increase was not statistically significant. This could confirm that when there is the presence of a control group, these groups feel the need to seek information on the topic because they are not involved in the interventions.

This work has several limitations, which must be acknowledged.

One limitation was the recruitment of participants to the study. Despite the strategies used, it was difficult to motivate students to agree to participate. Another possible limitation may have been the use of a questionnaire as a measurement instrument. Although this methodological choice was made in order to measure knowledge during all stages of the intervention, it may have contributed to participants dropping out of the intervention, since many students did not complete the questionnaire in the post-intervention and follow-up phases and therefore gave up continuing in the study. Studies with more than two follow-up phases generally have a high drop-out rate, especially if the participants do not receive a reward that interests them [9,11]. In this study, the drop-out rate was high, representing 63% of the initial sample. In this case, the representativeness of the sample is not fully accomplished, since the final results obtained cannot be generalizable.

However, the drop-out rate during the study did not impede the study, nor did it affect the results, as all four groups maintained an equivalent number of students. Although it is not possible to generalize the conclusions, the results found presuppose an initial step for future studies, in which a strategy should be considered to keep participants enrolled in the study for the duration of the intervention and thus reduce the drop-out rate.

Another limitation of this study was the fact that we could not 100% control the risk of contamination between groups. The choice of participants per group was random; we did not know and could not identify the participants due to the General Data Protection Regulation (GDPR). Alternatives to control the groups were not possible to implement because they would identify the participants; we only checked G1 for the number of views of each video during the time of the intervention.

It could also be considered a limitation of this work that G3 received only four news articles about depression in digital format during the intervention. In fact, this group differed both in content and format from the other groups, but this strategy was used to try to compare the audiovisual format of the digital intervention with the remaining formats, and thus find out if the DEEP intervention in audiovisual format would have more influence on participants' knowledge of depression.

Youth mental health literacy should be an area of further exploration, so that young people can recognize and respond appropriately to the signs and symptoms of depression or other mental disorders [3,4,9]. Future studies should focus on developing effective technology-linked interventions to improve knowledge and thus raise awareness among young university students about how to care for and maintain good mental health.

5. Conclusions

The DEEP digital intervention is based on an audiovisual strategy, grounded in a clinical-social approach, with the aim of improving the depression knowledge of Portuguese university students and with the intention of increasing quality of life and creating a state of full well-being.

The results of this study provide evidence that digital audiovisual content is more likely to increase depression literacy in university students than other formats. Young people learned more from the audiovisual content of the DEEP intervention than students who received the other formats with equivalent information. It is necessary that these interventions are evaluated by specialists before being delivered to the participants, because, as they deal with sensitive topics, information may be shared that is harmful to the participants.

Evaluating the DEEP intervention enriched the perception of the role of digital technologies to promote literacy in depression, highlighting the importance of complementing interventions with two different approaches: information videos (as a substitute for a specialist in the area) interspersed with videos of Sara's story (portraying the reality of a university student).

Digital technology and mental health together form a key partnership to address current public health challenges and are allies in improving the quality of mental health among university students, which is currently even more fragile due to the pandemic scenario. The DEEP digital intervention format highlighted the potential for videos as a vehicle to increase depression literacy, enabling the understanding of the disease, considering symptom identification and possible treatments. It is also important to note that digital interventions can be scaled up to all audiences and thus provide better health care whether for promotion/literacy/therapy or treatment of mental disorders.

Author Contributions: Methodology, L.D.D. and A.M.A.; validation, A.M.A. and A.C.L.; formal analysis, L.D.D.; investigation, L.D.D.; resources, A.M.A. and M.F.-B.; data curation, L.D.D.; writing—original draft preparation, L.D.D.; writing—review and editing, A.M.A., A.C.L. and M.F.-B.; visualization, A.M.A., A.C.L. and M.F.-B.; supervision, A.M.A. and M.F.-B.; project administration, A.M.A.; funding acquisition, L.D.D. All authors have read and agreed to the published version of the manuscript.

Funding: This paper is funded by the project eMental (ref 45-2019/393, funded by Ciência Viva) and the research grant reference B/UI73/8905/2021. Thanks are due to FCT/MCTES for the financial support to DigiMedia (UIDP/05460/2020 + UIBD/05460/2020), through national funds.

Institutional Review Board Statement: The study was conducted according to the guidelines of the Declaration of Helsinki, and approved by the Ethics Board of the University of Aveiro, Portugal (46-CED/2019 and date of approval: 1 April 2020).

Informed Consent Statement: Informed consent was obtained from all subjects involved in the study.

Data Availability Statement: The data that support the findings of this study are available from the corresponding author and the team involved in the project. Data are however available with upon reasonable request and with permission and autorizated the team.

Acknowledgments: To Ciência Viva, for the financial support of eMental Project "Assessing digital interventions for the promotion of literacy in depression and suicide". to Digital Media and Interaction research centre (DigiMedia) of the University of Aveiro and to the students involved in the development of the audiovisual intervention DEEP.

Conflicts of Interest: The authors declare that they have no conflict of interests.

Appendix A

This section presents the timetable used for sending the contents to each group. The sending occurred via email, and in Table A1, the days on which the groups received the contents are highlighted in bold.

Table A1. Calendar with the days when the contents were sent.

Mon	Tue	Wed	Thu	Fri
Day 1	**Day 2**	Day 3	Day 4	**Day 5**
Day 6	**Day 7**	Day 8	**Day 9**	**Day 10**
Day 11	Day 12	**Day 13**	**Day 14**	Day 15
Day 16	**Day 17**	Day 18	Day 19	**Day 20**
Day 21	Day 22	**Day 23**	Day 24	Day 25
Day 26	**Day 27**	**Day 28**	Day 29	**Day 30**
Day 31	Day 32	Day 33	**Day 34**	**Day 35**
Day 36	**Day 37**	**Day 38**	Day 39	**Day 40**

Table A2 shows the day, time and content sent to each group. The time varies between 4:00 p.m. and 7:00 p.m., generating a surprise factor when each content was sent.

Table A2. Timetable and contents sent to each group.

		Content Distribution Schedule		
Day	Hour	Content Group 1	Content Group 2	Content Group 3
Day 1	16:00	Teaser/PE-Video 1	Teaser/PE-Video 1	Article 1
Day 2	18:00	FS Video 1	FS text 1	
Day 5	19:00	PE Video 2	PE text 2	
Day 7	17:00	FS Video 2	FS text 2	
Day 9	16:00	PE Video 3	PE text 3	
Day 10	18:00	FS Video 3	FS text 3	
Day 11	19:00	PE Video 4	PE text 4	
Day 13	18:00	FS Video 4	FS text 4	Article 2
Day 14	19:00	PE Video 5	PE tex5	
Day 17	16:00	FS Video 5	FS text 5	
Day 20	19:00	PE Video 6	PE text 6	
Day 21	17:00	FS Video 6	FS text 6	
Day 23	16:00	FS Video 7	FS text 7	
Day 24	18:00	PE Video 7	PE text 7	Article 3
Day 27	17:00	FS Video 8	FS text 8	
Day 28	19:00	PE Video 8	PE text 8	
Day 30	16:00	FS Video 9	FS text 9	
Day 31	19:00	PE Video 9	PE text 9	
Day 34	17:00	FS Video 10	FS text 10	
Day 35	18:00	FS Video 11	FS text 11	
Day 37	16:00	FS Video 12	FS text 12	Article 4
Day 38	19:00	PE Video 10	PE text 10	
Day 40	17:00	FS Video 13	FS text 13	

FS video X: video of "the wound Sara", episode X; PE video X: psychoeducational video, episode X; FS text X: narrative text of "the wound Sara", episode X; PE text X: psychoeducational narrative texts; article X: news article from some Portuguese newspapers.

References

1. Carbonell, X.; Chamarro, A.; Oberst, U.; Rodrigo, B.; Prades, M. Problematic Use of the Internet and Smartphones in University Students: 2006–2017. *Int. J. Environ. Res. Public Health* **2018**, *15*, 475. [CrossRef]
2. Horgan, Á.; Sweeney, J. Young Students' Use of the Internet for Mental Health Information and Support. *J. Psychiatr. Ment. Health Nurs.* **2010**, *17*, 117–123. [CrossRef]
3. Burns, J.M.; Davenport, T.A.; Durkin, L.A.; Luscombe, G.M.; Hickie, I.B. The Internet as a Setting for Mental Health Service Utilisation by Young People. *Med. J. Aust.* **2010**, *192* (Suppl. 11), S22–S26. [CrossRef]
4. Chen, W.; Zheng, Q.; Liang, C.; Xie, Y.; Gu, D. Factors Influencing College Students' Mental Health Promotion: The Mediating Effect of Online Mental Health Information Seeking. *Int. J. Environ. Res. Public Health* **2020**, *17*, 4783. [CrossRef]
5. Christensen, H.; Griffiths, K. The Internet and Mental Health Literacy. *Aust. N. Z. J. Psychiatry* **2016**, *34*, 975–979. [CrossRef] [PubMed]
6. Mathews, S.C.; McShea, M.J.; Hanley, C.L.; Ravitz, A.; Labrique, A.B.; Cohen, A.B. Digital Health: A Path to Validation. *NPJ Digit. Med.* **2019**, *2*, 38. [CrossRef] [PubMed]
7. Cova Solar, F.; Alvial, S.W.; Aro, D.M.; Bonifetti, D.A.; Hernández, M.M.; Rodríguez, C.C. Problemas de Salud Mental En Estudiantes de La Universidad de Concepción. *Ter. Psicológica* **2007**, *25*, 105–112. [CrossRef]
8. Oliveira, C.; Varela, A.; Esteves, J.; Henriques, C.; Ribeiro, A. Programas De Prevenção Para A Ansiedade E Depressão: Avaliação Da Percepção Dos Estudantes Universitários. *Programas Prevenção Para A Ansiedade E Depress* **2016**, *111*, 96–111.
9. Frazier, P.; Meredith, L.; Greer, C.; Paulsen, J.A.; Howard, K.; Dietz, L.R.; Qin, K. Randomized Controlled Trial Evaluating the Effectiveness of a Web-Based Stress Management Program among Community College Students. *Anxiety Stress Coping* **2014**, *28*, 576–586. [CrossRef]
10. Hoare, E.; Collins, S.; Marx, W.; Callaly, E.; Moxham-Smith, R.; Cuijpers, P.; Holte, A.; Nierenberg, A.A.; Reavley, N.; Christensen, H.; et al. Universal Depression Prevention: An Umbrella Review of Meta-Analyses. *J. Psychiatr. Res.* **2021**, *144*, 483–493. [CrossRef]
11. Wongpakaran, N.; Oon-Arom, A.; Karawekpanyawong, N.; Lohanan, T.; Leesawat, T.; Wongpakaran, T. Borderline Personality Symptoms: What Not to Be Overlooked When Approaching Suicidal Ideation among University Students. *Healthc* **2021**, *9*, 1399. [CrossRef] [PubMed]
12. WHO. Depression. WHO, 2017. Available online: http://www.who.int/mental_health/management/depression/en/ (accessed on 16 June 2020).

13. Zhou, L.; Parmanto, B. Development and Validation of a Comprehensive Well-Being Scale for People in the University Environment (Pitt Wellness Scale) Using a Crowdsourcing Approach: Cross-Sectional Study. *J. Med. Internet Res.* **2020**, *22*, e15075. [CrossRef] [PubMed]
14. Pretorius, C.; Chambers, D.; Coyle, D. Young People's Online Help-Seeking and Mental Health Difficulties: Systematic Narrative Review. *J. Med. Internet Res.* **2019**, *21*, e13873. [CrossRef]
15. Griffiths, K.M.; Christensen, H.; Jorm, A.F.; Evans, K.; Groves, C. Effect of Web-Based Depression Literacy and Cognitive–Behavioural Therapy Interventions on Stigmatising Attitudes to Depression. *Br. J. Psychiatry* **2004**, *185*, 342–349. [CrossRef]
16. Warchoł, T. Przegląd Badań Edukacyjnych Educational Studies Review Tomasz Warchoł A Sense of the Role and Value of Non-Formal Education in the Opinion of Students Participating in Interactive Workshops. Przegląd Badań Eduk. *Educ. Stud. Rev.* **2018**, *2*, 71–84. [CrossRef]
17. Beck, A.; Rush, A.; Shaw, B.; Emery, G. Cognitive Therapy of Depression. *Aust. N. Z. J. Psychiatry* **1979**, *36*, 272–275. [CrossRef]
18. Garrido, S.; Millington, C.; Cheers, D.; Boydell, K.; Schubert, E.; Meade, T.; Nguyen, Q.V. What Works and What Doesn't Work? A Systematic Review of Digital Mental Health Interventions for Depression and Anxiety in Young People. *Front. Psychiatry* **2019**, *10*, 759. [CrossRef] [PubMed]
19. Frank, E.; Pong, J.; Asher, Y.; Soares, C.N. Smart Phone Technologies and Ecological Momentary Data: Is This the Way Forward on Depression Management and Research? *Curr. Opin. Psychiatry* **2018**, *31*, 3–6. [CrossRef]
20. Peng, Z.; Hu, Q.; Dang, J. Multi-Kernel SVM Based Depression Recognition Using Social Media Data. *Int. J. Mach. Learn. Cybern.* **2019**, *10*, 43–57. [CrossRef]
21. Wei, Y.; McGrath, P.J.; Hayden, J.; Kutcher, S. Mental Health Literacy Measures Evaluating Knowledge, Attitudes and Help-Seeking: A Scoping Review. *BMC Psychiatry* **2015**, *15*, 291. [CrossRef]
22. Giosan, C.; Mogoaşe, C.; Cobeanu, O.; Szentágotai Tătar, A.; Mureşan, V.; Boian, R. Using a Smartphone App to Reduce Cognitive Vulnerability and Mild Depressive Symptoms: Study Protocol of an Exploratory Randomized Controlled Trial. *Trials* **2016**, *17*, 609. [CrossRef]
23. Mohr, D.C.; Tomasino, K.N.; Lattie, E.G.; Palac, H.L.; Kwasny, M.J.; Weingardt, K.; Karr, C.J.; Kaiser, S.M.; Rossom, R.C.; Bardsley, L.R.; et al. IntelliCare: An Eclectic, Skills-Based App Suite for the Treatment of Depression and Anxiety. *J. Med. Internet Res.* **2017**, *19*, e10. [CrossRef] [PubMed]
24. Almeida, A.M.P.; Almeida, H.S.; Figueiredo-Braga, M. Mobile Solutions in Depression: Enhancing Communication with Patients Using an SMS-Based Intervention. *Procedia Comput. Sci.* **2018**, *138*, 89–96. [CrossRef]
25. Kerst, A.; Zielasek, J.; Gaebel, W. Smartphone Applications for Depression: A Systematic Literature Review and a Survey of Health Care Professionals' Attitudes towards Their Use in Clinical Practice. *Eur. Arch. Psychiatry Clin. Neurosci.* **2019**, *270*, 139–152. [CrossRef] [PubMed]
26. Durán, L.; Almeida, A.M.; Figueiredo-Braga, M. Digital Audiovisual Contents for Literacy in Depression: A Pilot Study with University Students. *Procedia Comput. Sci.* **2021**, *181*, 239–246. [CrossRef]
27. Sin, J.; Gillard, S.; Spain, D.; Cornelius, V.; Chen, T.; Henderson, C. Effectiveness of Psychoeducational Interventions for Family Carers of People with Psychosis: A Systematic Review and Meta-Analysis. *Clin. Psychol. Rev.* **2017**, *56*, 13–24. [CrossRef]
28. Khan, I.; Melro, A.; Oliveira, L.; Amaro, A.C. Internet of Things Prototyping for Cultural Heritage Dissemination. *J. Digit. Media Interact.* **2020**, *3*, 20–35.
29. Grigsby, T.J.; Unger, J.B.; Molina, G.B.; Baron, M. Evaluation of an Audio-Visual Novela to Improve Beliefs, Attitudes and Knowledge toward Dementia: A Mixed-Methods Approach. *Clin. Gerontol.* **2017**, *40*, 130–138. [CrossRef]
30. Uddin, S.; Al Mamun, A.; Iqbal, M.A.; Nasrullah, M. Internet Addiction Disorder and Its Pathogenicity to Psychological Distress and Depression among University Students: A Cross-Sectional Pilot Study in Bangladesh. *Psychology* **2016**, *7*, 1126–1137. [CrossRef]
31. Chu, J.T.; Wang, M.P.; Shen, C.; Viswanath, K.; Lam, T.H.; Chan, S.S.C. How, When and Why People Seek Health Information Online: Qualitative Study in Hong Kong. *Interact. J. Med. Res.* **2017**, *6*, e24. [CrossRef] [PubMed]
32. Pinto, L.T.; Figueiredo, V.A. Redes Sociais: Oportunidade de Buscar Evidências Nas Informações Compartilhadas Pelos Alunos. *Rev. Inf. Educ.* **2020**, *1*, 1–8.
33. Thornicroft, G.; Mehta, N.; Clement, S.; Evans-Lacko, S.; Doherty, M.; Rose, D.; Koschorke, M.; Shidhaye, R.; O'Reilly, C.; Henderson, C. Evidence for Effective Interventions to Reduce Mental-Health-Related Stigma and Discrimination. *Lancet* **2016**, *387*, 1123–1132. [CrossRef]
34. Michie, S.; Yardley, L.; West, R.; Patrick, K.; Greaves, F. Developing and Evaluating Digital Interventions to Promote Behavior Change in Health and Health Care: Recommendations Resulting from an International Workshop. Journal of Medical Internet Research. *J. Med. Internet Res.* **2017**, *19*, e232. [CrossRef]
35. Hollis, C.; Sampson, S.; Simons, L.; Davies, E.B.; Churchill, R.; Betton, V.; Butler, D.; Chapman, K.; Easton, K.; Gronlund, T.A.; et al. Identifying Research Priorities for Digital Technology in Mental Health Care: Results of the James Lind Alliance Priority Setting Partnership. *Lancet Psychiatry* **2018**, *5*, 845–854. [CrossRef]
36. Alkhaldi, G.; Hamilton, F.L.; Lau, R.; Webster, R.; Michie, S.; Murray, E. The Effectiveness of Prompts to Promote Engagement with Digital Interventions: A Systematic Review. *J. Med. Internet Res.* **2016**, *18*, e6. [CrossRef]

37. Duran, L.Q.; Almeida, A.M.P.; Figueiredo-Braga, M. Digital Audiovisual Narratives as Depression Literacy Promoters: Development of Psychoeducational Intervention DEEP. In Proceedings of the 15th Iberian Conference on Information Systems and Technologies (CISTI), Sevilla, Spain, 24–27 June 2020; pp. 1–6. [CrossRef]
38. Patel, S.; Akhtar, A.; Malins, S.; Wright, N.; Rowley, E.; Young, E.; Sampson, S.; Morriss, R. The Acceptability and Usability of Digital Health Interventions for Adults with Depression, Anxiety, and Somatoform Disorders: Qualitative Systematic Review and Meta-Synthesis. *J. Med. Internet Res.* **2020**, *22*, e16228. [CrossRef]
39. Hart, S.R.; Kastelic, E.A.; Wilcox, H.C.; Beaudry, M.B.; Musci, R.J.; Heley, K.M.; Ruble, A.E.; Swartz, K.L. Achieving Depression Literacy: The Adolescent Depression Knowledge Questionnaire (ADKQ). *Sch. Ment. Health* **2014**, *6*, 213–223. [CrossRef] [PubMed]
40. Spiker, D.A.; Hammer, J.H. Mental Health Literacy as Theory: Current Challenges and Future Directions. *J. Ment. Health* **2019**, *28*, 238–242. [CrossRef] [PubMed]
41. Farrer, L.; Gulliver, A.; Chan, J.K.Y.; Batterham, P.J.; Reynolds, J.; Calear, A.; Tait, R.; Bennett, K.; Griffiths, K.M. Technology-Based Interventions for Mental Health in Tertiary Students: Systematic Review. *J. Med. Internet Res.* **2013**, *15*, e101. [CrossRef]
42. Bona, R.J. Audiovisual Narratives Aimed at Children's Audience in the Early 1990s: Transmedia Intertextuality Practices in Cartoons. *Estud. em Comun.* **2018**, *1*, 215–229. [CrossRef]
43. Dowling, D.O.; Miller, K.J. Immersive Audio Storytelling: Podcasting and Serial Documentary in the Digital Publishing Industry. *J. Radio Audio Media* **2019**, *26*, 167–184. [CrossRef]
44. Naslund, J.A.; Bondre, A.; Torous, J.; Aschbrenner, K.A. Social Media and Mental Health: Benefits, Risks, and Opportunities for Research and Practice. *J. Technol. Behav. Sci.* **2020**, *5*, 245–257. [CrossRef]
45. Glick, G.; Druss, B.; Pina, J.; Lally, C.; Conde, M. Use of Mobile Technology in a Community Mental Health Setting. *J. Telemed. Telecare* **2015**, *22*, 430–435. [CrossRef]
46. Kutcher, S.; Bagnell, A.; Wei, Y. Mental Health Literacy in Secondary Schools: A Canadian Approach. *Child Adolesc. Psychiatr. Clin.* **2015**, *24*, 233–244. [CrossRef]
47. Ito-Jaeger, S.; Vallejos, E.P.; Curran, T.; Spors, V.; Long, Y.; Liguori, A.; Warwick, M.; Wilson, M.; Crawford, P. Digital Video Interventions and Mental Health Literacy among Young People: A Scoping Review. *J. Ment. Health* **2021**, 1–11. [CrossRef] [PubMed]
48. Hickie AM, I.B.; Davenport, T.A.; Luscombe, G.M.; Rong, Y.; Hickie, M.L.; Bell, M.I. The Assessment of Depression Awareness and Help-Seeking Behaviour: Experiences with the International Depression Literacy Survey. *BMC Psychiatry* **2007**, *7*, 48. [CrossRef]
49. Janoušková, M.; Tušková, E.; Weissová, A.; Trančík, P.; Pasz, J.; Evans-Lacko, S.; Winkler, P. Can Video Interventions Be Used to Effectively Destigmatize Mental Illness among Young People? A Systematic Review. *Eur. Psychiatry* **2017**, *41*, 1–9. [CrossRef]
50. Seedaket, S.; Turnbull, N.; Phajan, T.; Wanchai, A. Improving Mental Health Literacy in Adolescents: Systematic Review of Supporting Intervention Studies. *Trop. Med. Int. Health* **2020**, *25*, 1055–1064. [CrossRef]

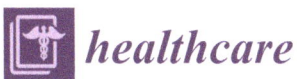

Article

Artificial Intelligence in Orthodontic Smart Application for Treatment Coaching and Its Impact on Clinical Performance of Patients Monitored with AI-TeleHealth System

Andrej Thurzo [1,*], Veronika Kurilová [2] and Ivan Varga [3]

[1] Department of Stomatology and Maxillofacial Surgery, Faculty of Medicine, Comenius University in Bratislava, 81250 Bratislava, Slovakia
[2] Faculty of Electrical Engineering and Information Technology, Slovak University of Technology, 81219 Bratislava, Slovakia; veronika.hanuskova@gmail.com
[3] Institute of Histology and Embryology, Faculty of Medicine, Comenius University in Bratislava, 81372 Bratislava, Slovakia; ivan.varga@fmed.uniba.sk
* Correspondence: Andrej@Thurzo.sk; Tel.: +421-903-110-107

Abstract: Background: Treatment of malocclusion with clear removable appliances like Invisalign® or Spark™, require considerable higher level of patient compliance when compared to conventional fixed braces. The clinical outcomes and treatment efficiency strongly depend on the patient's discipline. Smart treatment coaching applications, like strojCHECK® are efficient for improving patient compliance. Purpose: To evaluate the impact of computerized personalized decision algorithms responding to observed and anticipated patient behavior implemented as an update of an existing clinical orthodontic application (app). Materials and Methods: Variables such as (1) patient app interaction, (2) patient app discipline and (3) clinical aligner tracking evaluated by artificial intelligence system (AI) system— Dental monitoring® were observed on the set of 86 patients. Two 60-day periods were evaluated; before and after the app was updated with decision tree processes. Results: All variables showed significant improvement after the update except for the manifestation of clinical non-tracking in men, evaluated by artificial intelligence from video scans. Conclusions: Implementation of application update including computerized decision processes can significantly enhance clinical performance of existing health care applications and improve patients' compliance. Using the algorithm with decision tree architecture could create a baseline for further machine learning optimization.

Keywords: orthodontic treatment; clear aligners; smart application; AI; computerized learning; behavior change techniques; decision tree algorithm; telemedicine

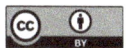

1. Introduction

Prevalence of malocclusion and orthodontic treatment need is well researched. Noticeable incisor irregularity occurs in the majority of all ethnic groups, with only 35% of adults having well-aligned mandibular incisors [1]. Irregularity is severe enough in 15% that both social acceptability and function could be affected, and major arch expansion or extraction of some teeth would be required for correction. About 20% of the population have deviations from the ideal bite relationship; in 2% these are severe enough to be disfiguring and are at the limit for orthodontic correction. Application of the Index of Treatment Need to the survey data reveals that 57% to 59% of each racial/ethnic group has at least some degree of orthodontic treatment need [1].

Both clear aligners and braces are effective in malocclusion treatment. Clear aligners had advantage in segmented movement of teeth and shortened treatment duration, but were not as effective as braces in producing adequate occlusal contacts, controlling teeth torque, and retention [2].

Clear Aligners therapy (CAT) is considered efficient orthodontic treatment. It aligns and levels the arches; and is effective in controlling anterior intrusion but not anterior extrusion; it is effective in controlling posterior buccolingual inclination but not anterior buccolingual inclination; it is effective in controlling upper molar bodily movements; and is less effective in controlling rotation of rounded teeth in particular [3].

However, CAT is currently under intense innovative technological pressure including new optimized attachment systems with high potential to use whole exposed tooth surface for application of forces to achieve proper tooth movements. This article is focused on support of modern CAT with smart mobile application and effect of its artificial intelligence (AI) upgrade.

1.1. Mobile Applications in Orthodontics

Mobile applications (apps) are to be a crucial tool in management of modern aesthetical and comfortable treatments where patient compliance is the key. They already play an increasingly important role in daily life and patients' social networks like Instagram represents an aid to the standard verbal motivation performed by orthodontists towards young patients under an orthodontic treatment [4]. With the number of orthodontic-related apps continuing to increase, and the rapid development of artificial intelligence, the potential to yield tremendous benefits to both clinicians and patients is apparent. More advanced features of artificial intelligence have been introduced to orthodontic applications recently. For example, three-dimensional convolutional neural networks (3D CNN) have high potential for automated 3D cephalometric evaluation directly from the Cone-Beam Computed Tomography (CBCT) or facial growth predictions [5].

These advanced forms of artificial intelligence can overtake also the process of orthodontic auxiliaries designing where currently dominates Finite Element Analysis (FEM) [6].

If orthodontic apps are to become mainstream and obtain greater acceptance, scientific validation and investigation of these apps are to be undertaken. The current situation in the clinical field shows only 20 publications about apps used in orthodontics. Their structure is expanded in the Table 1. In summary:

- 8 studies were Randomized Controlled Trials (RCTs) (35%)
- 10 were case-controls (53%)
- 1 was a cohort study (retrospective) (6%)
- 1 cross-sectional study was found (6%)

Seven studies (35%) were based on apps used for diagnostics, and all were cephalometric apps. 7 studies (41%) investigating apps used for reminders were present. 4 studies (24%) investigated dedicated remote monitoring apps and all four studied Dental Monitoring [7,8].

Table 1. The characteristics of current studies about apps used in orthodontics (n = 20).

Study Type	Author	Domain of Use	Focus Group of Apps
RCT	Alkadhi [9] 2017	Reminders	Patient
RCT	Deleuse [10] 2020	Reminders	Patient
RCT	Li [11] 2016	Reminders	Patient
RCT	Scheerman [12] 2020	Reminders	Patient
RCT	Zotti [13] 2016	Reminders; remote monitoring	Patient; clinician
RCT	Zotti [14] 2019	Reminders; remote monitoring	Patient; clinician
RCT	Al-Abdallah [15] 2021	Reminders	Patient; clinician
RCT	Ross [16] 2019	Reminders	Patient
Case-control	Abdul Khader [17] 2020	Diagnostics	Clinician
Case-control	Aksakalli [18] 2017	Diagnostics	Clinician
Case-control	Goracci [19] 2014	Diagnostics	Clinician
Case-control	Kumar [20] 2020	Diagnostics	Clinician

Table 1. *Cont.*

Study Type	Author	Domain of Use	Focus Group of Apps
Case-control	Kuriakose [21] 2019	Remote monitoring	Patient; clinician
Case-control	Livas [22] 2019	Diagnostics	Clinician
Case-control	Morris [23] 2019	Remote monitoring	Patient; clinician
Case-control	Moylan [24] 2019	Remote monitoring	Patient; clinician
Case-control	Sayar [25] 2017	Diagnostics	Clinician
Case-control	Caruso [26] 2021	Remote monitoring	Patient; clinician
Retrospective cohort study	Hansa [27] 2020	Remote monitoring	Patient; clinician
Cross-sectional	Underwood [28] 2015	Reminders	Patient

In comparison to app analyzed in this research paper (StrojCHECK®, Bratislava, Slovakia, 3Dent Medical, osim.sk (accessed on 1 November 2021)—Society for Medical Innovation (SMI)), most of the current apps used for orthodontic purposes, are simple apps without back-end or any Artificial Intelligence (AI) implementations. There is no publication about orthodontic apps other than simple reminders, basic diagnostics (cephalometry) or remote monitoring. Most of the app regarding orthodontic therapy are focused on oral hygiene status and coaching [12,29]. Despite the current weak scientific coverage, there are no doubts tele-orthodontics is the future of dental digitalization [30–33].

With the current situation described above, it is worth to highlight that over 90% of all apps used in orthodontics are single apps without any server back-end as well as they possess any truly intelligent behavior. Potential of implementations of machine learning algorithms and other levels of artificial intelligence features might bring significant leap in their clinical efficiency. This paper describes effect of an update of existing orthodontic app with AI algorithms of decision processes.

Technologies in our mobiles transformed almost every aspect of our lives. Smartphones enable patients to request, receive, and transmit information irrespective of the time and place. Also, the global pandemic has forced healthcare providers to employ TeleHealth technology to help handling this tense situation [34].

1.2. Tele-Orthodontics—Dental Monitoring and Other Aspects of TeleHealth

Tele-orthodontics—Dental Monitoring® (DM) (Dental Monitoring Co., Paris, France) with distant monitoring is current reality in orthodontics. We can, as the clinical orthodontists proactively monitor our patients with virtual examinations to supplement chairside appointments. Though this approach is tainted with negative connotations associated with the direct to patient business model [27,30], there are undisputable advantages of remote monitoring to the clinical practice of orthodontics [35].

Interesting aspect of this research paper is a true clinical evaluation of the impact of the app AI update. Performance of the app before and after the update was different. To evaluate clinical impact an AI Tele-Health system was used (DM). This system is capable to evaluate various clinical situations from the patients' home-made video-scans [26]. AI evaluation recognizes various clinical situations like: loss of attachment, loss of various accessories, gingivitis, caries and many other. In this paper this telemedicine system is used for frequent clinical evaluation of aligners tracking on the teeth. This AI TeleHealth system is frequently used in other studies and its accuracy and reliability is well evaluated [23,26,27,36–38]. How this study examined the true clinical performance of patients with this system is described in Material and methods chapter in more detail.

Dental Monitoring is reducing (not eliminating) the need for in-office visits. However, nearly half of the studies currently published on this topic comparing clinical treatment with DM and without DM, frequently misunderstand the focus of this technology. The spotlight of this AI-powered DM is not on reduction of patient's visits rather enhanced level of control over treatment development. As described earlier in this paper, the CAT in general, is prone to patients' indiscipline. Patient not wearing aligners properly (more than

22 h per day), results in situation called "non-tracking". This manifests as a discrepancy between shape of the aligner and real teeth position. This can be evaluated with DM. Possible lower frequency of physical visits to dental clinic is only secondary. However, it is beneficial for both the orthodontist and the patient, as the orthodontist can improve treatment and chairside efficiency, while the patients can avoid the extra financial and time costs of traveling to the practice [35,38]. The key point remains that DM setup protocol allows better control over the treatment despite they might result even in more frequent patient visits as every lost attachment is noticed and the alarms are triggered. In contrary the frequency of non-DM-patient checkups are defined by the orthodontist and loss of attachment might be overlooked and despite longer time between in-office visits of such a patient, the treatment with CAT with missing attachments will probably result in aligner non-tracking or even a necessity to restart the treatment.

Dental monitoring protocols are not paradigm shifting to older orthodontic techniques like fixed vestibular orthodontics treatments. These require a frequent chairside activation. On the other hand, customized appliances such as CAT may take full advantage of DM due to the preprogrammed tooth movement [38].

A typical implementation of TeleHealth systems like Dental Monitoring® (Dental Monitoring Co., Paris, France) require initial patient education. The patients' own mobile is used for the app and the scanning. First patient downloads the free Dental Monitoring app and activates the free DM app (Figure 1b). Then the first scan is performed with support of nurses in the clinic (Figure 1a). All consecutive video scans are created by patient usually in a home environment. Patient is provided with scan-box that improves quality of video scans (Figure 1a,b).

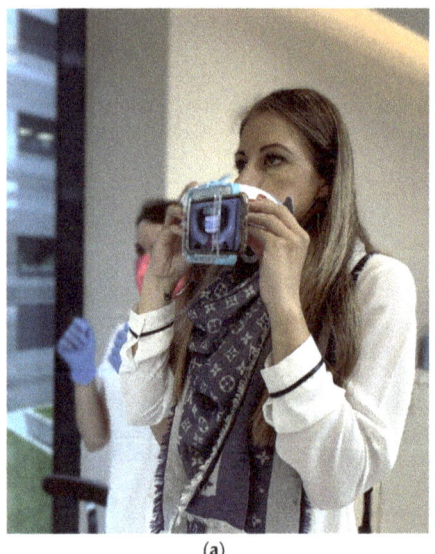
(a)

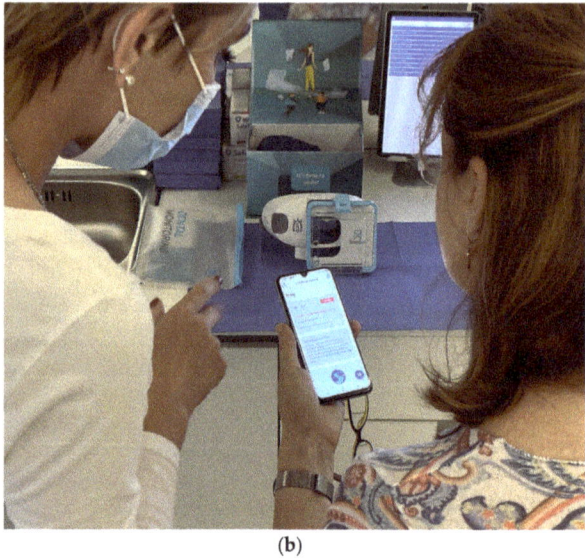
(b)

Figure 1. Introduction of Dental Monitoring® (DM): (**a**) Patient holding scan-box looking into the mirror, instructed by nurse, is scanning her first intraoral scan with her own mobile. (**b**) DM has its own app that is used for requests, uploading and reporting of the scans. Its first use is usually also instructed by nurse. The photo was taken for purposes of this article and is published with full written consent of the person.

Dental Monitoring® (Dental Monitoring Co., Paris, France) [39] is described as a software that allows patients to accurately capture their dentition using a patient's own smartphone and special cheek retractors. A special protocol with GoLive® (Dental Monitoring Co., Paris, France) option in DM is specifically targeted at CAT. Instead of conventional automatic aligner changes, the patients receive a weekly "GO" or "NO-GO" notification. "NO-GO" notification means the clinical situation was not evaluated as suitable for aligner change and patient is expected to stay on the current aligner without further step in the treatment. These notifications are paired with the orthodontists customized pre-recorded instructions. These indicate to patients whether they should proceed to the next aligner or remain in the current one for a few days more. The orthodontist is informed when a NO-GO notification is sent, and individual teeth tracking issues, poor oral hygiene, or broken attachments can be identified. The orthodontist can override a NO-GO if desired. DM has its own app; however, this app is different from the app StrojCHECK® (Bratislava, Slovakia, 3Dent Medical, osim.sk—Society for Medical Innovation (SMI)) analyzed in this research. The DM with its powerful AI capabilities can be used to clinically evaluate the patient clinical performance. Under clinical performance is meant the evaluation of patient's fit of aligners on teeth. Clinical accuracy of DM is well researched and validated [21,23,24].

Use of tele-orthodontics like DM can improve the monitoring of patients during the COVID-19 dissemination [40]. It allowed us to monitor all patients during pandemic lockdowns, reduced the costs and limited direct contact when was not necessary. With all these means it has decreased the risk of COVID-19 dissemination [41].

Attitude of dentists and patients towards the use of Dental Monitoring is positive. Both groups positively judged this tele-orthodontic approach, considering it a technologically advanced tool increasing the perception of quality and accuracy of the treatment [42].

The current state of the research, described above, reviewed aspects of orthodontic health issues, their prevalence and the TeleHealth technologies addressing them. Telemedicine based on orthodontics mobile apps with AI clinical evaluation with Dental Monitoring system is supportive backbone of the future orthodontic care. The next subchapter of introduction describes the researched subject of this research paper—the orthodontic mobile app (strojCHECK) and its AI update that implemented the computerized learning algorithms. And mathematical algorithms, provided by artificial intelligence, continuously boost new therapeutic paradigms [43].

1.3. Mobile Application StrojCHECK

Mobile application StrojCHECK® (Bratislava, Slovakia, 3Dent Medical, osim.sk—Society for Medical Innovation (SMI)) is a free smart app for orthodontic patients and doctors. Currently its further development drives the community of medical specialists and other enthusiasts associated under community—Society for Medical Innovation (www.OSIM.sk, accessed on 1 November 2021). The app was originally designed, in 2015 by an orthodontist—MUDr. Andrej Thurzo, PHD, MPH, MHA as simply a solo mobile app without any server background. Its original functions were mostly simple remainders and patient compliance observation. Further it has developed as a solution for complex treatment couching and motivation of orthodontic patients undertaking clear aligner therapy. Application now implements various functions dedicated to support patients on CAT. The app is free to use for everybody, and does not expose users to any form of commercial approach. It requires the clinic/dental office to be registered in the system to manage settings for its patients.

In general introduction of this app's purpose, it can be recapitulated that this smart-app is used for establishing proper treatment routines of orthodontic patients. This app evaluates activities registered by patient, motivates and educates patient enabling him to achieve proper behavioral patterns linked with successful therapy (Figure 1). Central screen is the "Main dashboard" (Figure 2a). This screen provides the complex view of the current day activities, remaining possible time of aligners removed, planned and all executed activities. In the lower chart of this screen there is a visualization of daily performance of time of aligners out-of-mouth. Above this is a current balance of earned points/treatment discount and current number of aligners. Remainder function is frequent feature of many orthodontic apps [10,11]. Remainders are frequently sent as a push notification to patient mobile and wearable either inquiring if the patient has ended an activity and forgot to return the aligners or is still performing the activity (Figure 2b). The activity can be finished by active patient interaction (with bonus) or automatically (with sanction) (Figure 2c). The settings side menu (Figure 2d) allows user to personalize the app and its communication. It provides a management screen for setting up scheduled routines or language. This is the section where patient can learn about his own performance or contact his doctor or nurses directly reporting an event. The events that can be possibly reported include situations of app malfunctions or attachment debonding. Smart functions of the app StrojCHECK® (Bratislava, Slovakia, 3Dent Medical, osim.sk—Society for Medical Innovation (SMI)) and their researched modifications are described in Materials and methods chapter.

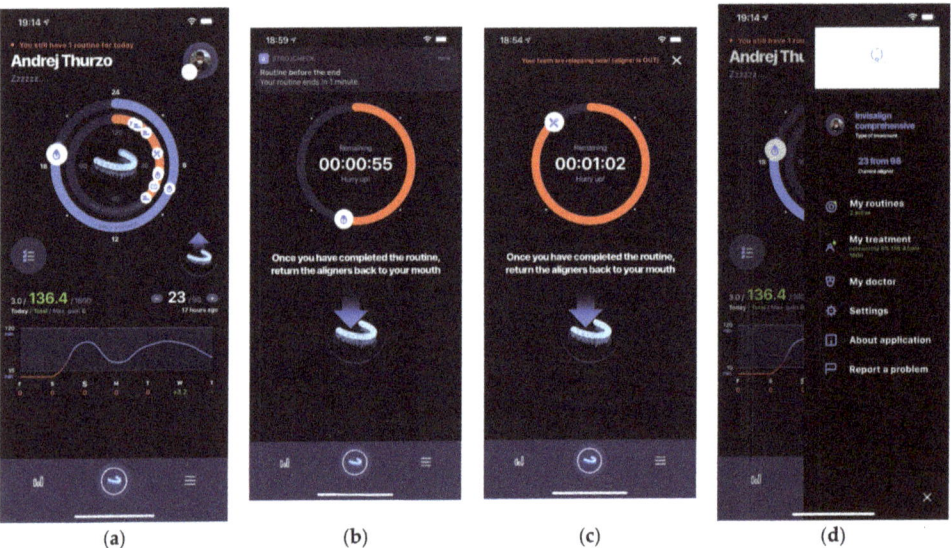

Figure 2. Main screens of orthodontic smart-app StrojCHECK®: (**a**) Main dashboard of the app provides complex view of the current day, remaining time, planned and executed activities, lower chart visualizes daily performance of time of aligners out-of-mouth, above it is current balance of earned points/treatment discount and current number of aligner (**b**) Remainders are frequently send as a push notifications to patient mobile and wearable either inquiring if the patient has ended an activity and forgot to return the aligners or is still performing the activity. (**c**) An activity can be finished by active patient interaction (with bonus) or automatically (with sanction) (**d**) Side menu allows user to personalize the app, set up scheduled routines, language, learn about his own performance or contact his doctor directly reporting an event.

1.4. Decision Tree Algorithm and Behavior Change Techniques (BCTs)

Smart algorithms that were subject of the app StrojCHECK update and their clinical impact is researched in this paper are introduced in this subchapter.

Mobile apps have been proven to be an effective tool in changing patients' behavior in orthodontics and can be used to improve their compliance with treatment [44]. In analysis of EU Google play and Apple App Store in August 2021 we have observed approximately 300 orthodontic apps. Some were not fully functional and was difficult to verify their full functionality. In approximately 30 of them the Behavior Change Techniques (BCTs) were observed. This well correlates with the recent findings in publication from September Siddiqui et al. 2021 [44].

The current availability of apps of sufficient quality for patient orthodontic coaching is very limited. There is therefore a need for high-quality orthodontic apps with appropriate BCTs to be created, which may be utilized to improve patients' compliance with treatment. This paper explores the usefulness and potential of implementation of AI algorithms for enhancing Behavior Change Techniques.

Decision Tree algorithm belongs to the family of supervised learning algorithms. Unlike other supervised learning algorithms, the decision tree algorithm can be used for solving regression and classification problems too.

The goal of using a Decision Tree in general is to create a training model that can be used to predict the class or value of the target variable by learning simple decision rules inferred from prior data (training data).

In Decision Trees, for predicting a class label for a record it begins from the root of the tree. The values of the root attribute are compared to the record's attribute. On the basis of comparison, the branch corresponding to that value is followed and algorithm jumps to the next node [45]. Types of decision trees are based on the type of target variable available. It can be of two types:

1. Continuous Variable Decision Tree: Decision Tree has a continuous target variable then it is called Continuous Variable Decision Tree.
2. Categorical Variable Decision Tree: Decision Tree which has a categorical target variable then it called a Categorical variable decision tree.

Practical examples of implemented decision tree process algorithms are described in more detail in Materials and methods chapter.

To keep this introduction comprehensible to scientists outside the field of orthodontic and AI-engineering research, it is necessary to clarify why personalization is currently ideal by means of patient and doctor computerized education. The system allows both groups to improve based on data gathered, evaluated, compared to other users of the system and calculating optimal suggestions. These are set by system autonomously, however from the clinical experience, these might be not optimal for every patient and personalization in this early stage is necessary.

1.5. Aim of This Research Paper

The goal of this research paper is to evaluate AI upgrade of an existing orthodontic mobile coaching app and clinical impact of such upgrade.

Secondary goal is to introduce the advantages of AI (decision tree process algorithm) implementation and method of clinical impact evaluation by means of tele-monitoring systems.

2. Materials and Methods

2.1. Participants, Statistical Analysis and Hypothesis

86 subjects (54 females and 32 males) in age between 12 and 68 years, were observed with DM 60 days before and 60 days after the AI update of the mobile app they were using. All patients were using the same orthodontic app for treatment coaching—StrojCHECK® (Bratislava, Slovakia, 3Dent Medical, osim.sk—Society for Medical Innovation (SMI)).

The research did not require any approval for human trials as the Dental Monitoring is well clinically established and certified technology [23,26,27,36–38] and patients' mobile application was modified in general (for all patients) with the central update on the official release hubs (App Store for iPhones and Google Play Store for Android mobiles). This was not an interventional study where some of the participants receive different treatment than others in order to evaluate it so there is no control group.

The statistical analysis was performed in Microsoft Office Excel 2016 (Microsoft Corporation, Redmond, WA, USA), Statistica 13.1 software (TIBCO Software Inc., Palo Alto, CA, USA) and StatsDirect 3.3.5 (StatsDirect Ltd., Cheshire, UK).

The collected demographic and clinical, as well as patient-generated data collected through mobile phones were summarized using descriptive statistics. Continuous variables are presented as means with the respective SD (standard deviation) as well as median and interquartile range.

Wilcoxon signed rank test was used to compare the difference in the outcome variables after the upgrading. After-before differences in the outcome variables were computed and regressed to age. The strength of the associations was evaluated by simple bivariate (Spearman's nonparametric) correlation coefficient.

All presented *p* values were two sided. Values of *p* < 0.05 were considered to indicate a statistically significant difference. Statistical analyses were performed using StatsDirect 3.3.5 (StatsDirect Ltd., Cheshire, UK) statistical software.

The basic hypothesis of this research paper is, that performance of patients interacting with the app (after AI update) will not be significantly different from the time prior to the update.

A possible controversial and diverging hypothesis could be a consideration of a patient using the app only virtually—lying about his true performance.

This would result in significant discrepancies between the app performance and clinical reality. Despite "lying" to the app is possible, it is extremely frustrating, time consuming and easily detectable.

2.2. Description of the Basic Functionality and Workflow Examples

The mobile app StrojCHECK® (Bratislava, Slovakia, 3Dent Medical, osim.sk—Society for Medical Innovation (SMI)) gathers patient data and helps to build a proper routine with focus on the first 120 days of treatment. After 4 months in the treatment, patient usually fixes the routines, even if they are wrong and inappropriate for the treatment. The app communicates with the patients even through their wearables like Apple watch® (Apple Inc., Cupertino, CA, USA), which is very practical. Modern mobile phones include a variety of sensors that can be used to gather data about the user's behavior [46]. The app functionality is based on these modalities. Mobile app, its back-end and technical background with statistical methods are described in later subchapters. Below are two examples of system intelligent workflows that became possible after the AI-update:

Example 1: Predictions

Let's say we have a problem to predict whether a patient will have his CAT interrupted with significant non-tracking of his removable aligners on his teeth (yes/no). Here we know that the "time-without-aligners" of patient is a key—significant variable but the doctor does not have exact time details for all his patients. Now, as we know this is an important variable, then we can build a decision tree to predict patient "time-without-aligners" based on treatment type, occupation, age, app-monitored-interactions, app-monitored-discipline, treatment difficulty and various other variables. In this case, we are predicting values for the continuous variables.

Example 2: Incentives

System regularly calculates the most frequent drop-out rate in the use of the app by patients, after 12 days of permanent use, it automatically suggests with push notification to every patient a special motivational badge for completing the continuous streak of daily proper use for another 7 days, however the patient psychology is much more complex and there are various reasons which can be addressed by clinician better who knows the patient personality. So, the doctor is allowed to bypass the system setting and can in particular cases employ a special clinical check-up or another, more suitable form, to bridge a difficult treatment period for the patient. Doctors' interactions in the system are recorded and will be used later to program separate decision tree algorithm.

2.3. Description of the Supportive Complex System (App StrojCHECK and Its Back-End)

The back-end, also called the server side, consists of the server which provides data on request, the application which channels it, and the database which organizes the information (Figure 3). The system consists of three parts:

- The first part is the patient interface in the form of a patient mobile smart application and a possible wearable device.
- The second part of this biomedical system is its "bioinformatic brain"—that is responsible for data gathering, sorting and processing. Also, for some autonomic decision processes and possible future machine-learning algorithms with its own top-admin interface.
- The third part of the system is the admin-interface (Figure 4) for clinical doctors and managers. Here is available the data gathered and processed from mobiles and

wearables of their patients. This back-end also allows them to fully customize their clinical set-ups, rules and patient motivation.

The 2nd and 3rd part are running as the software on the server and here is the platform where the future sophisticated AI algorithms will be trained and applied.

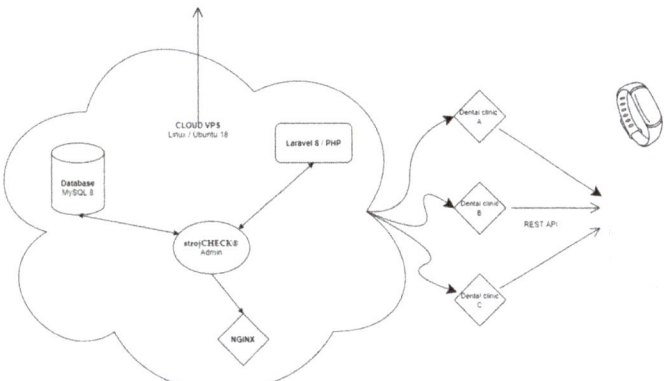

Figure 3. Global schematics of technological platforms fundamental to the complex system of StrojCHECK® from the back-end server through different dental clinics with their separate administrator portals up to end-user devices.

Methods of registration of complex patient behavior on clear aligner therapy depends on way too many variables to be simply programmed. Especially when their statistic evaluation could not be that straightforward. Sophisticated data mining algorithms in the future might be successful in extracting and discovering patterns in large data sets of patients' behaviors during CAT with other complementary data [47].

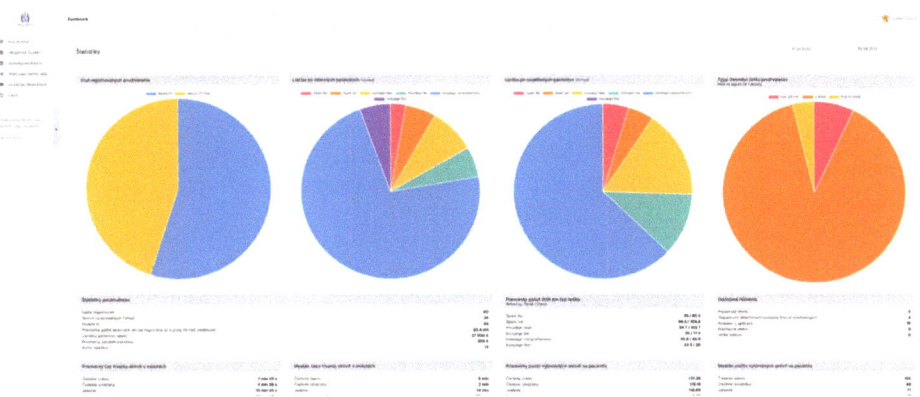

Figure 4. The view of the screen for administration. The portal of the server back-end for doctors and other administrators provides useful interface for statistical data processing and interactions with the system. Pie charts from left describe percentage of active users within the last 72 h (from all registered users), types of monitored appliances in the active users (Spark lite, Spark full, Invisalign teen, Invisalign lite, Invisalign comprehensive, Invisalign first), types of monitored appliances in the non-active users, types of daily limits of removed aligners (over 120 min, within 120 min limit and under 15 min). On the Figure bellow there are visualized user statistics, average times for various habits, Average time per aligner or frequency of patient reports.

Methods in apps processing with AI algorithms data images like X-ray, various sounds or ECG have regularly big datasets available that are essential to better training for deeper neural networks [48–51]. This is not situation for CAT. Variables include not only various behavioral patterns but also different biomechanical approaches on various types of malocclusions.

2.4. Description of the UPDATE (the Set of Computerized Methods Implemented in the Update)

The important part of this research paper is description of the set of computerized methods implemented in the update and later evaluated clinically with Dental Monitoring. All observed patients were using DM, which has its own positive clinical effect [36].

StrojCHECK app installed on the mobiles of the users collects tens of thousands of entries every day. This is not only information regarding their eating, drinking or brushing habits. System allows analysis of patterns of patients' dwindling discipline or their behavioral responses on the motivational events triggered by doctor(admin) or the system itself. We call these events "incentives".

The following three related parts with decision processes were implemented by the update (Figure 5):

(1) **System activation.** System learns when and where the patient does successfully perform her/his routines. When the system notices that the patient is underperforming daily routines or goals the app decides to push the notification in proper time and geo location. These responsivity functions are very simple yet and can be turned off by clinician or the user. System every day after midnight automatically recalculates the settings for various thresholds:

   (a) User drop-out rate (what day most users stop using the app)
   (b) First day of unfulfilled daily rules (what day most users have first discipline failure while using the app)
   (c) Incentives default settings (Badges) (Figure 6.)

   [1] Total domination Badge is achieved after more than X continuous days of proper app use (sum-up).
   [2] Badge of Sincere Hunger achieved after reaching at least X-th day average of more than 5 eating activities per day.
   [3] Badge of Huxley-Orwell, achieved after X-th day of using dental monitoring.
   [4] Badge of Mysophobia, achieved after X days with average aligner cleaning of 3 times per day and more.
   [5] Badge of the White Fang, achieved after X days with average teeth cleaning of 3 times per day and more.
   [6] Badge of compliance, achieved after X-th aligner change and XX days of continuous app use.

System sets the default settings for these stimuli according to recalculated system data. However, these can be changed and fixed by doctor led by his own clinical experience. Otherwise, the system automatically triggers the stimuli—motivational bonuses and rewards to prevent loss of users or their discipline deterioration.

(2) **Doctor activation.** Computerized calculation of various variables, especially time of aligners removed or non-fulfilling the basic criteria (described later) can result in evaluation of patient as underperforming user. 10% of the worse performing users are flagged and clinical team is educated about these patients on a regular basis. Human clinical response to such events most frequently results in extra call from the nurses or extra check-up by the doctor or a special motivational event triggered by doctor manually to prevent the anticipated negative event. The doctor's behavior in troubleshooting the underperforming patients and the results of such intervention is registered into the system and evaluated. Later the system will learn from it.

(3) **Patient activation.** Computerized analysis of patient performance in relation to all the compulsory clinician rules and also to performance of all other patients using

the app was formed as an important tool for patient education. Learning about own weaknesses is first step for improvement. The intelligent system generates and delivers an individualized email report to each patient every 7 days. The report explains the nonperformance events and their probable reasons. Computerized automatic recalculation of patient's performance can be delivered to patient email and possibly also email of his/her parents. This feature was supposed to help patient learn more about himself/herself and the reason of the failures to prevent them in the future.

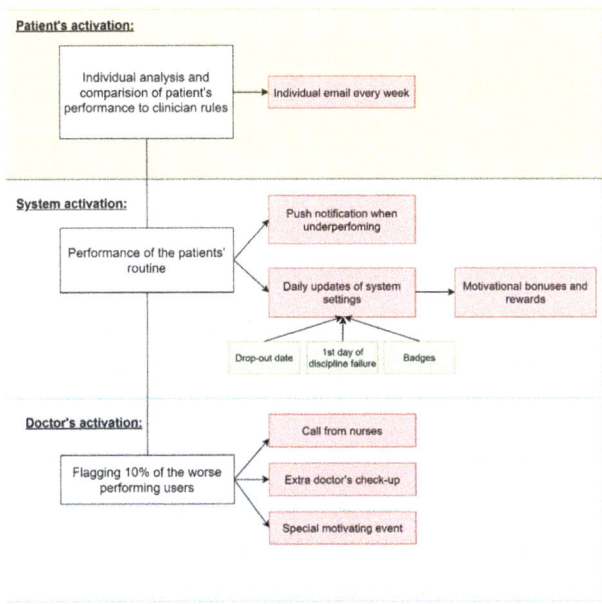

Figure 5. Scheme of three related parts with decision processes that were implemented by the update and represent three layers of system-user interaction.

Every day, after midnight, the system does calculations and analyses where it evaluates treatments during the previous day. It calculates how many times which patient removed aligners from his mouth, for how long, for what reason, if he returned them automatically within or after the limit, if he needed remainder or how many times the patient broke the rules and hundreds of other calculations for hundreds of patients. System finalizes the calculations by points allocation to each patient according to their performance and compliance with the rules. Points are allocated for each routine activity when interacting with the app (like eating, drinking, cleaning, monitoring etc.). Points can be gained also by special and rare events like computer-game achievements—called badges and also for sharing these badges on their social networks where the patient can boast about special treatment achievements. All previously mentioned points are credited after midnight only if the basic clinical requirements were met. These can be set differently for each participating clinic; however, default rules are required:

- clean the teeth at least twice a day (with a gap of 6 h between events)
- clean the appliance at least twice a day (with a gap of 6 h)
- at least one eating and one drinking
- and finally keep all the "aligners-time-out" between 15 and 120 min

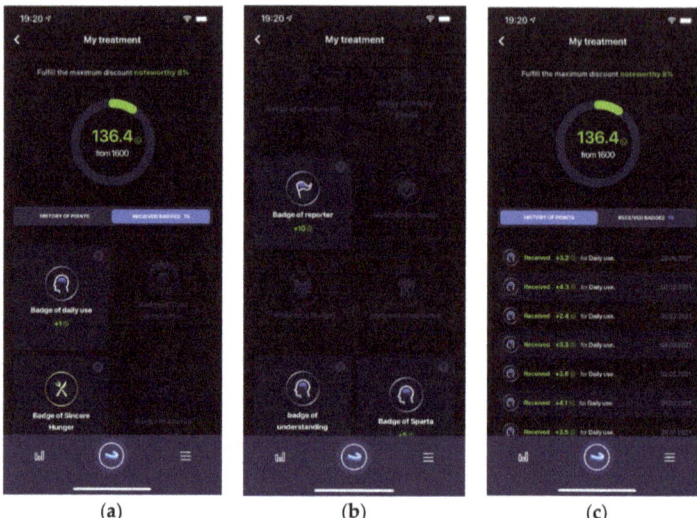

Figure 6. Screens of StrojCHECK® app regarding incentives: (**a**) Patient view of gained points that equal total discount from the treatment budget (**b**) Achieved incentives(badges) and other badges to be achieved are introduced grayed, dynamically introduced by the system. (**c**) List of gained points by following the rules and fulfilling motivational bonuses offered by the system (as special motivational events).

2.5. Technical Description of the Software Background

It is built on the latest and greatest available technologies which are popularly used nowadays for mobile app development. Our app architecture is divided into two main departments known as backend and frontend. Backend as the brain of our application, which stores all available data of our patients in the database, calculates and analyses their treatments, and many more logic operations which are necessary for a mobile application to work. Our CRM solution is running in the cloud on Ubuntu/Linux operating system. We use the latest relation database MySQL 8, the programming language is PHP 8 with help of Laravel framework 8, which is popular in the development of a large scale of CRM applications. Our frontend part of the application is running on Android and IOS mobile devices as a mobile application. We developed our mobile application on hybrid mobile app technology, which means we use one shared core of the application in both Ios and Android platforms. In other words, we do not need to develop two separate applications, which reduced the cost and development load of our developers. Our hybrid app is running on HTML5/CSS 3/Javascript and mainly VueJs 3 with the Ionic 5 framework.

3. Results

3.1. Age and Gender Impact

It is analyzed below whether age has an impact on how individual subjects have improved/deteriorated in the given parameters. Figure 7 shows correlation of Age vs. Interaction change after and before the AI update. Figure 8 shows correlation of Age vs. Discipline after and before the AI update. Figures 9 and 10 show correlation of aligner tracking AI evaluation with DM (GO and NO-GO scan evaluations). In short, the results shows that age does not affect the change in any of the monitored parameters.

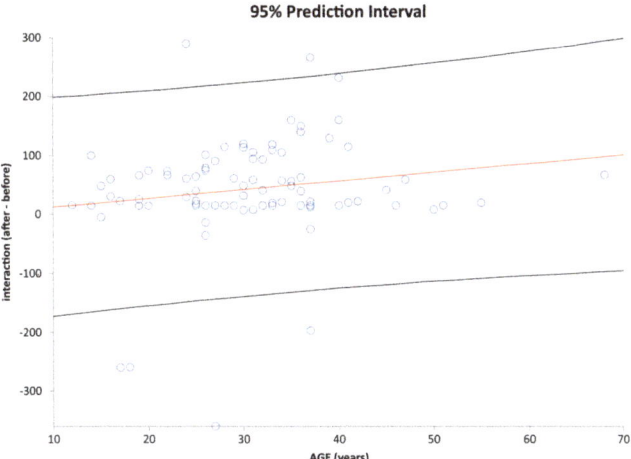

Figure 7. Prediction interval and linear regression line for Interaction (after-before) vs. Age in the investigated sample (correlation coefficient (r) = 0.160; p = 0.1416). Each circle represents a data point. The red line is the regression line (the linear model) and the black lines show the 95% prediction band for the forecasted Interaction (after-before).

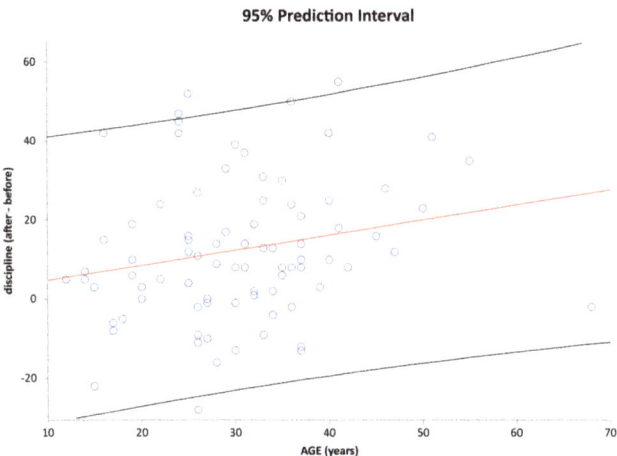

Figure 8. Prediction interval and linear regression line for Discipline (after-before) vs. Age in the investigated sample (r = 0.210; p = 0.0528). Regression line and 95% prediction interval are denoted as in Figure 7.

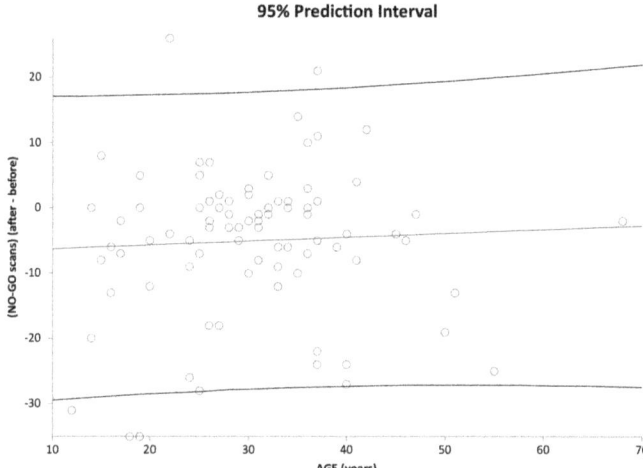

Figure 9. Prediction interval and linear regression line for No-go scans (after-before) vs. Age in the investigated sample (r = 0.0507; p = 0.6433). Regression line and 95% prediction interval are denoted as in Figure 7.

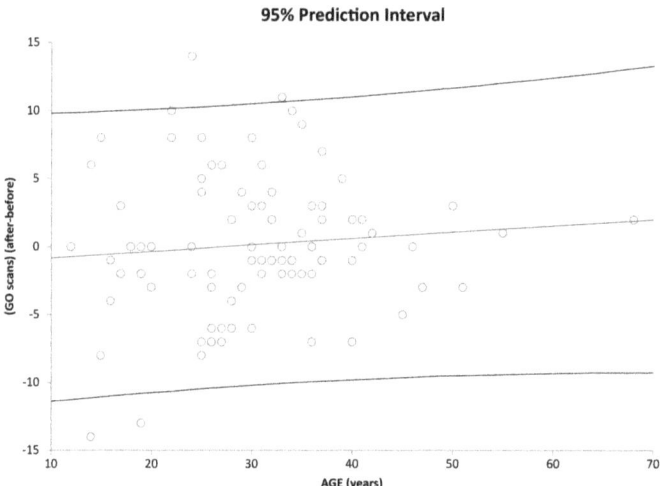

Figure 10. Prediction interval and linear regression line for Age vs. GO scans change (After-Before) vs. Age in the investigated sample (r = 0.0507; p = 0.6433). Regression line and 95% prediction interval are denoted as in Figure 7. Coefficient (r) = 0.089831 p = 0.4108.

The influence of gender and differences in individual parameters before vs after and their statistical significance (evaluated by Wilcoxon signed-rank test) is in the Table 2 below.

Table 2. The influence of gender and differences in individual parameters before vs after the AI update and their statistical significance (evaluated by Wilcoxon signed-rank test).

Parameter	Statistics	Females			Males			All		
		Before	After	Difference (After-Before)	Before	After	Difference (After-Before)	Before	After	Difference (After-Before)
Interaction	n	54	54	54	32	32	32	86	86	86
	Mean	166.7	204.8	38.07	99.71	151.5	51.78	141.8	185	43.17
	Std. Deviation	190.3	153.3	110	99.85	128.1	44.46	165.2	146	91.18
	Minimum	18	13.25	−359.3	15	35.75	8.25	15	13.3	−359.3
	25% Percentile	50	83.19	15	50	65	15	50	65	15
	Median	78.7	149.3	40.06	50	97.25	37.17	64.63	141	40.06
	75% Percentile	223.5	293.8	93.85	101.6	164.8	75.9	197.2	275	82
	Maximum	802.4	544.4	290.2	432.6	562.3	160.2	802.4	562	290.2
	p-value			<0.0001			<0.0001			<0.0001
Discipline	Mean	34.7	47.44	12.74	35.22	47.59	12.38	34.9	47.5	12.6
	Std. Deviation	19.44	16.57	19.7	18.46	17.83	15.07	18.97	17	18.02
	Minimum	0	2	−28	1	0	−16	0	0	−28
	25% Percentile	17.5	45.75	−2	19.25	42	3.5	18.75	45.8	0
	Median	34.5	55	11	37.5	56	9	36	55	10
	75% Percentile	55	59	25.5	51.75	59	18.75	53.25	59	24
	Maximum	60	60	55	60	60	50	60	60	55
	p-value			<0.0001			<0.0001			<0.0001
NO-GO scans	Mean	11.43	6.167	−5.259	11.44	6.813	−4.625	11.43	6.41	−5.023
	Std. Deviation	10.82	6.911	11.24	11.53	6.64	11.6	11.02	6.78	11.31
	Minimum	1	0	−35	1	0	−35	1	0	−35
	25% Percentile	3	1	−8.25	3.5	1.25	−10	3	1	−9.25
	Median	7	4	−3	6	5	−3	7	4	−3
	75% Percentile	19.75	11	1	15	12	2.75	15.25	12	1
	Maximum	45	30	26	50	25	14	50	30	26
	p-value			0.0002			0.0525			<0.0001
GO scans	Mean	10.87	11.15	0.2778	11.44	11.41	−0.03125	11.08	11.2	0.1628
	Std. Deviation	4.112	3.779	5.738	3.975	3.301	4.092	4.047	3.59	5.163
	Minimum	0	5	−14	2	5	−7	0	5	−14
	25% Percentile	7.75	8	−3	10.25	10	−2	9	9	−3
	Median	12	12	0	12	12	0	12	12	0
	75% Percentile	13	14	3.25	13	13	3	13	14	3
	Maximum	20	18	14	20	18	9	20	18	14
	p-value			0.7029			0.9207			0.7692

3.2. Differences of Evaluated Parameters before and after the Update

The graphs in this section present box differences caused by the AI update of the mobile app StrojCHECK® (Bratislava, Slovakia, 3Dent Medical, osim.sk—Society for Medical Innovation (SMI)). Figure 11a shows differences before and after the update in regard to app interaction parameter for all participants. Figure 11b shows differences before and after update regarding app interaction for all participants.

In short, the summary of the results is that there are significant differences in all parameters except GO scans for all and NO-GO scans for boys/men.

The Figure 12a shows differences before and after the app update regarding GO scans for all participants. Figure 12b shows NO-GO scans before and after the update, evaluated with Paired t test. Figure 13 shows in (a) females and (b) males' differences before and after the app AI-update in NO-GO Dental monitoring scans, where in (a) Females (is the difference significant) and in (b) Males is the difference not significant (despite were less frequent).

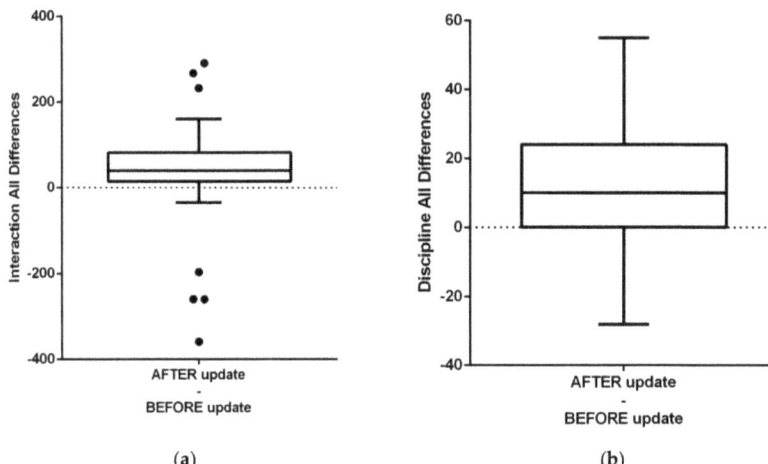

Figure 11. (**a**) Differences before and after update regarding app interaction for all participants. (Paired *t* test of variable Discipline) Measured parameter represented patient app interaction in easy and mostly fun interactions including sharing on social networks or achieving interesting badges. (**b**) Differences before and after update regarding app interaction for all participants (Paired *t* test of variable Discipline). Measured parameter represented patient app interaction in difficult and regular way fulfilling required rules of disciplined use that included teeth and appliance cleaning twice a day (separated by 180 min), at least once per day eating and drinking and as well as fitting the aligner out-of-mouth time between 15 and 120 min. This parameter improved significantly as well.

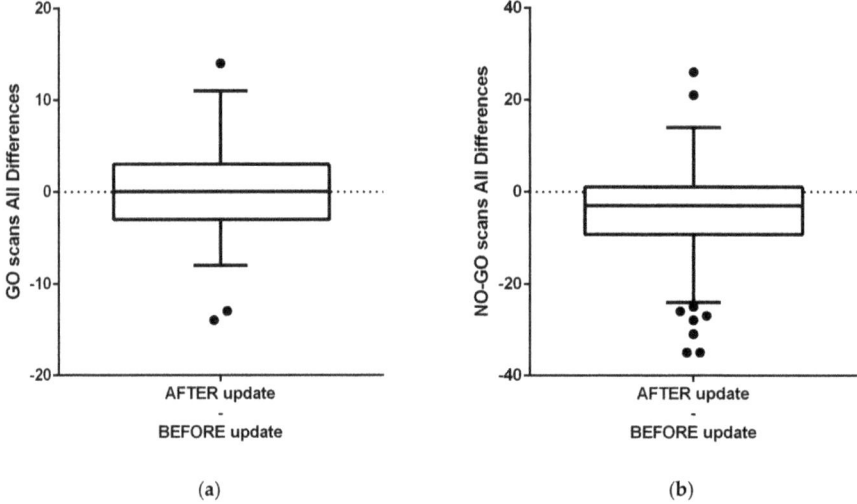

Figure 12. Differences before and after the app update regarding patient clinical performance observed with dental monitoring for all participants. (Paired *t* test) (**a**) Dental monitoring evaluated GO scans focused on proper aligner tracking, here is not a significant difference. (**b**) Dental monitoring evaluated NO-GO scans focused on proper aligner tracking, here is a significant improvement.

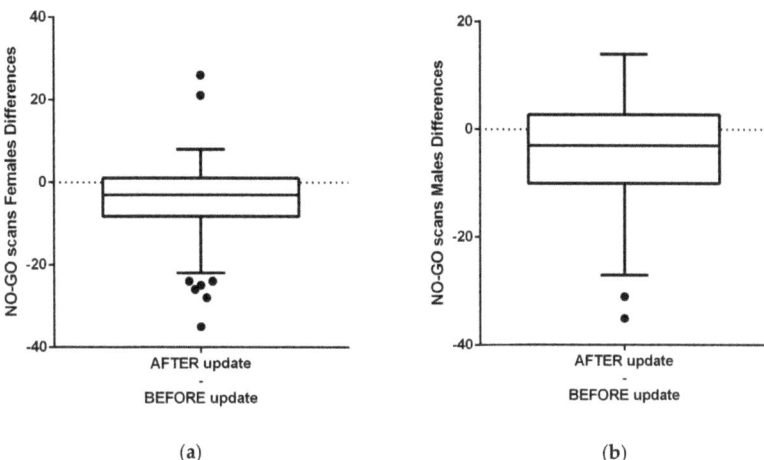

Figure 13. Differences before and after the app update in NO-GO Dental monitoring scans in (**a**) Females (significant) (**b**) Males. Difference, despite were less frequent, is not significant.

NO-GO scan is a clinical situation, for this research purposes focused only on "aligner non-tracking" evaluated by AI system of DM. Other reasons of NO-GO scans were not calculated as NO-GO scan, but it was counted into GO-scans group. Figure 14 shows differences before and after the app AI-update in frequency of GO Dental Monitoring scans that were not significant in (Figure 14a) in females (insignificant) and also insignificant in (Figure 14b) Males.

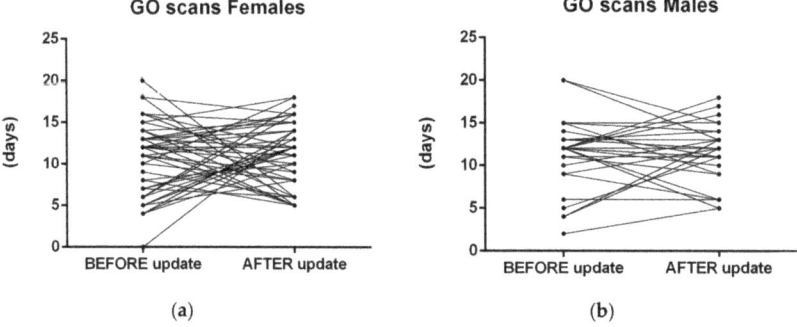

Figure 14. Differences before and after the app update in GO Dental monitoring scans were not significant (**a**) in females (insignificant) (**b**) Males (insignificant).

3.3. Collateral Interesting Findings

The use of the system and computerized statistical data processing revealed other interesting information, that were not main objectives of this research. To understand the power of such complex TeleHealth app providing support to many patients, is the realization of unprecedented knowledge about the users (patients and doctors). Table 3 shows some of the interesting collateral findings about patient behavior noticed by the system.

Table 3. Information from statistical data processing of the large set of patients.

Activity [1]	Median Session Length	Average Time
Teeth cleaning	6 min	8 min
Eating	14 min	
Drinking	6 min	
Appliance cleaning 2	3 min	
Dental monitoring	5 min	

[1] Activity describes only one uninterrupted session.

4. Discussion

This paper focuses on impact evaluation of Computer-based learning (CBL), Decision Tree Algorithms (DTA) and other computerized learning improvements to an existing mobile app—StrojCHECK® (Bratislava, Slovakia, 3Dent Medical, osim.sk—Society for Medical Innovation (SMI)).

The main aim of the research was to evaluate clinical impact of implementation of decision processes to an existing healthcare application for orthodontic treatment. The secondary goal was to use AI system (DM) to evaluate the clinical situation in high frequency established on video scans of patient teeth and their appliances.

The results invalidated the basic hypothesis of this research paper. That performance of patients interacting with the app (after the AI update) will not be significantly different from the time prior to the update.

With the use of decision processes methods applied in an existing healthcare app, unprecedented data about orthodontic patients' behavior are available for analysis. New technique for clinical research using patients' made video-scans has been presented as successful scientific tool [37]. The information about application StrojCHECK was never published before. It represents a complex healthcare system driven by computational methods.

Results show that impact of the app is significant in evaluation of patient—app interaction. The amount of GO scans is not significantly reduced and this might be explained due to the fact, that frequency of scans is defined by doctor and if everything goes well, the patient will go as prescribed and do the scan regularly.

The decrease of frequency of NO-GO scans is slightly significant only in women and not in man. This can be interpreted by fact that farther the patient goes into the treatment there is higher probability of discrepancy between teeth positions and aligners. So simply the clinical development shall deteriorate over time.

Results also confirmed that change in performance was significant in all observed parameters except the GO scans and NO-GO scans for males. Results also showed they are unrelated to the age. In general, the AI update of the app resulted significantly better clinical performance. The clinical variables like insignificant change in GO scans can be explained that first 60 days of treatment contains usually the better compliance and as well as the tracking of the patient that worsens in time. The clinical non-tracking gets worse over time naturally. It is the fact that GO scans frequency is defined by rigid doctor instruction and shall not change unless doctor indicates to speed up the protocol.

Result in insignificant improvement of NO-GO scans in males is showing the discrepancy of their increased app-activity regarding interactions with the app as well as the discipline, however without clinical effect. This might be explained by natural lag of clinical performance as well as rule described above regarding worsening clinical performance of tracking over-time.

In context to other publications, it is known the App update on the verge of AI can have a significant effect on its user behavior [28,44]. The success of further app development relies on understanding of the patient (user) behavior. CBL is a term used for any kind of learning with the help of computers. Computer-based learning makes the use of the interactive elements of the computer applications and software and the ability to present any type of information to the users. Authors of this paper have published their experience in smart learning algorithms implementation [52,53], albeit any sophisticated A.I. upgrade requires simple computerized learning features first.

TeleHealth solutions are currently driven with AI implementations in various medical fields from treatments of chronic pulmonary diseases, depressions or intellectual disabilities to other chronic diseases [54–61].

Another highlight of this study is that not necessarily a universal approach to modification of patient behavior would result in better clinical results as every patient behavior is unique and we need to differentiate between behavioral patterns of our patients first, program the proper motivational responses later. So, the concept was to invest the benefits of first intelligent features of the system into doctor module and patient module of the app. Under this we understand to provide the data of particular patient behavior to the doctor and allow him to adjust the motivational responses of the system as well as provide regularly the information about the patient's weaknesses to the patient himself.

Dentistry needs to expand its understanding of how dental apps; digital workflow models and digital health information are transforming dental practice in order to anticipate how this digital shift will impact the whole field of dentistry [62].

As has been stressed in this article repetitively—the CAT success strongly depends not only on patient motivation and discipline but also on patient's understanding of the basic treatment rules and his own weaknesses. These are frequently unknown to patient and often also to his doctor.

Recently published retrospective cohort study in the Journal of Clinical medicine presented interesting findings about factors influencing patient compliance during CAT [63]. These also can be used to guide practitioners towards limitedly compliant individuals, allowing early intervention and later to help program a sophisticated A.I. algorithms.

Clear aligners weakness is patient forgetfulness. As the CAT's effectivity is compromised when aligners are not on patient's' teeth for longer than 120 min per day. Patient removes them for cleaning the teeth and appliance, or during eating and drinking especially coloring food and drinks [64].

In wider context, authors of this paper were searching for a complex personalized solution that would significantly improve patient treatment compliance by the means of using a smart healthcare app. Today it seems impossible to achieve this without implementation of smart computerized data processing algorithms.

The big data automatically collected by the system is crucial for future machine learning. Analysis of the daily routines of CAT patients and understanding the patterns of their discipline, motivation, bad habits and behavioral responses to stimulus are foundation to successful future programming of more advanced AI algorithms. The goals of future AI implementation shall be:

1. Early identification of non-compliant patient
2. Anticipation of incoming drop of discipline according to app use pattern
3. Designing ideal treatment patterns for specific patient types upon their behavioral as well as clinical parameters
4. Designing ideal motivational impulses according to patient type, daily routines and specifics of his/her particular treatment

5. Conclusions

The principal conclusion of this research is that implementation of AI decision processes algorithm is not only the first step towards more sophisticated machine-learning decision optimization models, but also an already effective enhancement of an existing app with measurable benefits to patients. This conclusion is based on the results of this research as in all pairs of monitored variables was observed a significant improvement except for AI evaluation of clinical tracking of aligners in men.

Secondary conclusion is that Dental Monitoring is a useful tool in evaluation of clinical situation on the principles of telemedicine.

Author Contributions: Conceptualization, A.T. and V.K.; methodology, A.T.; software, A.T.; validation, V.K., I.V. and A.T.; formal analysis, A.T.; investigation, V.K.; resources, I.V.; data curation, A.T.; writing—original draft preparation, A.T.; writing—review and editing, V.K.; visualization, V.K.; supervision, A.T.; project administration, A.T.; funding acquisition, I.V. All authors have read and agreed to the published version of the manuscript.

Funding: This research was funded by the KEGA grant agency of the Ministry of Education, Science, Research, and Sport of the Slovak Republic (Grant No. 081UK-4/2021).

Institutional Review Board Statement: The study was conducted according to the guidelines of the Declaration of Helsinki, and no approval was necessary by the Ethics Committee. Ethical review and approval were waived for this study, due to the fact that no experimental materials or approaches were used.

Informed Consent Statement: Written informed consent was obtained from all subjects involved in the study.

Data Availability Statement: Data available in a publicly accessible repository that does not issue DOIs. Publicly available datasets were analyzed in this study. This data can be found here on the following link: https://bit.ly/3pPJCEr (accessed on 6 December 2021).

Acknowledgments: We acknowledge Peter Slezák and Iveta Waczulíková—Division of Biomedical Physics, Faculty of Mathematics, Comenius University for statistical data processing and technological support of digital Dental lab infrastructure of 3Dent Medical s.r.o company as well as dental clinic Sangre Azul s.r.o. We would like to thank also to team of programmers and designers for their valuable contribution, namely Marek Gogoľ, Juraj Karovič and Adrián Bortník.

Conflicts of Interest: The authors declare no conflict of interest.

Abbreviations

app	Mobile application
AI	Artificial Intelligence (A.I.)
BCT	Behavior Change Techniques (BCTs)
CBL	Computer-based learning
CAT	Clear Aligner Therapy
DTA	Decision Tree Algorithms
DM	Dental Monitoring
RCT	Randomized Controlled Trial

References

1. Proffit, W.; Fields, H.W., Jr.; Moray, L. Prevalence of Malocclusion and Orthodontic Treatment Need in the United States: Estimates from the NHANES III Survey. *Int. J. Adult Orthod. Orthognath. Surg.* **1998**, *13*, 97–106.
2. Ke, Y.; Zhu, Y.; Zhu, M. A Comparison of Treatment Effectiveness between Clear Aligner and Fixed Appliance Therapies. *BMC Oral Health* **2019**, *19*, 24. [CrossRef]
3. Rossini, G.; Parrini, S.; Castroflorio, T.; Deregibus, A.; Debernardi, C.L. Efficacy of Clear Aligners in Controlling Orthodontic Tooth Movement: A Systematic Review. *Angle Orthod.* **2015**, *85*, 881–889. [CrossRef] [PubMed]
4. Scribante, A.; Gallo, S.; Bertino, K.; Meles, S.; Gandini, P.; Sfondrini, M.F. The Effect of Chairside Verbal Instructions Matched with Instagram Social Media on Oral Hygiene of Young Orthodontic Patients: A Randomized Clinical Trial. *Appl. Sci.* **2021**, *11*, 706. [CrossRef]
5. Thurzo, A.; Kosnáčová, H.S.; Kurilová, V.; Kosmeľ, S.; Beňuš, R.; Moravanský, N.; Kováč, P.; Kuracinová, K.M.; Palkovič, M.; Varga, I. Use of Advanced Artificial Intelligence in Forensic Medicine, Forensic Anthropology and Clinical Anatomy. *Healthcare* **2021**, *9*, 1545. [CrossRef]
6. Thurzo, A.; Kočiš, F.; Novák, B.; Czako, L.; Varga, I. Three-Dimensional Modeling and 3D Printing of Biocompatible Orthodontic Power-Arm Design with Clinical Application. *Appl. Sci.* **2021**, *11*, 9693. [CrossRef]
7. Gupta, G.; Vaid, N. The World of Orthodontic Apps. *APOS Trends Orthod.* **2017**, *7*, 73. [CrossRef]
8. Vaid, N.R.; Hansa, I.; Bichu, Y. Smartphone Applications Used in Orthodontics: A Scoping Review of Scholarly Literature. *J. World Fed. Orthod.* **2020**, *9*, S67–S73. [CrossRef]
9. Alkadhi, O.H.; Zahid, M.N.; Almanea, R.S.; Althaqeb, H.K.; Alharbi, T.H.; Ajwa, N.M. The Effect of Using Mobile Applications for Improving Oral Hygiene in Patients with Orthodontic Fixed Appliances: A Randomised Controlled Trial. *J. Orthod.* **2017**, *44*, 157–163. [CrossRef] [PubMed]

10. Deleuse, M.; Meiffren, C.; Bruwier, A.; Maes, N.; le Gall, M.; Charavet, C. Smartphone Application-Assisted Oral Hygiene of Orthodontic Patients: A Multicentre Randomized Controlled Trial in Adolescents. *Eur. J. Orthod.* **2020**, *42*, 605–611. [CrossRef] [PubMed]
11. Li, X.; Xu, Z.-R.; Tang, N.; Ye, C.; Zhu, X.-L.; Zhou, T.; Zhao, Z.-H. Effect of Intervention Using a Messaging App on Compliance and Duration of Treatment in Orthodontic Patients. *Clin. Oral Investig.* **2015**, *20*, 1849–1859. [CrossRef] [PubMed]
12. Scheerman, J.F.M.; van Meijel, B.; van Empelen, P.; Verrips, G.H.W.; van Loveren, C.; Twisk, J.W.R.; Pakpour, A.H.; van den Braak, M.C.T.; Kramer, G.J.C. The Effect of Using a Mobile Application ("WhiteTeeth") on Improving Oral Hygiene: A Randomized Controlled Trial. *Int. J. Dent. Hyg.* **2020**, *18*, 73–83. [CrossRef]
13. Zotti, F.; Dalessandri, D.; Salgarello, S.; Piancino, M.; Bonetti, S.; Visconti, L.; Paganelli, C. Usefulness of an App in Improving Oral Hygiene Compliance in Adolescent Orthodontic Patients. *Angle Orthod.* **2016**, *86*, 101–107. [CrossRef] [PubMed]
14. Zotti, F.; Zotti, R.; Albanese, M.; Nocini, P.F.; Paganelli, C. Implementing Post-Orthodontic Compliance among Adolescents Wearing Removable Retainers through Whatsapp: A Pilot Study. *Patient Prefer. Adherence* **2019**, *13*, 609–615. [CrossRef]
15. Al-Abdallah, M.; Hamdan, M.; Dar-Odeh, N. Traditional vs. Digital Communication Channels for Improving Compliance with Fixed Orthodontic Treatment: A Randomized Controlled Trial. *Angle Orthod.* **2021**, *91*, 227–235. [CrossRef] [PubMed]
16. Ross, M.C.; Campbell, P.M.; Tadlock, L.P.; Taylor, R.W.; Buschang, P.H. Effect of Automated Messaging on Oral Hygiene in Adolescent Orthodontic Patients: A Randomized Controlled Trial. *Angle Orthod.* **2019**, *89*, 262–267. [CrossRef] [PubMed]
17. Khader, D.; Peedikayil, F.; Chandru, T.; Kottayi, S.; Namboothiri, D. Reliability of One Ceph Software in Cephalometric Tracing: A Comparative Study. *SRM J. Res. Dent. Sci.* **2020**, *11*, 35. [CrossRef]
18. Aksakallı, S.; Yılancı, H.; Görükmez, E.; Ramoğlu, S. Reliability Assessment of Orthodontic Apps for Cephalometrics. *Turk. J. Orthod.* **2016**, *29*, 98–102. [CrossRef]
19. Goracci, C.; Ferrari, M. Reproducibility of Measurements in Tablet-Assisted, PC-Aided, and Manual Cephalometric Analysis. *Angle Orthod.* **2014**, *84*, 437–442. [CrossRef] [PubMed]
20. Kumar, M.; Kumari, S.; Chandna, A.; Konark; Singh, A.; Kumar, H.; Punita. Comparative Evaluation of CephNinja for Android and NemoCeph for Computer for Cephalometric Analysis: A Study to Evaluate the Diagnostic Performance of CephNinja for Cephalometric Analysis. *J. Int. Soc. Prev. Community Dent.* **2020**, *10*, 286–291. [CrossRef] [PubMed]
21. Kuriakose, P.; Greenlee, G.M.; Heaton, L.J.; Khosravi, R.; Tressel, W.; Bollen, A.-M. The Assessment of Rapid Palatal Expansion Using a Remote Monitoring Software. *J. World Fed. Orthod.* **2019**, *8*, 165–170. [CrossRef]
22. Livas, C.; Delli, K.; Spijkervet, F.K.L.; Vissink, A.; Dijkstra, P.U. Concurrent Validity and Reliability of Cephalometric Analysis Using Smartphone Apps and Computer Software. *Angle Orthod.* **2019**, *89*, 889–896. [CrossRef] [PubMed]
23. Morris, R.; Hoye, L.; Elnagar, M.; Atsawasuwan, P.; Galang-Boquiren, M.; Caplin, J.; Viana, G.; Obrez, A.; Kusnoto, B. Accuracy of Dental Monitoring 3D Digital Dental Models Using Photograph and Video Mode. *Am. J. Orthod. Dentofac. Orthop.* **2019**, *156*, 420–428. [CrossRef] [PubMed]
24. Moylan, H.; Carrico, C.; Lindauer, S.; Tüfekçi, E. Accuracy of a Smartphone-Based Orthodontic Treatment-Monitoring Application: A Pilot Study. *Angle Orthod.* **2019**, *89*, 727–733. [CrossRef] [PubMed]
25. Sayar, G.; Kilinc, D.D. Manual Tracing versus Smartphone Application (App) Tracing: A Comparative Study. *Acta Odontol. Scand.* **2017**, *75*, 588–594. [CrossRef] [PubMed]
26. Caruso, S.; Caruso, S.; Pellegrino, M.; Skafi, R.; Nota, A.; Tecco, S. A Knowledge-Based Algorithm for Automatic Monitoring of Orthodontic Treatment: The Dental Monitoring System. Two Cases. *Sensors* **2021**, *21*, 1856. [CrossRef]
27. Hansa, I.; Semaan, S.J.; Vaid, N.R. Clinical Outcomes and Patient Perspectives of Dental Monitoring® GoLive® with Invisalign®—A Retrospective Cohort Study. *Prog. Orthod.* **2020**, *21*, 16. [CrossRef] [PubMed]
28. Underwood, B.; Birdsall, J.; Kay, E. The Use of a Mobile App to Motivate Evidence-Based Oral Hygiene Behaviour. *Br. Dent. J.* **2015**, *219*, E2. [CrossRef]
29. Farhadifard, H.; Soheilifar, S.; Farhadian, M.; Kokabi, H.; Bakhshaei, A. Orthodontic Patients' Oral Hygiene Compliance by Utilizing a Smartphone Application (Brush DJ): A Randomized Clinical Trial. *BDJ Open* **2020**, *6*, 24. [CrossRef]
30. Kravitz, N.; Burris, B.; Butler, D.; Dabney, C. Teledentistry, Do-It-Yourself Orthodontics, and Remote Treatment Monitoring. *J. Clin. Orthod.* **2016**, *50*, 718–726.
31. Bauer, J.; Brown, W. The Digital Transformation of Oral Health Care. Teledentistry and Electronic Commerce. *J. Am. Dent. Assoc.* **2001**, *132*, 204–209. [CrossRef] [PubMed]
32. Sfikas, P.M. Teledentistry: Legal and Regulatory Issues Explored. *J. Am. Dent. Assoc.* **1997**, *128*, 1716–1718. [CrossRef] [PubMed]
33. Lins, R.M.L.; Alves, G.F.; Costa, J.C.S.; Barbosa, M.S.M.; da Silva, C.B.V.; Santos, J.W.; Pugliesi, D.M.C.; Santos Junior, V.E. Development of a Mobile Application for Acquiring Clinical and Laboratory Skills and Abilities in Pediatric Dentistry and Orthodontics. *Pesquisa Brasileira em Odontopediatria e Clínica Integrada* **2020**, *20*, 1–8. [CrossRef]
34. Park, J.H.; Rogowski, L.; Kim, J.H.; al Shami, S.; Howell, S.E.I. Teledentistry Platforms for Orthodontics. *J. Clin. Pediatric Dent.* **2021**, *45*, 48–53. [CrossRef]
35. Mandall, N.; O'Brien, K.; Brady, J.; Worthington, H.; Harvey, L. Teledentistry for Screening New Patient Orthodontic Referrals. Part 1: A Randomised Controlled Trial. *Br. Dent. J.* **2005**, *199*, 659–662. [CrossRef] [PubMed]
36. Hansa, I.; Katyal, V.; Ferguson, D.J.; Vaid, N. Outcomes of Clear Aligner Treatment with and without Dental Monitoring: A Retrospective Cohort Study. *Am. J. Orthod. Dentofac. Orthop.* **2021**, *159*, 453–459. [CrossRef]

37. Impellizzeri, A.; Horodinsky, M.; Barbato, E.; Polimeni, A.; Salah, P.; Galluccio, G. Dental Monitoring Application: It Is a Valid Innovation in the Orthodontics Practice? *Clin. Ter* **2020**, *171*, 260–267. [CrossRef]
38. Roisin, L.-C.; Brézulier, D.; Sorel, O. Remotely-Controlled Orthodontics: Fundamentals and Description of the Dental Monitoring System. *J. Dentofac. Anom. Orthod.* **2016**, *19*, 408. [CrossRef]
39. Official Web Site—Home—DentalMonitoring. Available online: https://dental-monitoring.com/ (accessed on 1 November 2021).
40. Giudice, A.; Barone, S.; Muraca, D.; Averta, F.; Diodati, F.; Antonelli, A.; Fortunato, L. Can Teledentistry Improve the Monitoring of Patients during the COVID-19 Dissemination? A Descriptive Pilot Study. *Int. J. Environ. Res. Public Health* **2020**, *17*, 3399. [CrossRef] [PubMed]
41. Maspero, C.; Abate, A.; Cavagnetto, D.; El Morsi, M.; Fama, A.; Farronato, M. Available Technologies, Applications and Benefits of Teleorthodontics. A Literature Review and Possible Applications during the COVID-19 Pandemic. *J. Clin. Med.* **2020**, *9*, 1891. [CrossRef] [PubMed]
42. Dalessandri, D.; Sangalli, L.; Tonni, I.; Laffranchi, L.; Bonetti, S.; Visconti, L.; Signoroni, A.; Paganelli, C. Attitude towards Telemonitoring in Orthodontists and Orthodontic Patients. *Dent. J.* **2021**, *9*, 47. [CrossRef] [PubMed]
43. Soares dos Santos, M. What Can Mathematics Say about Unsolved Problems in Medicine? *Insights Biol. Med.* **2018**, *2*, 1–2. [CrossRef]
44. Siddiqui, N.R.; Hodges, S.J.; Sharif, M.O. Orthodontic Apps: An Assessment of Quality (Using the Mobile App Rating Scale (MARS)) and Behaviour Change Techniques (BCTs). *Prog. Orthod.* **2021**, *22*, 25. [CrossRef]
45. Chauhan, N.S. Decision Tree Algorithm, Explained—KDnuggets. Available online: https://www.kdnuggets.com/2020/01/decision-tree-algorithm-explained.html (accessed on 1 November 2021).
46. Castro, L.A.; Favela, J.; Quintana, E.; Perez, M. Behavioral Data Gathering for Assessing Functional Status and Health in Older Adults Using Mobile Phones. *Pers. Ubiquitous Comput.* **2015**, *19*, 379–391. [CrossRef]
47. Chang, P.-Y.; Cheng, C.-Y.; Hon, J.-S.; Kuo, C.-D.; Yen, C.-L.; Chai, J.-W. Traditional versus Microsphere Embolization for Hepatocellular Carcinoma: An Effectiveness Evaluation Using Data Mining. *Healthcare* **2021**, *9*, 929. [CrossRef]
48. Almalki, Y.E.; Qayyum, A.; Irfan, M.; Haider, N.; Glowacz, A.; Alshehri, F.M.; Alduraibi, S.K.; Alshamrani, K.; Basha, M.A.A.; Alduraibi, A.; et al. A Novel Method for COVID-19 Diagnosis Using Artificial Intelligence in Chest X-ray Images. *Healthcare* **2021**, *9*, 522. [CrossRef]
49. Soto-Murillo, M.A.; Galván-Tejada, J.I.; Galván-Tejada, C.E.; Celaya-Padilla, J.M.; Luna-García, H.; Magallanes-Quintanar, R.; Gutiérrez-García, T.A.; Gamboa-Rosales, H. Automatic Evaluation of Heart Condition According to the Sounds Emitted and Implementing Six Classification Methods. *Healthcare* **2021**, *9*, 317. [CrossRef] [PubMed]
50. Wu, L.; Xie, X.; Wang, Y. ECG Enhancement and R-Peak Detection Based on Window Variability. *Healthcare* **2021**, *9*, 227. [CrossRef] [PubMed]
51. Gómez-Quintana, S.; Schwarz, C.E.; Shelevytsky, I.; Shelevytska, V.; Semenova, O.; Factor, A.; Popovici, E.; Temko, A. A Framework for AI-Assisted Detection of Patent Ductus Arteriosus from Neonatal Phonocardiogram. *Healthcare* **2021**, *9*, 169. [CrossRef]
52. Kurilová, V.; Goga, J.; Oravec, M.; Pavlovičová, J.; Kajan, S. Support Vector Machine and Deep-Learning Object Detection for Localisation of Hard Exudates. *Sci. Rep.* **2021**, *11*, 16045. [CrossRef] [PubMed]
53. Thurzo, A.; Stanko, P.; Urbanova, W.; Lysy, J.; Suchancova, B.; Makovnik, M.; Javorka, V. The WEB 2.0 Induced Paradigm Shift in the e-Learning and the Role of Crowdsourcing in Dental Education. *Bratisl. Med. J.* **2010**, *111*, 168–175.
54. Mucchi, L.; Jayousi, S.; Gant, A.; Paoletti, E.; Zoppi, P. Tele-Monitoring System for Chronic Diseases Management: Requirements and Architecture. *Int. J. Environ. Res. Public Health* **2021**, *18*, 7459. [CrossRef] [PubMed]
55. Mühlensiepen, F.; Kurkowski, S.; Krusche, M.; Mucke, J.; Prill, R.; Heinze, M.; Welcker, M.; Schulze-Koops, H.; Vuillerme, N.; Schett, G.; et al. Digital Health Transition in Rheumatology: A Qualitative Study. *Int. J. Environ. Res. Public Health* **2021**, *18*, 2636. [CrossRef] [PubMed]
56. Donner, C.F.; ZuWallack, R.; Nici, L. The Role of Telemedicine in Extending and Enhancing Medical Management of the Patient with Chronic Obstructive Pulmonary Disease. *Medicina* **2021**, *57*, 726. [CrossRef] [PubMed]
57. Jang, S.; Kim, Y.; Cho, W.K. A Systematic Review and Meta-Analysis of Telemonitoring Interventions on Severe COPD Exacerbations. *Int. J. Environ. Res. Public Health* **2021**, *18*, 6757. [CrossRef]
58. Krysta, K.; Romańczyk, M.; Diefenbacher, A.; Krzystanek, M. Telemedicine Treatment and Care for Patients with Intellectual Disability. *Int. J. Environ. Res. Public Health* **2021**, *18*, 1746. [CrossRef] [PubMed]
59. Corea, F.; Ciotti, S.; Cometa, A.; De Carlo, C.; Martini, G.; Baratta, S.; Zampolini, M. Telemedicine during the Coronavirus Disease (COVID-19) Pandemic: A Multiple Sclerosis (MS) Outpatients Service Perspective. *Neurol. Int.* **2021**, *13*, 25–31. [CrossRef]
60. Pradana, A.; Sahar, J.; Kesehatan, H.P.-J. Utilization of Information Technology in Prevention of Depression in Older Adults. *J. Kesehat.* **2021**, *14*, 14–20. [CrossRef]
61. Alghamdi, S.M.; Rajah, A.M.A.; Aldabayan, Y.S.; Aldhahir, A.M.; Alqahtani, J.S.; Alzahrani, A.A. Chronic Obstructive Pulmonary Disease Patients' Acceptance in E-Health Clinical Trials. *Int. J. Environ. Res. Public Health* **2021**, *18*, 5230. [CrossRef]
62. Neville, P.; van der Zande, M. Dentistry, e-Health and Digitalisation: A Critical Narrative Review of the Dental Literature on Digital Technologies with Insights from Health and Technology Studies. *Community Dent. Health* **2020**, *37*, 51–58. [CrossRef]

63. Timm, L.H.; Farrag, G.; Baxmann, M.; Schwendicke, F. Factors Influencing Patient Compliance during Clear Aligner Therapy: A Retrospective Cohort Study. *J. Clin. Med.* **2021**, *10*, 3103. [CrossRef] [PubMed]
64. Bowman, S.J. Improving the Predictability of Clear Aligners. *Semin. Orthod.* **2017**, *23*, 65–75. [CrossRef]

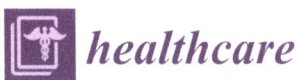

Article

Detecting a Stroke-Affected Region in the Brain by Scanning with Low-Intensity Electromagnetic Waves in the Radio Frequency/Microwave Band

Ibrahim El rube' [1], David Heatley [2,*] and Mohamed Abdel-Maguid [3]

1. Computer Engineering Department, Taif University, Taif 21944, Saudi Arabia; Ibrahim.ah@tu.edu.sa
2. Heatley Consulting, Ipswich IP5 3RE, UK
3. Faculty of Science, Engineering & Social Sciences, Canterbury Christ Church University, Canterbury CT1 1QU, UK; mohamed.abdel-maguid@canterbury.ac.uk
* Correspondence: consulting@davidheatley.co.uk

Abstract: There is a compelling need for a new form of head scanner to diagnose whether a patient is experiencing a stroke. Crucially, the scanner must be quickly and safely deployable at the site of the emergency to reduce the time between a diagnosis and treatment being commenced. That will help to improve the long-term outlook for many patients, which in turn will help to reduce the high cost of stroke to national economies. This paper describes a novel scanning method that utilises low-intensity electromagnetic waves in the radio frequency/microwave band to detect a stroke-affected region in the brain. This method has the potential to be low cost, portable, and widely deployable, and it is intrinsically safe for the patient and operator. It requires no specialist shielding or power supplies and, hence, can be rapidly deployed at the site of the emergency. That could be at the patient's bedside within a hospital, at the patient's home or place of work, or in a community setting such as a GP surgery or a nursing home. Results are presented from an extensive programme of scans of inanimate test subjects that are materially valid representations of a human head. These results confirm that the scanning method is indeed capable of detecting a stroke-affected region in these subjects. The significance of these results is discussed, as well as ways in which the efficacy of the scanning methodology could be further improved.

Keywords: stroke detection; portable head scanner; low-intensity EM waves; intrinsically safe; low carbon footprint

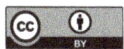

1. Introduction

Strokes are the 4th most prevalent cause of death and the leading cause of long-term invalidity in the UK [1]. Globally, the statistics are considerably worse with strokes being the 2nd most prevalent cause of death, although they are only the 3rd leading cause of long-term invalidity [2]. In the UK, around 110,000 people experience a stroke each year and around 1.2 M survivors are living with the consequences today. The treatment and rehabilitation for these patients, including the loss of productivity in the workplace and the high volume of benefit claims, costs the UK economy around GBP 26bn annually [1]. That figure is projected to reach GBP 75bn by 2035 if the current trajectory is sustained.

Given that the total healthcare expenditure in the UK for 2018 was GBP 214.4bn, which accounted for about 10.0% of GDP that year [3], it is clear that the cost of stroke alone is a significant percentage. That cost is intimately linked to the survivability of stroke patients and the proportion who require protracted treatment and long-term rehabilitation. The percentage figure for that proportion is influenced by the time between the occurrence of their stroke and treatment being commenced. The often-quoted mantra in medical circles, "time is brain", perfectly sums up the criticality of stroke patients receiving treatment promptly in order to save as much healthy brain tissue as possible and lessen the long-term consequences. Stroke patients who receive treatment within the first hour following their stroke—the so called "golden hour"—have the highest probability of a good recovery requiring little, if any, rehabilitation (assuming there are no pre-existing underlying health issues that dominate the outcome). However, once past the golden hour, the long-term outlook for surviving patients begins to decline, and beyond around 3–4 h the outlook rapidly diminishes, with some degree of long-term invalidity becoming inevitable. Typically, around 66% of these patients leave hospital with a long-term disability [1].

The current pathway for stroke patients requires them to be transported from the site of the emergency, which in many cases is their own home or place of work, to the nearest acute stroke unit to receive a CT and/or MRI scan. Only then can a conclusive diagnosis be made on whether the patient has indeed experienced a stroke and about which type of stroke they experienced (ischaemic: i.e., a clot, haemorrhagic: i.e., a bleed). Only then can the appropriate treatment be administered. Delays, sometimes significant, can occur at several points in the pathway, between the emergency call being made and treatment commencing. In the UK, thrombolysis treatment for ischaemic strokes, which are about 85% of all cases [1], is only licensed to be administered to patients within 4.5 h from the onset of their symptoms [1]. If the time when symptoms began is unknown, or it is known that more than 4.5 h have elapsed since symptoms began, the treatment cannot be provided. The outlook for those patients is inevitably compromised given that thrombolysis reportedly increases the chance of a good outcome by 30% [1].

If a diagnosis can be made at the site of the emergency and the stroke is confirmed to be ischaemic, there is the potential for many more patients to fall within the eligibility window for thrombolysis if it can be administered at that location. That will help to increase the proportion of stroke survivors who require little or perhaps even no long-term care and rehabilitation. Statistics show that the number of patients who survive a stroke and are able to return to their normal lives without any added assistance increases by 2% when thrombolysis is given within 3 h [1]. Besides that being of huge benefit to those patients, it will also help to reduce the enormous cost of stroke to the nation. However, administering thrombolysis at the site of the emergency is not yet approved in the UK. Furthermore, there is not yet a widely available capability to determine the type of stroke at the site of the emergency. Trials are underway in some countries with specially adapted ambulances that contain a CT scanner to deliver a diagnostic capability for stroke at the site of the emergency [4,5]. These vehicles will always be extremely few in number due to their high cost, and hence, they will only be available to an extremely small number of cases that happen to arise in a favourable location. This resource, although of immense benefit to the few stroke patients involved, will nevertheless have a negligible impact on the national statistics for stroke.

However, there is also the potential for time to be saved elsewhere in the patient pathway, specifically, by shortening the door-to-needle time (i.e., the time between the patient arriving at the hospital door and treatment being commenced). Although this is not as profound a saving of time compared with commencing treatment at the site of the emergency, shortening the door-to-needle time is readily implementable within the current pathway procedures and will make an important contribution to increasing the proportion of ischaemic stroke patients who are eligible to receive thrombolysis. Figure 1 illustrates how this can be achieved by equipping the attending paramedics at the site of the emergency with a new form of head scanner that is capable of reliably determining whether the patient is or is not experiencing a stroke, regardless of the type. This is the motivation for the authors' research reported in this paper. If the diagnosis is positive, the attending paramedics can alert the acute stroke unit's clinicians that a confirmed case of a stroke is now in transit. In addition, diagnostic data and images could be shared with these clinicians in real time during the journey via 4G/5G mobile connections, enabling the stroke unit to be more fully prepared to fast track the patient upon arrival. To quote a seminal review of this topic published in The Lancet [6], "Stroke physicians should be engaged not only in the in-hospital phase, but also in the pre-hospital phase of acute stroke management".

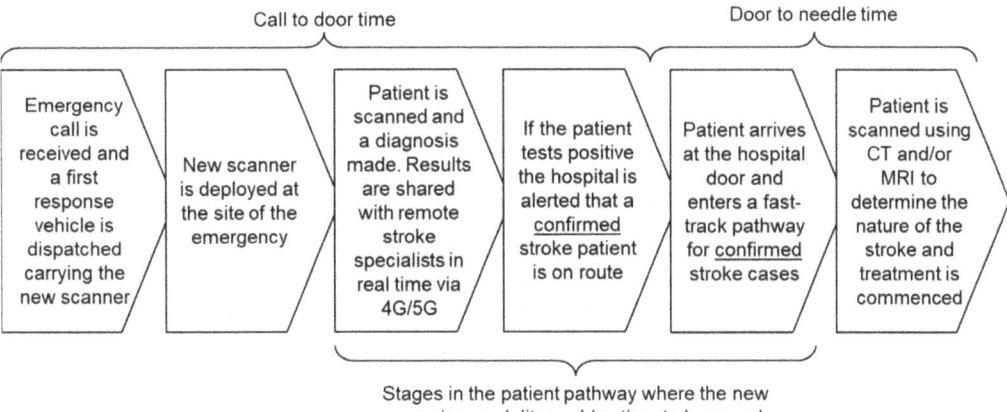

Figure 1. Reducing delay in the patient pathway for stroke.

Clearly there is a compelling need and significant benefits to be gained from a new form of head scanner for stroke diagnosis that can be carried in all present-day ambulances and other first response vehicles and quickly and safely deployed at the site of the emergency. The authors are researching a new method of scanning that has the potential to meet this challenge. It uses low-intensity electromagnetic waves in the radio frequency/microwave band to detect the presence of a stroke-affected region in the brain. No specialist shielding or bespoke high-voltage power supply are required, which enables the new scanning modality to be operated almost anywhere with no prior planning. The use of low-cost COTS devices throughout the experimental apparatus and a compact, lightweight, portable construction provides a credible blueprint for a future commercially developed scanner that could be carried in ambulances and first response vehicles and operated on-scene in complete safety. Such a scanner could also be widely deployed in hospitals on crash trolleys and operated at the bedside in emergency departments and high-dependency wards, and similarly in nursing and care homes where there is a localised elderly population at an increased risk of stroke. The material and operational carbon footprint of the scanner would be intrinsically low, and the absence of any form of ionizing radiation and toxic materials avoids costly end-of-life disposal directives.

In this paper, the authors describe their research into the new scanning modality and report the latest results from a comprehensive programme of scans of inanimate test subjects that are materially valid representations of a human head. The results are presented in a visual format that illustrates how a diagnosis could be displayed to the scanner operator. This serves to highlight the simplicity in interpreting these images, which enables the operator to quickly form a diagnosis. It is clear from these results that the new modality is indeed capable of detecting the presence and location of a stroke-affected region in the test subjects. At this stage of development, it is not yet known whether the new modality has the ability to reliably determine the type of stoke—ischaemic or haemorrhagic. However, discussions with stroke specialists have revealed that the ability to reliably confirm a stroke/no-stroke diagnosis at the site of the emergency, and then to alert the acute stroke unit ahead of arrival, would be a significant and welcome advance over the current protocols. That is the focus of the authors' current research and the results reported in this paper.

2. Related Work in This Field

Methods of scanning and imaging human anatomy with low-intensity radio frequencies/microwaves are being researched by other institutions across the world. For example, researchers at the University of Queensland at Brisbane, Australia [7–9], are investigating a scanning modality for stroke diagnosis that has some similarities with that reported in this paper. Their scanning apparatus acquires data across a similar range of frequencies, although they use a different approach to reconstruct an image of a stroke inclusion in their test subjects. They have also avoided the need for mechanical movements in their scanning apparatus by implementing a ring of stationary antennas encircling the subject that electronically translate the scanning beam in a circular path. Their results demonstrate that a stroke inclusion can be detected using their particular scanning modality, which is consistent with the findings from the different scanning modality reported in this paper.

Other institutions have taken their research in this area to commercialisation. Medfield Diagnostics (Gothenburg, Sweden) is commercialising in their Strokefinder product [10,11] with work undertaken by researchers at the Chalmers University of Technology in Gothenburg, Sweden and partner institutions [12,13]. They are also targeting stroke diagnosis using low-intensity radio/microwave frequencies; however, their approach differs from the authors of this study in several key areas. Firstly, their scanning modality uses a pulsed beam and the acquired data from the scanning chamber contains time-of-flight information, akin to radar. Secondly, their scanning beam does not translate around the phantom in a circular orbit. Instead, an array of stationary antennas is arranged in a bowl-shaped geometry that fits over the patient's head. One antenna is assigned as the pulse transmitter at any moment while the others are receivers, then a different antenna is assigned as the transmitter while the others are receivers. That sequence progresses around all of the antennas in a defined but noncircular sequence.

Micrima (Bristol, UK) is commercialising in their Maria product [14] work that was originally undertaken at the University of Bristol [15,16]. Maria also uses low-intensity radio/microwave frequencies in a radar-like modality; however, its application is exclusively breast screening. It also uses an array of stationary antennas arranged in a bowl-shaped geometry but designed to accommodate a woman's breast. The scanning modality and the manner in which it has been implemented in Maria affords a number of advantages over conventional breast screening, in particular, a greatly increased degree of safety for the patient and operators through the absence of X-rays, and a much-improved degree of comfort for the patient during the examination. These and other advantages are described in the referenced articles.

A common thread running through these examples and the authors' work reported in this paper is the intrinsic safety of the scanning modalities as well as the potential for some of the scanners to be portable and deployed at the patient's location with no prior planning. This is a profound departure from their equivalents that use X-rays or intense magnetic fields.

3. Materials and Methods

3.1. Considerations in Computed Tomography

In X-ray CT, the scanning beam is arranged to penetrate the whole subject, from front to back, then detected as it emerges on the far side. Information about the scanned subject is contained within the characteristics of the detected signal. That form of propagation and detection is labelled S21 according to scattering parameters convention (S-parameters) [17]. The extremely short wavelength of X-rays (0.01–10 nm) and the intensity of the beam ensure that the projection (i.e., shadow) cast by the subject on the detectors has a well-defined outline with little diffusion around the edges. An image of the scanned subject is reconstructed from the data delivered by the detectors using an algorithm based on the Inverse Radon Transform [18], which is well suited to the sharply defined edges of the projection and the low level of diffusion.

Initially the authors adopted the S21 configuration in their new scanning modality in deference to the well-established convention in X-ray CT. However, it was found that the Inverse Radon Transform is not suited to the new implementation because the wavelength of the scanning beam is many orders of magnitude longer than that of X-rays. In addition, the beam undergoes significantly more attenuation, diffusion, and scatter during its passage through the scanned subject. Consequently, the outline of the projection is highly blurred and feint against the naturally occurring background noise. Reconstructing an image from the acquired data is therefore significantly more challenging than the case with X-rays.

Attention is now being given to the data acquired from the reflected portion of the scanning beam, labelled S11 in the S-parameters convention. Although the scanning beam is still subjected to attenuation, diffusion, and scatter, the typically shorter path length that the reflected portion undergoes ensures that data quality is improved, particularly if the stroke-affected region in the brain happens to be close to the surface. In addition, whereas S21 requires two antennas to translate around the subject multiple times in a co-ordinated pattern, S11 requires only one antenna to orbit the subject just once. Consequently, S11 facilitates a shorter scanning duration as well as a simpler construction of scanning chamber that surrounds the subject. Details are given in the next section.

It is important to note that S11 data, although derived from the reflected portion of the scanning beam, are not the same as pulsed radar in which discrete pulses are emitted from an antenna and the reflected signals are detected. S11 data in the context of the new scanning modality derive from a continuous-wave signal—not a pulsed signal, and S11 data characterise the dielectric properties of the static environment in close proximity to the antenna—not the round-trip propagation time of pulses.

S11 data are implicit in all of the experimental results reported in this paper.

3.2. Experimental Scanning Apparatus

To ensure that the experimental scanning apparatus affords maximum flexibility and ease of modification, its construction employs readily available materials and devices, and a simple mechanical movement. Figure 2 shows the totality of the apparatus. It comprises a scanning chamber in which an antenna, labelled Tx, mechanically translates around the test subject, labelled phantom, under the action of a stepper motor. While the antenna is in motion, the phantom is stationary. This is the same convention used in CT. The antenna employs a compact Vivaldi design that is rated to operate across 5–18 GHz, although in reality, the operating range extends down to 1 GHz.

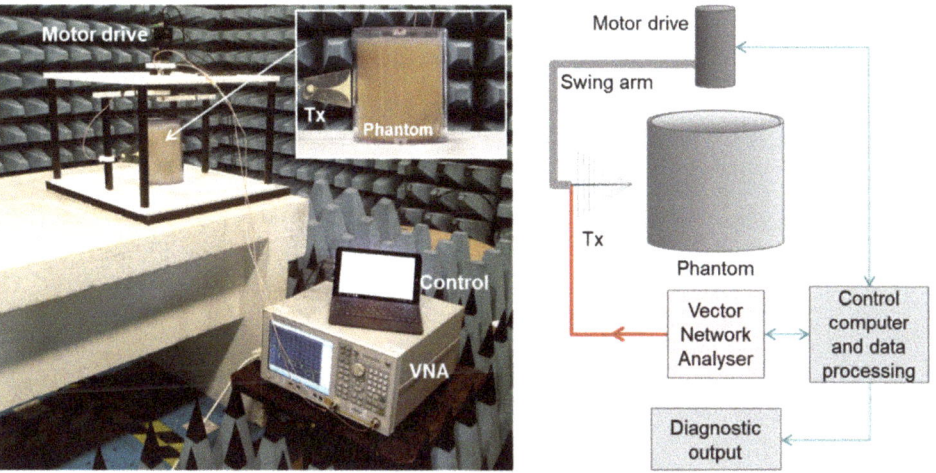

Figure 2. Components of the experimental scanning apparatus.

The antenna is connected to a Vector Network Analyser (VNA model P9374A, manufactured and supplied by Keysight Technologies, Santa Rosa, CA, USA), which measures S11 over a broad range of frequencies. The VNA, as well as the stepper motor, are under the control of a bespoke script running on a laptop PC, which also stores and processes the acquired data. It is evident that the scanning apparatus is minimalist, comprising only the scanning chamber, a VNA, and a controller. This supports the view that, in due course, a commercial version of the scanner could be compact, lightweight, and portable, as well as relatively low cost, particularly if the full-featured benchtop VNA in the photograph is replaced with a low-profile version that delivers only the required features. Preferably, the mechanically translated single antenna would also be replaced with a ring of stationary, electronically switched antennas.

During the scans reported in this paper, the antenna translates through 360 degrees in 100 equal steps (3.6 degrees per step), pausing for a brief moment at each step while the VNA measures S11 at 1601 spot frequencies between 1 GHz and 20 GHz. At each frequency, the S11 data include the magnitude and phase of the signal detected at the antenna. Consequently, each scan acquires 320,200 data points. These data and the frequency range are more than is needed for a reliable diagnosis; however, the current priority is to acquire as much data as are available to facilitate later work on refining the operation and performance of the scanner.

The use of a VNA ensures that the apparatus is highly immune to electromagnetic interference (EMI) in the surrounding environment, from sources such as Wi-Fi hubs, mobile phones, and masts, as well as other wireless services. This benefit stems from the fact that the detector side of the VNA is internally locked in frequency and phase to the transmitter side. Consequently, only the transmitted signal is recognised and accepted by the receiver. All other sources are effectively ignored. It is plausible that a future commercial development of this scanning apparatus would embed a low-profile VNA in its construction, thereby ensuring a high degree of EMI immunity. In addition, the scanning chamber that encloses the patient's head and houses the antenna system would be designed to function as an electromagnetic screen.

A primary goal of the new scanning modality is that it must be fundamentally safe for the patient and operators and requires no specialist shielding or other safety precautions. To achieve that goal the intensity of the scanning beam must be very low. In the absence of formal regulatory guidance on the approved beam intensity for the kind of scanning modality being researched, the decision was taken early on to adopt a beam power of only 1 mW, 0 dBm. That is 100× lower than the radiated power of domestic Wi-Fi hubs (typically 100 mW, +20 dBm). At such low power levels, patients could be continuously scanned on a 24/7 basis with no safety concerns. There is no practical reason for that to be done, but it nevertheless serves to highlight the unparalleled safety margin that the new scanning modality affords compared with X-ray CT. In due course, when guidance for the new scanning modality is formally ratified by the regulatory authorities, it is reasonable to expect that the approved beam intensity will be at least 100× or even 1000× greater than the level being used because of the very short exposure period during a scan, while still remaining within the guidance limits for non-scanning wireless applications such as mobile telecommunications. However, for the time being, the authors' research will continue with a conservative power level of 1 mW, 0 dBm. That level is implicit in all of the results reported in this paper.

3.3. Test Subjects (Phantoms)

The test subjects used in the scans, commonly referred to as phantoms, are constructed using fluids that closely replicate the dielectric properties of the anatomical constituents of a human head. These fluids are contained in the polycarbonate vessels shown in Figure 3. That material is used because of its high transparency at the beam frequencies. The phantoms have a cylindrical geometry in order to maintain a constant gap of 3–4 mm between the antenna and the outer edge of the phantom while the antenna is in motion around the stationary phantom. The cylindrical geometry also simplifies data interpretation by limiting the acquired data to a single slice in the horizontal X-Y plane, located at the mid-point of the vertical Z axis. Future work will use 'head-shaped' phantoms and will acquire data at multiple X-Y planes along the Z axis.

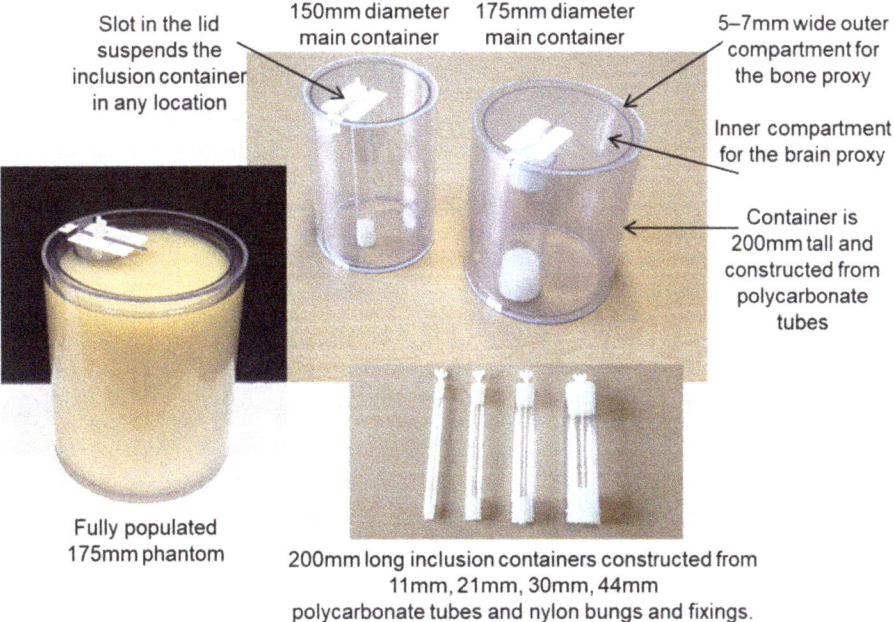

Figure 3. Polycarbonate vessels used in the construction of the phantoms.

The 175 mm diameter container in Figure 3 represents an adult head, while the 150 mm diameter container represents an adolescent. Both containers have a 5–7 mm wide outer compartment that is filled with a proxy fluid for skull bone. The large inner compartment is filled with a proxy fluid for brain matter. Stroke-affected regions are implemented by placing one of the inclusion containers in the brain proxy fluid, anchored to the top lid of the outer container. The different diameters of the inclusion containers (11 mm, 21 mm, 30 mm, 44 mm) represent strokes of different severity and stage of progression, while their fluid contents are selected to represent an ischaemic or haemorrhagic stroke. By moving the top anchorage point of these containers along the slot in the top lid, strokes at different depths within the brain are represented. The use of nylon bungs and fixings with these containers ensures that they have minimal influence on the data acquired during scans. The photograph at the left in Figure 3 shows an example fully populated 175 mm phantom with the 44 mm stroke inclusion installed and located close to the surface of the brain. The comprehensive program of scans that produced the results reported in this paper used both phantom sizes and all four stroke inclusions at a variety of locations between the surface of the brain and the centre.

The anatomical simplicity of these phantoms contrasts with the steps taken by some of the other researchers in this field in the construction of their phantoms. For example, the University of Queensland group elected to create discrete anatomical structures within their phantoms, each with a distinct set of dielectric properties for that particular anatomical element [19]. Similarly, Micrima employed phantoms that contained a degree of anatomical geometry. Notwithstanding the undoubted validity of these approaches to phantom construction, the authors of this paper decided instead to favour an intrinsically simpler construction for several important reasons. Firstly, the wavelength of the scanning beam inside a phantom head (or a human head alike) ranges from several mm to several cm. Consequently, fine structural details within the phantom are inherently smeared out in the data, leaving just the macro-level details. It is therefore sufficient that the phantoms used in this study incorporate a simple geometry while still being a materially valid representation of a human subject. Secondly, for the purposes of a triage diagnosis at the site of the emergency, fine detail of the kind displayed in CT images is not required. The priority is firmly on determining whether the patient has or has not experienced a stroke. The simplicity of the authors' phantoms is consistent with that priority. Thirdly, in order to physically assemble and sustain a detailed anatomical structure within a phantom, the proxy materials must have a solid, or at least a semi-solid consistency. Consequently, individual phantoms must be constructed from scratch for every different size/severity and location of the stroke-affected region that needs to be studied. That could amount to a great many phantoms if the study is wide ranging, as is the authors' study reported herein. In contrast, the simpler anatomy favoured by the authors coupled with the use of fluid proxies enables a broad range of stroke size/severity and location to be represented with ease in just a single construction of a phantom for each head size: one for an adult and one for an adolescent.

Sourcing the correct proxy fluids is vital for the material validity of the phantoms. The dielectric properties of the fluids, and particularly their relative permittivity as a function of frequency, define how they interact with the scanning beam of the new modality. These parameters are therefore central to selecting fluids that have a relative permittivity that is closest to the human material(s) they represent. The proxy fluid selected for brain matter is produced by the National Physical Laboratory [20] to an international standard and supplied to the telecoms industry for use in specific absorption rate (SAR) tests associated with the safety of mobile phones and the influence of their emissions on brain tissue [21]. Its relative permittivity characterises that of grey and white matter and cranial fluids (blood, CSF, ECF, ISF, etc.) in a single unified medium. This off-white opaque fluid is evident in the fully populated phantom in Figure 3. Figure 4 shows plots of its relative permittivity against frequency (measured by the supplier) and compares those plots with measured and computed plots for the individual constituents of a human body that are widely available in the literature and frequently referenced by researchers in this field [22–27]. Figure 4 also includes a single data point for Ethylene Glycol, which serves as a proxy fluid for skull bone. It too is a single unified medium that characterises cancellous and cortical bone and marrow.

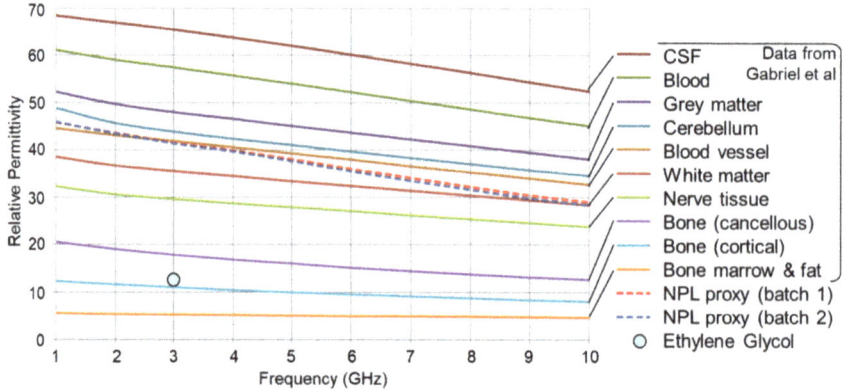

Figure 4. Relative permittivities of the proxy fluids obtained from NPL and published plots for other human anatomical constituents.

The proxy fluids for an ischaemic inclusion and a haemorrhagic inclusion are RS-I fluid [28] and defibrinated sheep blood [29], respectively. Given that 85% of all diagnosed strokes are ischaemic [1], this paper focusses on the results obtained with RS-I fluid representing an ischaemic stroke. The results from defibrinated sheep blood representing a haemorrhagic stroke will be reported in due course, together with the authors' investigation into whether the two types of stroke can be discriminated by the new scanning modality.

3.4. Data Processing

During a scan, the real and imaginary components of the detected S11 signal, denoted $Sr[tx,k]$ and $Si[tx,k]$, respectively, are acquired by the VNA at each of 100 stationary locations of the antenna tx as it steps around the phantom through 360 degrees. At each location, the VNA measures $Sr[tx,k]$ and $Si[tx,k]$ at up to 1601 spot frequencies between 1 GHz and 20 GHz, where $tx = 1:100$ is the antenna location index and $k = 1:1601$ is an index that corresponds to the spot frequencies actually used.

The signature of the stroke cannot be easily identified within this complex data for several reasons, but principally the following:

- The beam intensity launched from the antenna is very low (1 mW, 0 dBm) for the reasons given earlier. In addition, the attenuation of the beam as it propagates through the phantom is significant, particularly towards the upper end of the range of frequencies. Consequently, the signal-to-noise ratio of the acquired data is low.
- The beam undergoes significant scatter and diffusion during its passage through the phantom. This greatly reduces the definition of the signature of the stroke in the data against the naturally occurring background fluctuations and noise in the data.

To resolve these challenges several processes are performed on the dataset to facilitate a more effective search for features in the data that signify a stroke. The complex S11 signal $Sc[tx,k]$ detected at the antenna at each measurement instant is thus expressed as follows:

$$S_c[tx,k] = S_r[tx,k] + jS_i[tx,k] \qquad (1)$$

Using this expression, Figure 5a shows the magnitude of the totality of raw data acquired from the antenna during a scan of the 175 mm phantom containing a 44 mm stroke inclusion located close to the surface. The actual phantom is shown in the photo in Figure 3 in the previous section. All of the results reported in this section derive from a scan of that particular phantom, which is henceforth referred to as 'scan #1' for brevity. The results from scans of a broad range of phantoms and inclusions of different sizes and locations are presented in the next section.

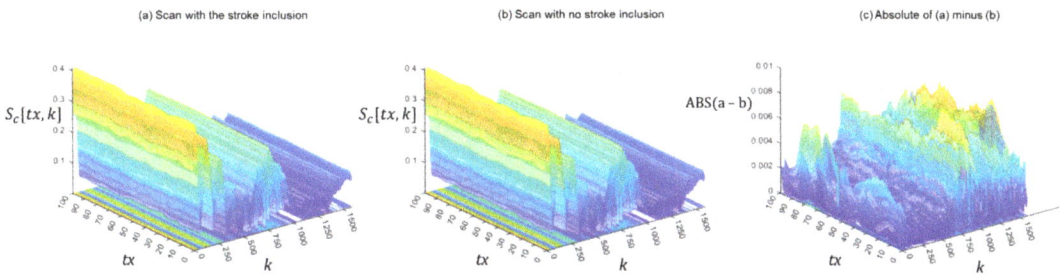

Figure 5. Magnitude of the raw data acquired during scan #1: (**a**) with the stroke inclusion, (**b**) without the inclusion, and (**c**) the absolute (ABS) of the difference between (**a**,**b**).

Interestingly, when the same scan is repeated with the stroke inclusion removed from the phantom vessel, the resulting raw data in Figure 5b are superficially unchanged. This highlights the challenge faced in extracting the signature of the stroke inclusion from the raw data. It is at an extremely low level relative to the surrounding data. One potential solution explored by the authors involved subtracting the 'no inclusion' data from the 'with inclusion' data to accentuate information about the stroke inclusion and its location. This method was ultimately rejected for two primary reasons. Firstly, in a practical setting, it is all but impossible to envisage a scenario when clinicians will have two recent scans of the same patient: one taken shortly before the onset of their stroke and the other taken while their stroke is occurring. Consideration was given to utilising publicly accessible libraries of scans of healthy patients and developing a method to use those data as a generalised 'no inclusion' scan. However, the challenges in ensuring that these scans not only accurately represented a stroke patient prior to the onset of their stroke, but that they can also be formatted in a way that precisely replicates the output of the new scanning modality had it actually been used, were felt to be insurmountable. Secondly, subtracting the two scans from each other produces the highly complex data field in Figure 5c. Reliably identifying and extracting the low-intensity signature of the stroke inclusion from within a data field containing such extreme variability is challenging, particularly for stroke inclusions that are small in size and deeply seated within the brain. The decision was therefore taken to develop the following robust and computationally efficient method that reliably extracts the signature of a stroke inclusion in the raw data from just a single scan of the patient while they are experiencing their stroke.

The Inverse Fast Fourier Transform (IFFT) is used to transform the dataset in Figure 5a from the frequency domain to the time domain. Given that the S11 scanning modality that underpins this paper uses only one antenna, the data acquired at each stationary location of the antenna as it steps around the phantom are not influenced by a second nearby antenna, as was the case in the previous S21 scanning modality that was briefly alluded to earlier. It is therefore sufficient to perform a 1D IFFT on the complex signal $S_c[tx,k]$ in Equation (1) at each antenna location, which produces:

$$s[tx,n] = \frac{1}{N} \sum_{k=1}^{N} S_c[tx,k] e^{j2\pi(n-1)(k-1)/N} \qquad (2)$$

where $N = 1:1601$, $tx = 1:100$, and $n = 1:1601$. If only real data are applied to the transformation, the output data are reflected around its centre. However, for the purposes of this study, the real and imaginary components of the acquired data are applied to the transformation, which yields values in just the first half (i.e., left half) of the transform domain, as is evident in Figure 6.

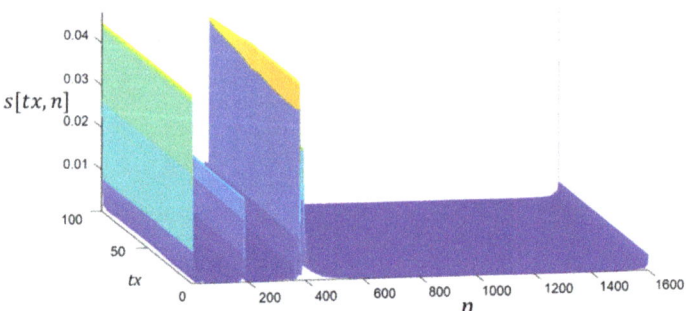

Figure 6. IFFT transformed data acquired from scan #1.

The output of the IFFT, denoted $s[tx,n]$ in Equation (2), comprises N complex 1D sequences that are computed independently in accordance with the structure of the data acquired during a scan. Therefore, at each antenna location as it steps around the phantom, the average of the transformed sequence over the temporal domain is calculated by averaging the sequence $s[tx,n]$, and thus:

$$s_{av}[tx] = \frac{1}{N} \sum_{n=1}^{N} s[tx, n] \qquad (3)$$

This 1D averaged data $s_{av}[tx]$ describes the S11 signal at the antenna for all frequencies that are the input to the IFFT at each antenna location. However, for each antenna location, $s_{av}[tx]$ does not yield a distinct unmistakable signature of the stroke inclusion because of the strong influence of unwanted values on it. This is evident in Figure 7, which shows multiple peaks and troughs computed from Equation (3), rather than a single distinct signature.

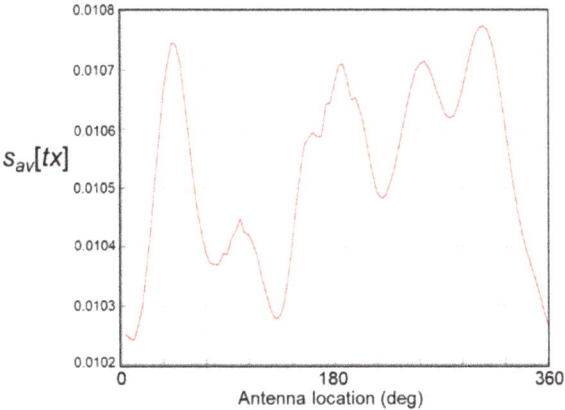

Figure 7. Magnitude values computed from Equation (3).

Further study of the transformed series $s[tx,n]$ in Figure 6 using scans of several different phantoms in which the inclusion is present in some while is absent in others, reveals that the position of $n = N/4$ is dominant when the inclusion is present but not when the inclusion is absent. The data sequence around the $n = N/4$ index can therefore be summed to resolve a more distinct signature of the stroke inclusion. Equation (3) can then be rewritten as:

$$\hat{s}_{av}[tx] = \frac{1}{2a+1} \sum_{n=\frac{N}{4}-a}^{\frac{N}{4}+a} s[tx, n] \qquad (4)$$

where $a \geq 0$ represents the width of the span centred on $n = N/4$. The value of a is selected in accordance with the strength of the signature of the inclusion. For example, in instances when the strength is high, the value of a is not critical, whereas when the strength is low, studies have found that $a = 2$ returns optimum results. Throughout the results presented in this paper, a is assumed to be 2. The real and imaginary components of the complex data sequence represented by Equation (4) are shown in Figure 9.

Both components carry vital information about the presence and location of the stroke inclusion. It is therefore prudent to use both. They can be combined by computing the absolute value of the averaged data sequence in Equation (4), expressed thus as:

$$s_{Mag}[tx] = |\hat{s}_{av}[tx]| \tag{5}$$

Figure 8 shows the data computed by Equation (5). The signature of the stroke inclusion is visible in the form of a distinctive peak, the location of which corresponds with the location of the inclusion on the horizontal axis.

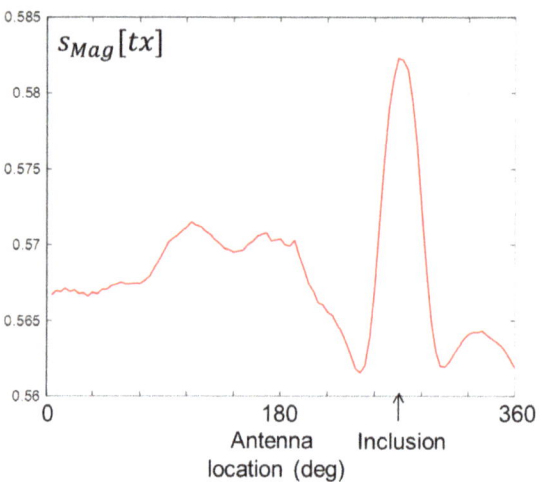

Figure 8. $s_{Mag}[tx]$ computed from Equation (5) for scan #1.

To reduce the intensity of the data on either side of the peak in Figure 8, and thereby increase the distinctiveness of the signature, $s_{Mag}[tx]$ in Equation (5) can be differentiated as follows:

$$s_d[tx] = s_{Mag}[tx+1] - s_{Mag}[tx] \tag{6}$$

Figure 10 shows the differentiated data computed by Equation (6). The presence of the stroke inclusion is evidenced by the distinctive double peak, while the location of the inclusion on the horizontal axis coincides with the zero crossing between the two peaks.

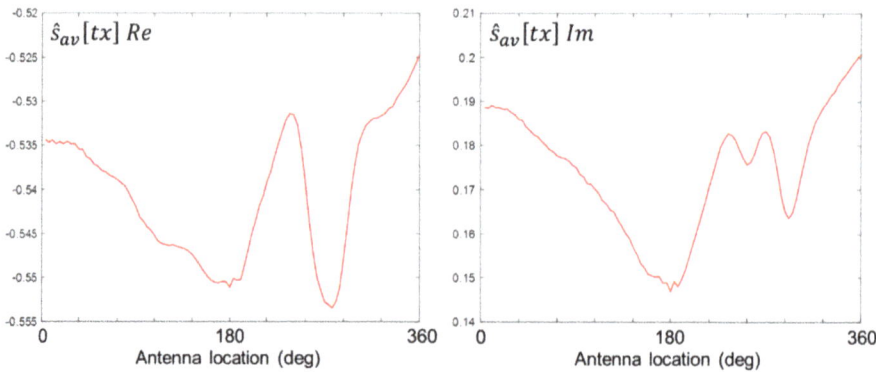

Figure 9. Real (**left**) and imaginary (**right**) values of $\hat{s}_{av}[tx]$ for scan #1.

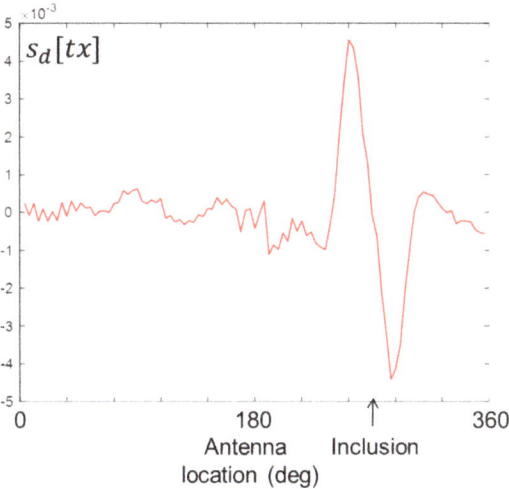

Figure 10. $s_d[tx]$ computed from Equation (6) for scan #1.

The above results confirm that the method of data analysis devised for this study successfully extracts the signature of a stroke inclusion from the raw data acquired during a scan. The next section presents the results from a comprehensive programme of scans of phantoms of different sizes and inclusions of different sizes and locations. In this way, the results are representative of a population of adults and adolescents who are experiencing strokes of different severity and depth within the brain.

4. Results and Analysis

To ensure consistency across the scans reported in this paper, the majority were carried out with the stroke inclusion at the 9 o'clock position on a clock face, as illustrated in Figure 11 for the 44 mm inclusion in the 175 mm phantom.

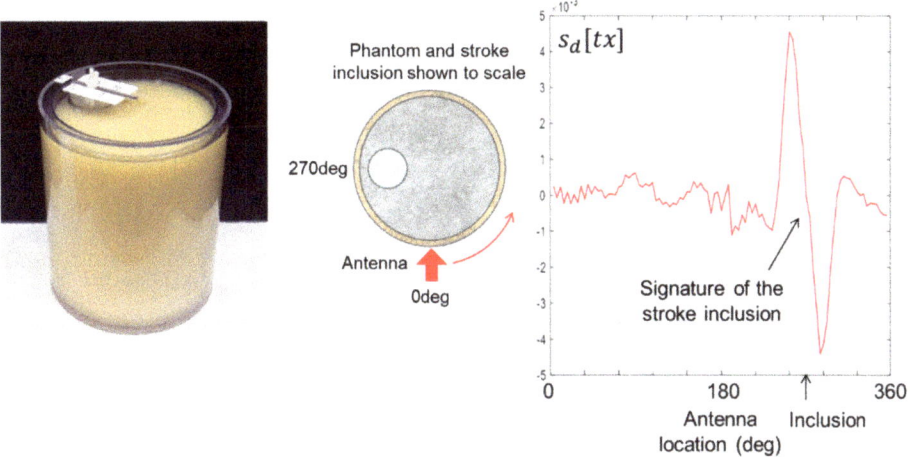

Figure 11. Signature of a 44 mm inclusion in the 175 mm phantom.

The antenna begins and ends every scan at the 6 o'clock position and translates anticlockwise around the phantom. The 6 o'clock position can therefore be designated 0 degrees, as shown, in which case the inclusion is located at 270 degrees. As the antenna translates around the phantom, the signature of the stroke inclusion is highly visible as the double peak (i.e., differentiated pulse) first observed in Figure 10. The middle zero crossing between the two peaks corresponds to the location of the inclusion. This result and those that follow confirm that the new scanning modality is indeed capable of detecting the presence and location of a stroke inclusion.

The data plots in Figure 12 show that progressively smaller inclusions in the 175 mm phantom are detectable down to 22 mm in size; however, the smallest 11 mm inclusion is beyond the sensitivity threshold of the apparatus. However, Figure 13 shows that the smallest 11 mm inclusion is detectable in the 150 mm phantom, which indicates that the sensitivity threshold of the apparatus is in fact at or close to 11 mm for both phantom sizes.

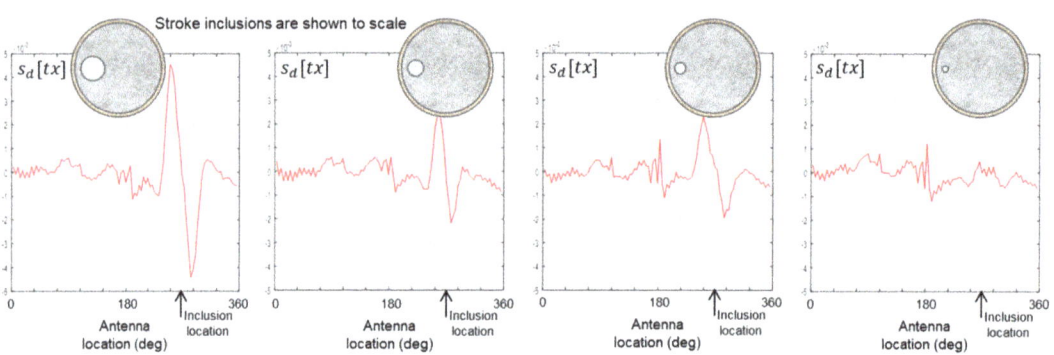

Figure 12. Data from scans of the 175 mm phantom with inclusion sizes of 44 mm (**left**), 30 mm, 21 mm, 11 mm (**right**).

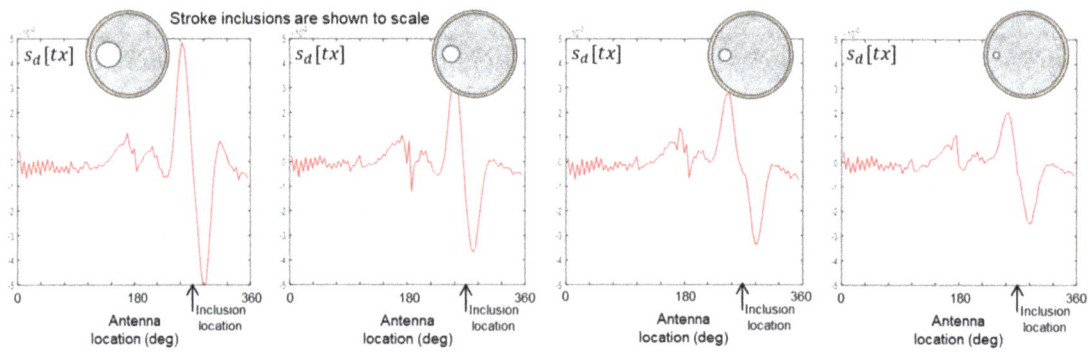

Figure 13. Data from scans of the 150 mm phantom with inclusion sizes of 44 mm (**left**), 30 mm, 21 mm, and 11 mm (**right**).

It is important to remember that the power level in the scanning beam is only 1 mW, 0 dBm, for the reasons outlined earlier. Had these scans been carried out at a higher beam intensity of the magnitude that could be approved by regulatory authorities in due course, it is reasonable to assume that the 11 mm inclusion, and perhaps even smaller, would be consistently detectable.

During the scans in Figures 12 and 13, the inclusion is located close to the surface of the proxy brain. The scans in Figure 14 show the impact of locating the inclusion more deeply within the proxy brain of the 175 mm phantom. Scans of the 150 mm phantom reveal the same trend, so they need not be included. It is clear that the scanning beam is unable to penetrate to a depth approximately half-way between the surface and centre of the proxy brain. Again, it is important to note the low intensity of the scanning beam and the likelihood that an approved higher intensity will penetrate more deeply and be more detectable by the apparatus.

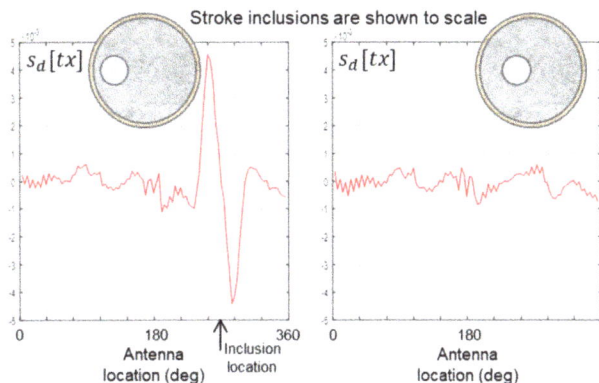

Figure 14. Data from scans of progressively deeper 44 mm inclusions in the 175 mm phantom.

The data plots reported thus far all derive from scans in which the stroke inclusion is located at 9 o'clock on a clock face. As stated at the start of this section, that was done to ensure consistency across those data plots and to facilitate valid comparisons between the plots. However, in order to confirm that the signature is indeed caused by the stroke inclusion and is not an artefact of the scanning apparatus or the surrounding environment that just happens to be at the correct location, the additional scans in Figure 15 were carried out with the inclusion located at 12 o'clock and 3 o'clock. The resulting data plots confirm that the location of the signature correctly tracks the actual location of the inclusion.

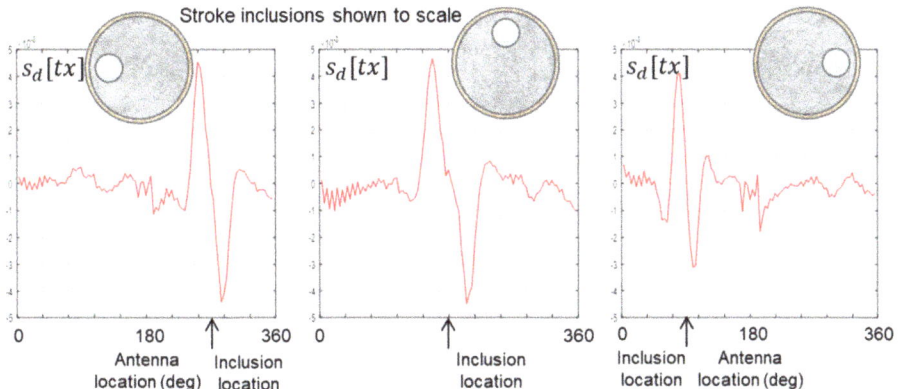

Figure 15. Data from scans in which the 44 mm inclusion is at different locations relative to the start of each scan.

Scans were also carried out in which there is no stroke inclusion in the phantom, as well as scans in which there is no phantom present in the scanning apparatus. The data from some of these scans are shown in Figure 16. The absence of any form of signature provides further confirmation that neither the framework of the phantom (i.e., the structural vessel excluding any inclusion) nor the scanning apparatus and the surrounding environment influenced the results reported throughout this paper.

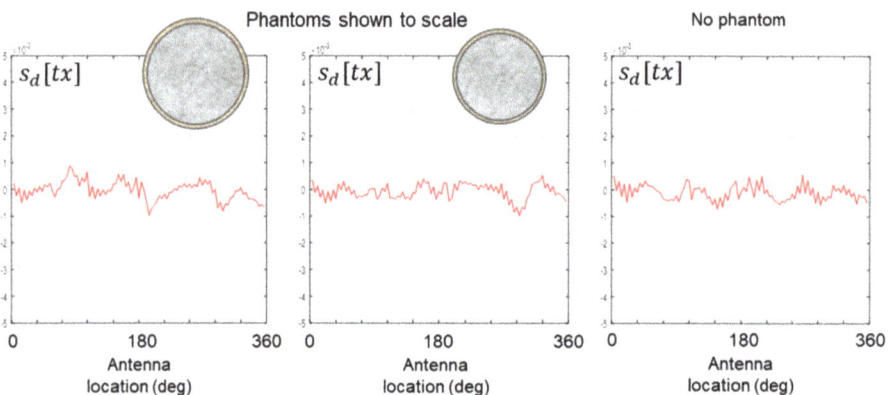

Figure 16. Data from scans of the 175 mm and 150 mm phantoms with no stroke inclusion present, and a scan of just the scanning apparatus.

5. Discussion

The results confirm that the new scanning modality is capable of detecting the presence and location of a proxy for an ischaemic stroke. The clarity of the signature of the stroke in the data is testament to the efficacy of the analytical procedure devised specifically for this application. Besides being computationally efficient, which helps to minimise the time to display a diagnosis, the simplicity of the signature it produces lends itself to rapid, unambiguous interpretation with minimal training. It should, however, be noted that the phantoms used in the scans are simplified, idealised versions of a human subject. Notwithstanding that the phantoms were constructed from proxy materials that closely replicate the dielectric properties of human tissue, fluids, and bone, the complexities of a vascular structure and the anatomy of different tissue types and fluid-filled cavities are absent in the phantoms. In justification of that, the simplification of the phantoms should be viewed as an 'averaged' human subject in which the boundaries between different anatomical regions are blurred to the point of completely merging into one medium. Indeed, the proxy medium used in the phantoms for brain matter is a single fluid specifically manufactured by NPL [20] to a materially valid formula that represents the unified dielectric properties of white and grey matter and all brain fluids. Furthermore, given that the wavelength of the beam inside a phantom or a human subject alike ranges from several mm to several cm, fine structural details present in the subject are inherently smeared out in the data, leaving just the macro-level details, which are manifest in the signature of the stroke. It is therefore consequential, as well as beneficial, that the phantoms used in this study need only incorporate a simple geometry while still being a valid representation of a human subject.

The long wavelength of the scanning beam also speaks to an important distinction between the new scanning modality and X-ray CT. For the purposes of a triage diagnosis at the site of the emergency, the fine detail in CT images is not required. Indeed, even the location of the stroke is not essential. The priority is firmly on determining whether the patient is or is not experiencing a stroke. The new scanning modality has demonstrated its suitability in that role. The fact that it also indicates the location of the stroke is an added benefit.

In a further simplification of the anatomy of the stroke inclusion, the authors assumed that any previous or non-vascular cerebral lesions that the patient might have experienced are closely co-located with the stroke-affected region itself. Consequently, the anomalous region that is detected is assumed to be a singular amorphous mass. However, in practical settings that assumption is not always valid. Previous or non-vascular cerebral lesions could be present in locations removed from the stroke-affected region. To take account of this, the next phase of the study will include phantoms that contain multiple inclusions to represent stroke patients whose ongoing stroke and previous cerebral lesions are dispersed throughout the brain.

Beam intensity has been shown to be a critical factor in the ability to detect a deeply seated stroke inclusion. Striking the optimum balance between having sufficient intensity to penetrate the patient's brain to a useful depth while remaining safe to the patient and scanner operator is a fundamental objective of the new scanning methodology promoted in this paper. It is creditable that the current experimental apparatus, despite using a very low-beam intensity, is achieving sufficient penetration for stroke inclusions close to the surface to be detected, even for inclusions as small as 11 mm. However, given that the current beam intensity of 1 mW (0 dBm) is some $100\times$ lower than that emitted by a domestic Wi-Fi hub, there is scope to increase the beam intensity by $100\times$ or even $1000\times$ while still remaining within the guidance limits for non-scanning applications such as mobile telecommunications. In due course, it is reasonable to expect that medical regulatory authorities will approve beam powers significantly higher than those used in this study given the very short exposure period. The next phases of the project will employ higher powers to assess the performance of the new scanning modality under more realistic conditions.

It is important to emphasise that the new scanning modality will not replace nor displace X-ray CT or MRI; quite the contrary. Its purpose is to add a valuable new capability for stroke diagnosis that complements X-ray CT and MRI in settings where they are unsuited, particularly when the scanner needs to be brought to the patient's location.

The whole life cost is a further important consideration that favours the new scanning modality. The end-of-service disposal costs of X-ray CT and MRI scanners can be a significant proportion of their whole life cost. In contrast, the scanning modality described in this paper does not use radioactive devices nor does it produce any form of toxic long-term contamination. In addition, its energy carbon footprint is significantly lower since it does not require a specialist high-voltage power supply and, indeed, has the potential to be battery operated.

It should be noted that all of the results presented in this paper relate to an ischaemic stroke. Approximately 85% of all strokes are ischaemic [1], hence, why it was prioritised in this paper. The authors also carried out preliminary scans of phantoms with the proxy fluid for the inclusion is defibrinated blood to represent a haemorrhagic stroke. The results are very similar to those in this paper for an ischaemic stroke, which is to be expected since, as is evident in Figure 4, the relative permittivity of blood and CSF are very similar. It has yet to be determined whether the new scanning modality in its current experimental form is able to reliably distinguish between both types of stroke. Without that determination the correct treatment for the particular stroke cannot be commenced. Consequently, an on-scene diagnosis can only be a stroke or no-stroke determination. Nevertheless, as mentioned earlier, discussions with stroke specialists revealed that the ability to reliably confirm a stroke/no-stroke diagnosis at the site of the emergency, and then to alert the acute stroke unit ahead of arrival, would be a significant and welcome advance over the current protocol. Notwithstanding that trials are underway in some countries with specialist ambulances that contain a mobile CT unit [4,5] that can differentiate the two types of stroke, these units will always be extremely few in number due to their high cost and are therefore not a scalable solution. The hope is that new scanning modalities, such as the modality described in this paper, which have the potential to be carried in all ambulances and first response vehicles and used in complete safety, will pave the way for on-scene diagnosis and treatment if the ability to differentiate the two types of stroke can be developed and proven. Meeting that challenge is a priority supported by The Lancet article [6], which states, "The strategy of treatment directly at the emergency site (mobile stroke unit concept), could contribute to more efficient use of resources and reduce the time taken to instigate treatment to within 60 min—the golden hour—of the onset of the symptoms of stroke". The authors' work towards differentiating the two types of stroke will be reported in due course.

6. Conclusions

The results presented in this paper conclusively show that low-intensity electromagnetic waves in the radio frequency/microwave band can detect the presence of a stroke-affected region in a materially valid phantom of a human head. A key step in achieving that outcome is the computationally efficient method of data analysis devised for the purposes of this study, which makes the signature of a stroke inclusion highly visible in the raw data from the experimental scanning apparatus. The performance of this method will continue to be improved as the project progresses. Alternative methods that show good promise will also be investigated.

There is scope in the next development phases of the project to increase the intensity of the scanning beam used in this study by $100\times$ or even $1000\times$ and still remain within the safety guidelines for mobile communications and other non-scanning applications. That is certain to enable smaller and more deeply seated stroke inclusions to be detected. The results from that work will be reported in due course.

The next development phases will also employ more complex phantoms that represent patients who have multiple anomalous regions in their brain caused by previous or non-vascular cerebral lesions in addition to the stroke that is occurring at that moment.

It is certain that being able to administer stroke treatment at the site of the emergency has the potential to reduce the time expired from the occurrence of a stroke to the absolute minimum. However, for that fundamental departure from the current patient pathway to be approved by all of the relevant regulatory authorities and clinical and patient advisory groups, it is vital that the scanning methodology deployed at the site of the emergency is proven to be capable of reliably differentiating between ischaemic and haemorrhagic strokes. Achieving that with the scanning modality described in this paper in its current form has been shown to be challenging due to the very similar dielectric properties of the fluids involved in both types of stroke. However, given that this scanning modality undoubtedly has the potential to deliver a reliable stroke/no-stroke diagnosis at the site of the emergency, that alone will help to shorten the time to treatment by enabling the acute stroke unit to be alerted that a confirmed stroke patient is in transit. That patient can then be fast tracked upon arrival to shorten the door-to-needle time. That will make a valuable contribution towards minimising the overall time from the occurrence of the stroke to treatment being administered in hospital. That will be a highly beneficial interim measure for stroke patients until such a time in the future when new scanning modalities of the kind reported in this paper are able to reliably discriminate between both types of stroke, and treatment is approved to be administered at the site of the emergency.

There is no doubt that the new scanning modality has the potential to be simple and low cost to implement, and it is therefore suited to manufacture at scale. Such scanners could be carried in all first response emergency vehicles and be in situ in hospitals and acute stroke units, GP surgeries, and residential care homes. It is that kind of coverage that is needed to transform the outlook for stroke patients and have a significant positive impact on the current stroke statistics and the enormous cost of stroke to national economies.

Author Contributions: Conceptualization, D.H.; methodology, I.E.r., D.H. and M.A.-M.; software, I.E.r.; formal analysis, D.H. and I.E.r.; investigation, D.H.; writing—original draft preparation, D.H. and I.E.r.; writing—review and editing, D.H., I.E.r. and M.A.-M.; project administration, D.H. All authors have read and agreed to the published version of the manuscript.

Funding: An earlier phase of this research was partially funded by Innovate UK (then the Technology Strategy Board), grant number 710830.

Institutional Review Board Statement: Not applicable.

Informed Consent Statement: Not applicable.

Data Availability Statement: Not applicable.

Acknowledgments: The authors acknowledge the contributions of past colleagues in Scannerfutures Ltd, UK. and TTP plc UK during an earlier phase of this project.

Conflicts of Interest: The authors declare no conflict of interest.

References

1. *State of the Nation—Stroke Statistics February 2018.* Published by the Stroke Association, a UK Registered Charity. Available online: www.stroke.org.uk (accessed on 6 July 2021).
2. Johnson, W.; Onuma, O.; Owolabi, M.; Sachdev, S. Stroke: A global response is needed. *Bull. World Health Organ.* **2016**, *94*, 633–708. [CrossRef] [PubMed]
3. Healthcare Expenditure. *UK Health Accounts: 2018*; Published by the UK Office of National Statistics: 2020. Available online: www.ons.gov.uk (accessed on 6 July 2021).
4. Cerejo, R.; John, S.; Buletko, A.B.; Taqui, A.; Itrat, A.; Organek, N.; Cho, S.-M.; Sheikhi, L.; Uchino, K.; Briggs, F.; et al. A Mobile Stroke Treatment Unit for Field Triage of Patients for Intra-arterial Revascularization Therapy. *J. Am. Soc. Neuroimaging* **2015**, *25*, 940–945. [CrossRef] [PubMed]
5. Calderon, V.J.; Kasturiarachi, B.M.; Lin, E.; Bansal, V.; Zaidat, O.O. Review of the Mobile Stroke Unit Experience Worldwide. *Interv. Neurol.* **2018**, *7*, 347–358. [CrossRef] [PubMed]
6. Fassbender, K.; Balucani, C.; Walter, S.; Levine, S.R.; Haass, A.; Grotta, J. Streamlining of prehospital stroke management: The golden hour. *Lancet Neurol.* **2013**, *12*, 585–596. [CrossRef]
7. Mohammed, B.J.; Abbosh, A.M.; Mustafa, S.; Ireland, D. Microwave System for Head Imaging. *IEEE Trans. Instrum. Meas.* **2014**, *63*, 117–123. [CrossRef]
8. Abbosh, A.M.; Zamani, A.; Mobashsher, A.T. Real-time Frequency-Based Multistatic Microwave Imaging for Medical Applications. In Proceedings of the IEEE MTT-S 2015 International Microwave Workshop Series on RF and Wireless Technologies for Biomedical and Healthcare Applications (IMWS-BIO), Taipei, Taiwan, 21–23 September 2015.
9. Mobashsher, A.T.; Abbosh, A. Microwave Imaging System to Provide Portable Low-Powered Medical Facility for the Detection of Intracranial Hemorrhage. In Proceedings of the 1st Australian Microwave Symposium, Melbourne, Australia, 26–27 June 2014.
10. Medfield Diagnostics—Strokefinder™. Available online: www.medfielddiagnostics.com/products/ (accessed on 6 July 2021).
11. Strokefinder MD100 Microwave Tomography for Early Diagnosis of Stroke Type. March 2014. Publication of the National Institute for Health Research. Available online: http://www.io.nihr.ac.uk/wp-content/uploads/migrated/2569.8dda16ee.StrokefinderMD100AlertFinal2.pdf (accessed on 6 July 2021).
12. Persson, M.; Fhager, A.; Trefna, H.; Yu, Y.; McKelvey, T.; Pegenius, G.; Karlsson, J.; Elam, M. Microwave-Based Stroke Diagnosis Making Global Prehospital Thrombolytic Treatment Possible. *IEEE Trans. Biomed. Eng.* **2014**, *61*, 2806–2817. [CrossRef] [PubMed]
13. Ljungqvist, J.; Candefjord, S.; Persson, M.; Jönsson, L.; Skoglund, T.; Elam, M. Clinical Evaluation of a Microwave-Based Device for Detection of Traumatic Intracranial Hemorrhage. *J. Neurotrauma* **2017**, *34*, 2176–2182. [CrossRef] [PubMed]
14. Micrima—Evolving Medical Imaging. Available online: https://micrima.com/ (accessed on 6 July 2021).
15. *New Technology Could Revolutionise Breast Cancer Screening*; University of Bristol Press: Bristol, UK, 2008.
16. Klemm, M.; Craddock, I.; Leendertz, J.; Preece, A.; Benjamin, R. Experimental and clinical results of breast cancer detection using UWB microwave radar. In Proceedings of the IEEE Antennas and Propagation Society International Symposium, San Diego, CA, USA, 5–11 July 2008.
17. Carlson, A.B. *Communication Systems: An Introduction to Signals and Noise in Electrical Communication*, 3rd ed.; University of Michigan: Ann Arbor, MI, USA; McGraw-Hill: New York, NY, USA, 1986.
18. Pan, X. Tomographic Image Reconstruction. In Proceedings of the 41st Annual Meeting of the American Association of Physicists in Medicine, Nashville, TN, USA, 25–29 July 1999.
19. Mobashsher, A.T.; Wang, Y. Microwave System to Detect Traumatic Brain Injuries Using Compact Unidirectional Antenna and Wideband Transceiver with Verification on Realistic Head Phantom. *IEEE Trans. Microw. Theory Tech.* **2014**, *62*, 1826–1836. [CrossRef]
20. *Tween-Based Tissue-Equivalent Liquid, Manufactured and Supplied by National Physical Laboratory (NPL England) as per IEEE 1528 Standard*; IEEE: Piscataway, NJ, USA, 2016.
21. *IEEE Standard 1528-2013: IEEE Reccommended Practice for Determining the Peak Spatial Average Specific Absorption Rate (SAR) in the Human Head for Wireless Communications Devices: Measurement Techniques*; IEEE: Piscataway, NJ, USA, 2013.
22. Gabriel, C.; Gabriel, S. Compilation of the Dielectric Properties of Body Tissues at RF and Microwave Frequencies. 1997. Available online: http://niremf.ifac.cnr.it/docs/DIELECTRIC/home.html (accessed on 6 July 2021).
23. Calculation of the Dielectric Properties of Body Tissues in the Frequency Range 10 Hz–100 GHz. Publication of the Italian National Research Council, Institute for Applied Physics. Available online: http://niremf.ifac.cnr.it/tissprop/htmlclie/htmlclie.php (accessed on 6 July 2021).

24. Gabriel, C.; Gabriel, S.; Corthout, E. The dielectric properties of biological tissues: I. Literature survey. *Phys. Med. Biol.* **1996**, *41*, 2231–2249. [CrossRef] [PubMed]
25. Gabriel, S.; Lau, R.W.; Gabriel, C. The dielectric properties of biological tissues: II. Measurements in the frequency range 10 Hz–20 GHz. *Phys. Med. Biol.* **1996**, *41*, 2251–2269. [CrossRef] [PubMed]
26. Gabriel, S.; Lau, R.W.; Gabriel, C. The dielectric properties of biological tissues: III. Parametric models for the dielectric spectrum of tissues. *Phys. Med. Biol.* **1996**, *41*, 2271–2293. [CrossRef] [PubMed]
27. Peyman, A.; Holden, S.J.; Watts, S.; Perrott, R.; Gabriel, C. Dielectric properties of porcine cerebrospinal tissues at microwave frequencies: In vivo, in vitro and systematic variation with age. *Phys. Med. Biol.* **2007**, *52*, 2229–2245. [CrossRef] [PubMed]
28. AQIX. RS-I Fluid. Supplied by Aqix Ltd, UK. 2016. Available online: www.aqix.com (accessed on 6 July 2021).
29. Defibrinated sheep blood supplied by TCS Biosciences Ltd, UK. Available online: www.tcsbiosciences.co.uk (accessed on 6 July 2021).

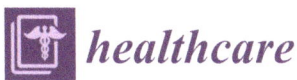

Review

A Blockchain and Artificial Intelligence-Based, Patient-Centric Healthcare System for Combating the COVID-19 Pandemic: Opportunities and Applications

Mohamed Yaseen Jabarulla and Heung-No Lee *

School of Electrical Engineering and Computer Science, Gwangju Institute of Science and Technology, Gwangju 61005, Korea; yaseen@gm.gist.ac.kr
* Correspondence: heungno@gist.ac.kr

Abstract: The world is facing multiple healthcare challenges because of the emergence of the COVID-19 (coronavirus) pandemic. The pandemic has exposed the limitations of handling public healthcare emergencies using existing digital healthcare technologies. Thus, the COVID-19 situation has forced research institutes and countries to rethink healthcare delivery solutions to ensure continuity of services while people stay at home and practice social distancing. Recently, several researchers have focused on disruptive technologies, such as blockchain and artificial intelligence (AI), to improve the digital healthcare workflow during COVID-19. Blockchain could combat pandemics by enabling decentralized healthcare data sharing, protecting users' privacy, providing data empowerment, and ensuring reliable data management during outbreak tracking. In addition, AI provides intelligent computer-aided solutions by analyzing a patient's medical images and symptoms caused by coronavirus for efficient treatments, future outbreak prediction, and drug manufacturing. Integrating both blockchain and AI could transform the existing healthcare ecosystem by democratizing and optimizing clinical workflows. In this article, we begin with an overview of digital healthcare services and problems that have arisen during the COVID-19 pandemic. Next, we conceptually propose a decentralized, patient-centric healthcare framework based on blockchain and AI to mitigate COVID-19 challenges. Then, we explore the significant applications of integrated blockchain and AI technologies to augment existing public healthcare strategies for tackling COVID-19. Finally, we highlight the challenges and implications for future research within a patient-centric paradigm.

Keywords: digital healthcare; patient-centric; blockchain; artificial intelligence; federated learning; coronavirus (COVID-19); pandemic management; healthcare transformation; public health strategies

Citation: Jabarulla, M.Y.; Lee, H.-N. A Blockchain and Artificial Intelligence-Based, Patient-Centric Healthcare System for Combating the COVID-19 Pandemic: Opportunities and Applications. *Healthcare* 2021, 9, 1019. https://doi.org/10.3390/healthcare9081019

Academic Editor: Marco P. Soares dos Santos

Received: 30 June 2021
Accepted: 28 July 2021
Published: 8 August 2021

Publisher's Note: MDPI stays neutral with regard to jurisdictional claims in published maps and institutional affiliations.

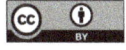

Copyright: © 2021 by the authors. Licensee MDPI, Basel, Switzerland. This article is an open access article distributed under the terms and conditions of the Creative Commons Attribution (CC BY) license (https://creativecommons.org/licenses/by/4.0/).

1. Introduction

The novel coronavirus disease (COVID-19) has spread to almost every country since the outbreak in December 2019 from Wuhan, China. The severity of this epidemic became extensive within a month of the virus's widescale spread. Thus, a Public Health Emergency of International Concern (PHEIC) was declared by the World Health Organization (WHO) [1]. The outbreak forced several nations to close their borders, maintain lockdowns, and practice social distancing to limit the spread of COVID-19. These led to massive interruptions in the economy of many sectors, such as industry, insurance, agriculture, supply chains, transport, and tourism [2]. The pandemic has had an unexpected impact at the global level, not just on an economic scale, but also pushing healthcare systems around the world to their limits, such as through a lack of personal protective equipment (PPE) for healthcare workers and by causing difficulties in diagnosing and monitoring large populations [3]. In general, the healthcare system has operated in a closed ecosystem of siloed institutions, where healthcare professionals (i.e., doctors, radiologists, clinicians, and researchers) have served as the primary stakeholders of medical information. The flow of information has gone in one direction, i.e., healthcare expert to patient. However, in the era of digitized patient health records, data are growing and flowing across a closed healthcare system faster than ever before. The one-to-one flow of information is giving way to a multiplicity of information, sharing relationships with many-to-many, one-to-many, and many-to-one [4]. In such cases, most coronavirus information collected from the public, hospitals, and clinical laboratories may not be faithful, since the data are not gathered according to set guidelines [5] and are not monitored or stored appropriately because of the vastness of digitized patient health records. The existing healthcare technology requires trustable data, which is crucial to providing the correct widespread information about the novel coronavirus. Furthermore, the virus test procedure using medical tools for detecting coronavirus infections often takes several days to complete because of the inaccuracy and manual processing of large volumes of data. Finally, tracking or surveilling infected patients or their contacts raises several privacy issues [6]. These insufficiencies exposed by COVID-19 have prompted healthcare organizations to transform the existing digital healthcare system to combat pandemic situations. Overall, the digital healthcare ecosystem needs to facilitate clinical trials, frontline care, data surveillance, medical billing, telemedicine, drug delivery, treatment facilities, and strategy discovery. In addition, it is essential to design a more patient-centric and democratized digital healthcare ecosystem for combating COVID-19 and future pandemics by using digital platforms.

Recently, several researchers have focused on utilizing disruptive technologies, such as blockchain and artificial intelligence (AI), to provide solutions for these ongoing COVID-19 crises [7,8]. Blockchain is a peer-to-peer (P2P) distributed and shared ledger, where transactions are digitally recorded into blocks. The nodes (miners) of the blockchain network are responsible for linking the blocks to each other in chronological order. Blockchain nodes contain a copy of the stored information and keep their network active [9]. Thus, blockchain provides the entire history or provenance of data. It is possible to store sample test results, patient records, discharge summaries, and vaccination statuses in a blockchain digital ledger. These will support clinical laboratories, patients, hospitals, and government-funded healthcare organizations in a decentralized way to manage healthcare information using self-executing contracts called "smart contracts" [8]. Smart contracts are computer programs that execute the predefined terms of an agreement between participants when certain conditions are met within the blockchain network [10]. Furthermore, smart contracts based on blockchain technology could automate auditing processes, medical supply chain management, outbreak tracking, and remote patient monitoring [10]. On the other hand, AI technologies, such as machine learning and deep learning, have been used as powerful tools for enhancing COVID-19 detection, diagnosis, and vaccination/drug discovery, and for performing extensive data analysis [11]. In addition, the federated learning paradigm [12,13] has gained traction for healthcare applications to solve the data privacy and governance problems by training AI models collaboratively without sharing the raw datasets. Thus, AI could process an enormous amount of data in less time and at a fraction of the cost by performing tasks that are difficult to achieve manually. Meanwhile, the blockchain could promote secure data access and interoperability while protecting the privacy and security of health data [14]. Integrated blockchain and AI technology could reshape the healthcare ecosystem by advancing the patient-centric approach [15–17]. A patient-centric approach could provide a viable solution to cope with the coronavirus epidemic for disseminating treatment and managing pandemic situations.

Although researchers have reviewed blockchain and AI to combat COVID-19 [18], these reviews mainly focused on the role of blockchain, such as the development of data storage, managing big data, and security issues for COVID-19 patients [14]. Other reviews focused on analytics and decision tools for healthcare professionals to combat COVID-19 using AI technologies [11]. However, these reviews lacked a concrete and comprehensive study on integrating blockchain and AI for COVID-19 responses based on a patient-centric approach in the healthcare ecosystem, a limitation that was the primary driver for conducting our research. This paper aimed to provide and explore insight into combined blockchain and AI technology to mitigate the COVID-19 pandemic's challenges by transforming the traditional healthcare ecosystem. Then, we discuss the services and practical applications of using these innovative technologies to facilitate COVID-19 healthcare strategies. The contributions of this article are as follows:

1. We conceptually redefined the traditional healthcare model by integrating blockchain and AI for tackling COVID-19 in a patient-centric paradigm.
2. We exploited the existing public health strategies, such as patient information sharing, data management for diagnosing the infection, contact tracing, monitoring, and mitigation of the impact on healthcare, using the proposed decentralized, patient-centric frameworks.
3. Based on the study, we discussed the challenges, solutions, and future research directions that are anticipated to be of significant value for patients and healthcare organizations.

This work is organized as follows: Section 2 includes related research work and recent trends in healthcare systems that utilize blockchain and AI technologies. Section 3 provides an overview of digital healthcare services and describes the background of blockchain and AI technologies. In Section 4, we exploit a blockchain- and AI-based conceptual framework for delivering patient-centric healthcare services to combat COVID-19. Section 5 explores the potential applications of the decentralized, patient-centric framework to facilitate pandemic healthcare strategies. In Section 6, we discuss the relevant open issues, possible solutions, and further research directions. Finally, we conclude the paper in Section 7.

2. Related work
2.1. Blockchain and AI in Healthcare Systems

In this section, state-of-the-art research related to healthcare systems based on blockchain and AI is presented. The key risks and issues in a traditional healthcare system include a single point of failure, data alterations, high chances of malicious cyberattacks, centralized authority, high data management cost, and databases that are not transparent. To address these issues, researchers have proposed numerous blockchain-based solutions. The authors of [19] addressed the security and privacy concerns by using a blockchain-based server–client architecture network to store the hashed patients' data. However, these server–client architectures are prone to a single-point failure. Thus, a blockchain-based distributed mechanism for data accessibility between patients and doctors in a healthcare system is presented in [20]. The authors of [10] designed a smart contract-based, real-time patient monitoring system to record wearable device data as events and share that information with healthcare professionals. The primary goal of this system is to eliminate third parties and resolve the vulnerability issues in remote monitoring. In other studies [21,22], researchers created a secure and trusted digital environment using a smart contract-based healthcare system to prevent data breaches in electronic health records (EHRs). To attain decentralized data management in healthcare, the authors of [16] proposed a framework to store patient EHRs in a decentralized, patient-centric framework that allows patients to control their data using a rule-based smart contract. On the other hand, healthcare systems based on AI [23] require more computational power due to the exponentially increased parameter numbers, complex architectures, and sufficient data to achieve accurate deep learning solutions. Meanwhile, the data are accumulated from different sources and stored on the central server to find a global model. Therefore, researchers have proposed distributed AI approaches based on blockchain that leverages parallel computing power, as well as focuses on distributed data storage. One such effective distributed learning solution is federated learning that trains locally stored data with local computational power while protecting privacy [12]. The federated learning approach allows researchers to obtain decent insight from patient data without revealing any sensitive information (medication history of patients, text messages, and patient names, etc.). Researchers are typically looking for statistical results rather than raw data, and researchers can achieve unbiased statistical insight without even having access to the data itself. Jonathan et al. [24] proposed a conceptual framework based on blockchain-orchestrated federated learning for healthcare consortia. Their architecture provides a privacy-preserving audit trail that logs events in the network without revealing identities.

2.2. Trends in Related Research

More recently, the massive outbreak of the COVID-19 pandemic has prompted various researchers, scientists, and organizations around the world to conduct large-scale research to help develop efficient pandemic management and response strategies. Several patient-centric approaches [15,17] have been studied in the context of the COVID-19 pandemic, such as facilitating pharmaceutical care [25], clinical trials [26], conducting ethical research [27], and health system restructuring [28]. The emergence of disruptive technologies like AI and blockchain leveraged several healthcare applications [11,14,18,29] that emphasized COVID-19 data analysis, data security, data privacy, authenticity, and data sharing at various levels. In this regard, Samuel et al. [30] have reviewed the role of AI in the arena of predicting, contact tracing, forecasting, screening, and drug development for coronavirus and its related epidemic. The authors of [14] reviewed the existing literature on blockchain technology in solving challenging problems due to the COVID-19 pandemic. The authors proposed a blockchain-based platform that discussed significant blockchain applications for solving issues arising from the COVID-19 pandemic. Nguyen et al. [18] introduced a new conceptual architecture that integrates blockchain and AI for combating the COVID-19 pandemic. However, this article only consists of an extensive survey about the latest research efforts on blockchain and AI applications for combating COVID-19. In addition, none of these works provided an overall architecture of the blockchain and AI framework based on a patient-centric paradigm.

From the abovementioned works, we concluded that, although several studies were focused on the current scenario of the COVID-19 outbreak, they provided only a limited idea about integrating blockchain and AI technologies to combat COVID-19. To the best of our knowledge and at the time of writing, no study has provided a decentralized, patient-centric framework that emphasizes the COVID-19 pandemic and its potential implications using converged blockchain and AI technologies. To this end, our present work has more potential to address the research gaps while presenting the conceptual framework with a detailed explanation of each layer and its functionalities. The purpose of our study was to provide the readers with an initial systematic framework of how integrated blockchain and AI are able to facilitate traditional public healthcare strategies, such as patient information sharing, data management for diagnosing the infection, contact tracing, monitoring, and the mitigation of the impact on healthcare, using the envisioned decentralized, patient-centric frameworks.

3. Overview

3.1. Digital Healthcare Services during the COVID-19 Pandemic

Digital health can improve pandemic strategies and responses by increasing access to healthcare-related services for individuals and enhancing the experience of delivering or receiving care [31]. Digital health is an umbrella term that includes mobile health (mHealth), electronic health (eHealth), and emerging technologies, such as the use of blockchain, medical internet of things (MIoT), AI, and big data [32,33]. Although some digital technologies, such as telemedicine and telehealth, have existed for decades, they have poor penetration into the healthcare market due to the sparsity of supportive payment structures and heavy regulations [34]. A nationwide surge of COVID-19 cases forced healthcare organizations to transform healthcare delivery by leveraging the power of digital technologies [33,35]. The use of telemedicine for diabetic patients in fighting the COVID-19 pandemic has already been demonstrated [36,37]. Various technologies, such as biosensors, multi-drone systems, and industry 4.0 [29,38,39], could be employed for combating the coronavirus disease. The viewpoint of the authors of [40] represents pandemic management and response strategies based on a methodological application of digital technologies. Their framework highlights the ways in which successful countries (e.g., South Korea,

Australia, Germany, Singapore, and Taiwan) have adopted digital technologies in the real world for pandemic healthcare services, such as contact tracing, testing, surveillance, pandemic planning, and quarantine. Table 1 summarizes specific healthcare services [14] by highlighting the functions, challenges, and digital technologies utilized for the pandemic's management and response strategies.

Table 1. Summary of the COVID-19 pandemic's management and response strategies [40,41].

Strategies	Functions	Digital Technologies	Challenges
Contact Tracking	Identifies and monitors individuals that come into contact with an infected person within a specific duration of time.	Bluetooth Low Energy technology, mobile phone applications, wearables, and IoT devices.	Security and privacy issues, since individuals' data are analyzed and stored in a centralized cloud system.
Quarantine and Self-Isolation	In quarantine, individuals are requested to stay in a place (i.e., home or government facilities) for 14 days after being exposed to a COVID-19-infected person. In self-isolation, an infected person isolates within a house or other location to prevent contacting uninfected persons.	AI, a global positioning system, cameras, and recorders.	Breaches civil liberties, restricted access to essential services, and fails to track the individual who runs away from a quarantine facility without their device, like a mobile phone.
Automated Surveillance	To identify and monitor individuals without facemasks, social distancing, and accidental touching in public gathering places. Detects symptoms, such as breathing difficulties, coughing, and fever, using self-tracking digital technologies.	Facial recognition, digital thermometers, surveillance cameras, and thermal cameras.	Security attacks, operational cost.
Clinical Data Management	Used to diagnose infected individuals and provides the capacity for telemedicine services and virtual care, prediction of clinical outcomes, and monitoring of clinical status by clinicians.	Picture archiving and communications system (PACS).	Not cost efficient, privacy breaches may occur, failure in diagnosis.
Patient Information Sharing	Patient health and medical information sharing could decrease the possibility of duplicate testing and avoid medication errors. Furthermore, sharing patient data among the global research community plays an essential role in coronavirus research by formulating powerful raw data sets.	AI, web-based toolkits, and PACS.	Satisfying Health Insurance Portability and Accountability Act (HIPAA) compliances, lack of anonymity, security, privacy, and data management issues.
Contactless Delivery	During the lockdown, contactless delivery of essential supplies, such as medicine, food, and sanitizers, prevents direct interactions with people, since doorstep delivery might not be safe during a high transmission rate.	Robots and drones.	Security attacks, operational costs, and legal issues in the case of an accident.
Supply Chain Management	Identify and secure logistics capacity based on the type of goods, such as medical equipment and vaccines/drugs or other pharmaceutical medicines.	Mobile platforms, data analytics, cloud, and IoT.	Procuring medical equipment, pharmaceutical medicines, and household essentials are difficult due to the surge in demand.
Disaster Relief and Insurance	Financial organizations and governments have to help the public by providing unemployment insurance relief, loans to protect their business losses, and health insurance that covers treatment costs during the COVID-19 outbreak.	Web-based toolkits and mobile applications.	Time-consuming and ineffective due to paper-based procedures and centralized authority.

Figure 1 illustrates a representation of a complex healthcare ecosystem with multiple stakeholders who constantly integrate, interrelate, and interoperate with digital technologies during pandemic situations. The key stakeholders of the healthcare ecosystem are described below:

- Patient—anyone who seeks medical care can be termed a patient, and their data play a crucial role in pandemic preparedness and response.
- Providers—Includes physician groups, hospitals, laboratories, doctors, and other healthcare professionals and medical facilities that deliver medical care to patients. Patient data, such as electronic medical records (EMRs), are stored, organized, and managed in a large-scale centralized clinical repository. Providers contribute to clinical teams and researchers by providing health information to combat diseases.
- Payers—A payer is a company (for example, an insurance company) that pays people or bodies, other than the patient, to finance or refund the cost of the medicinal products and healthcare services. A payer is responsible for processing payments, patient eligibility, enrollment, and claims.
- Pharma—Pharmaceutical companies are the makers of vaccines prescribed by healthcare providers. They supply medicines and provide other supporting services, such as patient disease and medication management.
- Researchers—Conduct pharmaceutical and biomedical research. Digital healthcare can augment researchers' insights by analyzing the healthcare data, clinical trials, and public health research.
- Regulators—Healthcare industries and government agencies that oversee industry standards, enforce and write regulations, and set healthcare policy.
- Government—Handles public safety and emergencies. It implements stay-at-home orders or lockdown to reorganize, rebalance resources, and protect health workers while combating COVID-19. They execute policies that encourage and support innovators to create healthcare solutions based on information technologies where information flows securely to the required parties. Involved in the management of the procurement of PPE kits, medicinal supplies, and appliances/oxygen condensers. Provides staff training on COVID-19 prevention and provision of patient counseling on medicines.

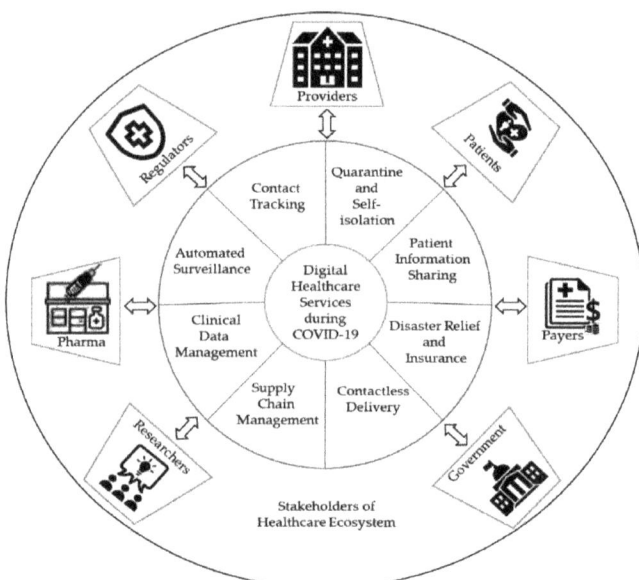

Figure 1. Healthcare ecosystem and digital services for pandemic preparedness and response during COVID-19.

Health services need trustable data to provide the correct information about the novel coronavirus's spread or outbreak. Multiple efforts are being made around the world to cultivate a patient-centric culture by using ever-growing volumes of research, patient data, and applications of digital technologies [4,42–44]. Specifically, disruptive technologies, such as AI and blockchain, are emerging in digital healthcare, which uses the greater availability of health data to identify high-risk patients, track the spread of COVID-19, predict mortality risk, manage healthcare data, and fight against coronavirus and other pandemics [11,14,18]. AI gives us the unprecedented capability to decouple complex variables and reach a nuanced understanding of the effect and cause at the population as well as the individual levels. AI allows organizations to understand what their data are depicting and use that to develop targeted interventions. Blockchain plays a vital role in health information exchange by facilitating the healthcare transition to patient-driven and patient-mediated interoperability [45]. In this article, we propose a decentralized, patient-centric framework that integrates AI and blockchain technologies for tackling COVID-19. We explore the potential applications and use cases of these combined technologies for facilitating the healthcare response to the COVID-19 pandemic [16,41].

3.2. Blockchain and Artificial Intelligence Technologies

Blockchain is a promising and revolutionary technology, mainly used where centralization is unnatural and privacy is essential [46,47]. Blockchain [8,48] has a particular interest in health data, with an emphasis on sharing, distribution, and encryption. Decentralization and cryptographic hashing are the fundamental concepts of a blockchain. The contents or databases stored in a blockchain are shared across the network. The network creates a decentralized distributed chain that allows every participant to access the blockchain's contents. The security of the network is protected by a mechanism called consensus. A consensus mechanism is a fault-tolerant mechanism that uses a set of rules to achieve necessary agreement on the status of the blockchain ledger among all participants. Blockchain consists of three key components: blocks, nodes, and miners. Here, a block is like a record book page that records some or all of the recent transaction data that have not been stored in any prior blocks. Each time a block is completed or mined, it gives way to the next block in the blockchain. Starting from the genesis block, each block consists of data, its own unique nonce, and hash value that links to the previous block via a hash label, which creates a chain of blocks and prevents any modification risks [49]. Nodes are responsible for the functioning of a blockchain network, and ensure the storage of the given data in the distributed ledger. Each node has its copy of the blockchain, and the participating node creates new blocks in the chain for which participants receive a reward. The consensus mechanism provides equal rights to all participants in the network to access the distributed ledger and protect the chain from third-party entities to avoid security issues, such as double-spending attacks [50]. There are several consensus mechanisms available, such as proof-of-work (PoW), Byzantine faulty tolerant (BFT), zero-knowledge proof, and proof-of-stake (PoS) [49]. Furthermore, smart contracts are used to enhance the transparency and trust between two parties by using blockchain technology to enable the creation of accessible and immutable contracts. In a blockchain network, each participant has a unique alphanumeric identification number that shows their transactions. Therefore, every action can be easily monitored and viewed by the participants in the distributed ledger. The smart contract makes secure transactions that help to avoid disruption from centralized authorities. Ethereum Virtual Machine or Solidity platforms [51,52] could be used to build smart contracts for automatizing auditing processes, providing time-bound access to distributed patients' data, and improving the supply chain management of pharmaceutical products. The healthcare industry has become overloaded by data, and blockchain can provide solutions to healthcare stakeholders to handle this enormous data in reality. In addition, blockchain establishes reliable and privacy-preserving data exchange protocols within the healthcare ecosystem. Blockchain's immutable and decentralized nature [53] has demonstrated its promising potential in healthcare applications, such as secure data management [54], transparent medical data storage [55], and healthcare data privacy [16,56].

Artificial intelligence (AI) technology appears in every technology field, and is becoming inseparable from daily life activities. Moreover, Accenture researchers [57] predicted that the application of AI in the healthcare market is expected to increase from $600 million to $6.6 billion between the years 2014 and 2021. Recent studies show that AI-based ML and DL models are utilized for solving coronavirus-related issues [11]. ML plays an important role in AI research, and has a huge potential to detect patterns and anomalies of medical image data. Then, it matches those data into learning models to automate decision-making processes for healthcare specialists [58]. For example, ML can be used to perform an automated facial recognition framework to detect temperature on the human body for mitigating coronavirus-infected people [58,59]. Meanwhile, DL models consist of multiple neural network layers to form a deep learning architecture [60]. A deep neural network architecture consists of an input layer, output layer, and a single hidden layer for receiving data samples, training data samples, and generating training outcomes. Here, the depth of the DL architecture depends on the number of hidden layers. Either unsupervised or supervised learning techniques are used to estimate the desired output using unlabeled or labeled data samples, which are associated with the adjustment of the hyper-parameters. Several AI companies have created DL-based models to predict and analyze coronavirus infection [61]. For example, DarwinAI developed a COVID-Net framework using a convolutional neural network architecture to detect COVID-19 from chest radiography images, and Google uses neural network software to predict patient outcomes, such as the length of a visit, odds of death, and readmission possibilities. However, AI algorithms require large, varied, high-quality, and confidential coronavirus datasets that may be siloed across different healthcare institutions. Thus, obtaining patient coronavirus data securely for training the datasets with a global AI model for the detection of positive COVID-19 cases is a challenging task. To address this data security problem, McMahan et al. [12] proposed federated learning frameworks to train an AI model securely by analyzing a broad range of data located at multiple sites. Federated learning secures data and aggregates only the AI model parameters from multiple organizations [13,62,63]. However, several federated learning approaches are based on a centralized server, which raises concerns about the privacy of sensitive data. Thus, researchers proposed blockchain-based federated learning approaches for several applications [63–65] to implement asynchronous collaborative AI models between a distributed network. Hence, the blockchain-based federated learning method enables collaborations between several healthcare organizations to train the ML or DL models without relying on any centralized server and avoids the direct sharing of sensitive clinical data with each other. A blockchain smart contract, such as Ethereum, is used to realize the automated management of the entire federal learning method with an incentive mechanism. For instance, Microsoft researchers [66] are developing a system that collaboratively improves ML algorithms hosted on a public blockchain. The collaboration through the system is incentivized, since blockchain makes it possible to reward people who provide data for improving AI models using smart contracts. This decentralized approach to train models preserves privacy and security and ensures the immutability of uploaded AI models via computing and recording their quality in the blockchain.

The patient-centric approach aims to facilitate the democratization of ever-growing volumes of patient data and effectively uses it for the application of AI and blockchain to mitigate COVID-19 challenges. Figure 2 depicts the important features of blockchain and AI technology that are essential in combating COVID-19. AI and blockchain are catalyzing the pace of innovation in digital healthcare, which directly impacts patients and service providers. Moreover, these two technologies have their degree of technical complexity as well as ethical concerns, but converging both technologies may be able to redesign the entire traditional healthcare paradigm into a decentralized, patient-centric paradigm to mitigate COVID-19. In summary, the advantages of utilizing blockchain and AI technologies in healthcare to mitigate COVID-19 challenges are as follows:

- Blockchain helps to improve interoperability among different healthcare organizational platforms, such as pharmaceutical needs, hospital databases, supply chain logistics, and insurance claims.
- Storage and management of health record data using blockchain platforms offer patients the protection of their data and provides access to their health records based upon request.
- Blockchain improves information management among stakeholders in the healthcare ecosystem.
- Blockchain reduces centralized control over patient datasets. Thus, it helps to boost medical research and treatment.
- A smart platform can be developed using AI for the automated surveillance, monitoring, detection, and prediction of the spread of this virus.
- The use of AI in reviewing and analyzing radiology images, such as CTs and X-rays, could help to increase COVID-19 detection accuracy.
- AI could automatically estimate the number of positive COVID-19 cases and death cases in any region. In addition, AI helps to determine the most virus-exposed countries, regions, and people to take measures accordingly in advance.
- The application of artificial intelligence (AI) in medication development can help pharmaceutical companies streamline drug repurposing and discovery.

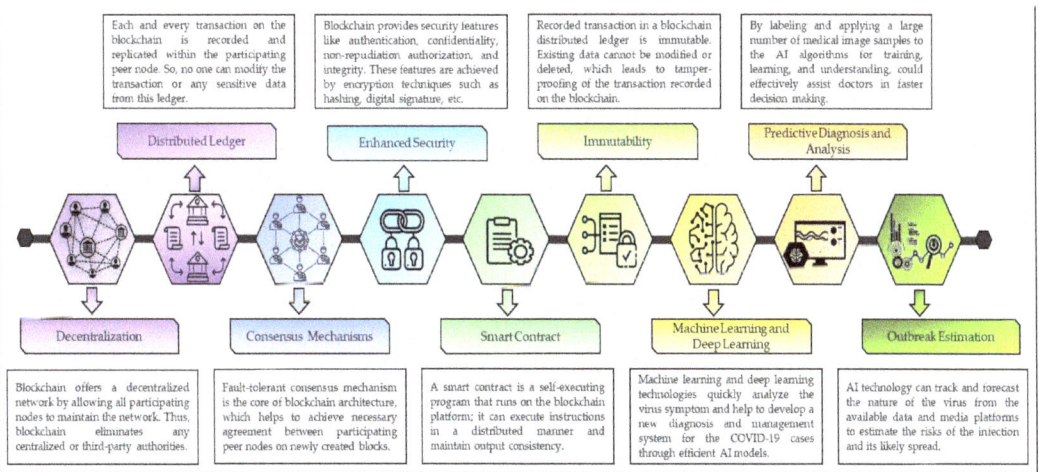

Figure 2. Key features to mitigate COVID-19 challenges using blockchain and AI.

4. The Proposed Patient-Centric Framework

In this section, we present a patient-centric digital healthcare framework by integrating AI and blockchain technology. Figure 3 illustrates the schematic representation of the envisioned patient-centric framework using blockchain and AI for COVID-19. The framework is conceptually organized into three layers: blockchain, AI, and decentralized storage layers. These three layers are integrated with the smart contract to make decisions and maintain accessibility within the patient-centric healthcare ecosystem. The blockchain as a decentralized technology enables multiple healthcare participants, such as regulators, researchers, providers, pharma, payers, and government, to benefit from the patient-centric healthcare services and applications.

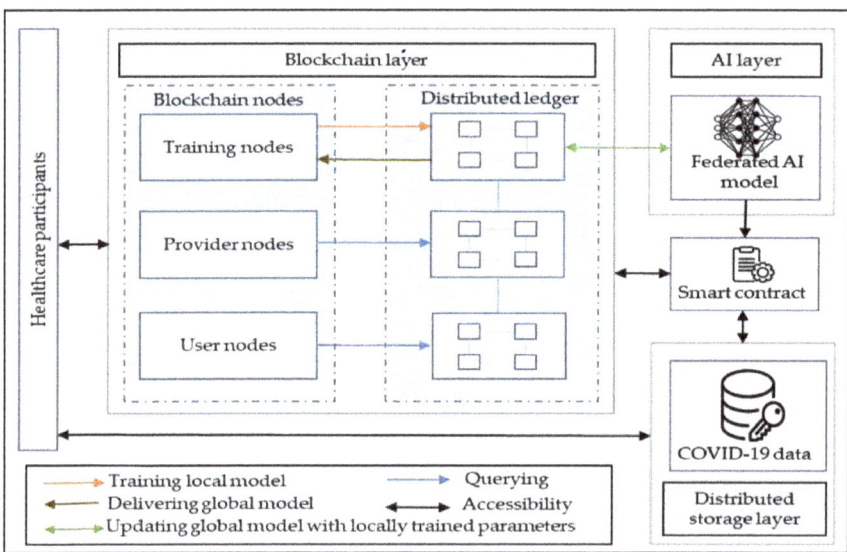

Figure 3. Schematic representation of the envisioned patient-centric framework using blockchain and AI technologies.

The decentralized storage layer consists of the P2P storage system. All the coronavirus data from hospitals, clinical labs, patient-generated data (IoT sensors and mobile operators), and several other sources are combined to construct a primary dataset that subsequently leads to big data. These big data are encrypted and stored in a decentralized storage system by utilizing privacy and security features [67,68]. In a decentralized storage system, the data are distributed into different chunks and stored inside various nodes of a P2P network, instead of storing all the coronavirus-related data in a centralized server. The advantages of utilizing a decentralized storage system include security, privacy, no single point of failure, and cost effectiveness [69]. There have been a few successful distributed file-sharing systems, like IPFS, storj, swarm, orbitDB, GUN, skeps, and sia [69,70]. These file-sharing systems combined blockchain technology to enable off-chain and on-chain storage mechanisms. In off-chain storage, data are not publicly accessible, and the transaction agreement happens outside of the blockchain. An on-chain storage mechanism refers to blockchain transactions that are valid when transacted on the publicly distributed ledger. The significant purpose of a decentralized storage system is to enable the distributed and immutable off-chain and on-chain storage networks to facilitate patient-centric management for coronavirus data. For instance, an infected X-ray image has been encrypted for privacy purposes by a doctor and uploaded to the IPFS network to store the image data off-chain. The stored encrypted image returns an IPFS hash value, and this hash value is stored on-chain in the blockchain ledger after being verified by the key participants of the healthcare ecosystem [70]. Key participants can be a doctor, clinicians, and hospital administrators. Thus, combining on-chain and off-chain data storage mechanisms allows the building of a permanently addressable decentralized storage system that could be connected securely to other crucial databases or systems in the world to form a global healthcare network [16,71].

The blockchain layer consists of provider nodes, user nodes, and training nodes. The provider node includes participants, such as hospitals, clinics, or healthcare organizations, to store and update every patient information (name, patient's unique ID, prescribed medicines, and discharge summaries) in the blockchain ledger. Furthermore, provider nodes assign ownership to the patient medical data in the on-chain blockchain distributed ledger, as well as store coronavirus-related electronic health records, such as CT scans, chest X-rays, and medical reports, in off-chain decentralized storage networks. The user node consists of patients who manage and control their coronavirus-related datasets on blockchain platforms. This operation can be achieved by implementing an Ethereum-based smart contract protocol, such as patient-centric access control (PCAC-SC), to enable a distributed and trustworthy access control policy [16]. The smart contract ensures access to the control and safety of patient-sensitive data without using a centralized infrastructure. The participants in the patient-centric healthcare ecosystem are synchronized with the provider blockchain network to share communications between them regarding accessing the patient data for establishing pandemic management and response strategies. The patient-centric approach allows patients to protect and give access to COVID-19 data based upon the healthcare entities' requests. The blockchain-based, patient-centric framework could offer a number of feasible solutions for coronavirus-related services and applications with improved interoperability among different healthcare platforms, such as insurance claims, pharmaceutical needs, hospital databases, supply chains, and clinical data management.

The AI layer is integrated with blockchain and a decentralized storage network using the smart contract protocol. The AI layer consists of federated machine learning and deep learning models, where data providers, such as hospitals or clinics, train an AI model locally using the private data obtained from patients and upload only the locally trained AI model parameters to the decentralized storage network. The reference to the parameters of the locally trained AI model is stored in the distributed blockchain ledger to update the global model. For example, let us consider a scenario where two hospitals and one research institute teamed up to build an AI model that can automatically analyze CT scan data for detecting COVID-19 infections. The team employs a blockchain-based federated learning approach to maintain the global deep neural network. Each hospital would receive a copy of the AI model to train the model with a CT scan dataset available in their healthcare infrastructure. Once the AI model has been trained locally in the hospital for a couple of iterations, the participants would send only their updated version of the AI model back to the blockchain network. The contributions from all participants would then be aggregated from the decentralized storage network. The updated AI model parameters are shared with participating healthcare organizations, such as hospitals, to continue the local training. Thus, hospitals only share weights and gradients by keeping their patients' sensitive data privately within their healthcare infrastructure. Here, blockchain technology distributes the AI model parameters among hospitals. The decentralized architecture for hospitals can share their data among multiple healthcare organizations without any leakage of the patients' privacy. The smart contract in the framework ensures a decentralized trust among the involved participants by defining rules for the model training agreement and automatically enforcing those obligations [72]. Smart contracts record agreements as a computer code with certain rules. When the rules are satisfied, the agreement is enabled. Smart contracts not only facilitate rule-based accessibility, but also provide flexibility to implement custom federated learning solutions. In addition, smart contracts enable different incentives based on participants' contributions, restrict operations, and define new rules consisting of upcoming requirements. The trained model in the blockchain network provides better and more accurate predictions, because it holds the most up-to-date information about COVID-19 symptoms. These models are deployed to disseminate and analyze data, which can directly impact patients, service providers, and other participants of the patient-centric healthcare ecosystem. Furthermore, blockchain can accelerate the development of data-hungry AI applications using rule-based smart contract protocols [73], since, in healthcare, patients' archival data need to be immutable and accessible only to specific researchers for privacy purposes.

The use of smart contracts for rule-based model training is a novel concept, and blockchain is an ideal platform for standardizing health data structures for AI training, clinical trials, and regulatory purposes. The summary of various technical aspects and their benefits for implementing the conceptually proposed framework over traditional healthcare systems are presented in Table 2. The proposed blockchain-based, patient-centric healthcare system could facilitate AI models and large datasets to be widely shared, updated, and trained to increase the rate of AI adoption and effectiveness. AI implication procedures were developed in the healthcare industry for fighting the COVID-19 pandemic by performing accurate analysis and reliable predictions on vast data collected from coronavirus sources. The blockchain and AI technology that supports patient-centered care has to coordinate the flows of COVID-19 data that are coming from a variety of sources through services and applications, such as outbreak estimation, coronavirus detection, drug/vaccine development, coronavirus analytics, future case projections, and performing automated surveillance.

Table 2. Comparison between traditional healthcare systems over proposed healthcare system based on various technical aspects and their benefits.

Aspects	Standard Healthcare System	Proposed Healthcare Platform
Source Data Storage	The COVID-19 data are stored in a centralized cloud-based storage system, like PACS.	The COVID-19 data are stored in decentralized storage systems, such as IPFS.
Database Sharing Mechanism and Integrity	Depends on a cloud-based mechanism and EHR databases managed by a third-party clearinghouse. Thus, there are possibilities of data tampering.	Depends on a blockchain-based sharing mechanism and EHR databases managed by the participants of the healthcare ecosystem. Thus, databases are immutable.
Administration Performance and Scalability	More transactions are processed per second and enable great scalability.	Process minimal transactions per second, and there are scalability issues since the framework is at its developing stage.
Implementation Cost	Easy to implement and maintain due to its large-scale adoption.	Uncertainty in the operating costs.
Incentive Mechanism for Sharing Data	Not available.	The patient can receive an incentive for sharing their medical data for research purposes.
Data Accessibility	Depend on healthcare entities.	Patients have complete access to and control over their data.
Anonymity	High risk of privacy leakage and identity theft.	The identity of the patients and the transactions between healthcare participants remain anonymous since blockchain public addresses do not link to anyone's identity.
Data Auditability	Always depends on administrators to audit the data.	The moment the blockchain reaches a predetermined state, any node in the blockchain network can track and trace the data right from its origin based on cryptography technology.
Computational Performance of AI	Computationally expensive for training large datasets acquired from different sources in a centralized server.	The federated learning approach reduces the computational power by enabling collaborations between several healthcare organizations to train the distributed global AI models without relying on any centralized server.
Decision Making	Human involvement.	Human involvement, AI, and a smart contract.
Fault Tolerance	Risk of a single point of failure.	A distributed blockchain ledger is highly fault-tolerant because of the consensus mechanism.

5. Applications for Healthcare Management and Response Strategies during COVID-19

In this section, we explore the digital service opportunities and applications of the blockchain- and AI-based, patient-centric framework for facilitating COVID-19 healthcare strategies. Figure 4 shows the possible decentralized digital healthcare services and applications offered by the converged blockchain and AI technologies to participants in a patient-centric healthcare ecosystem. The traditional healthcare system has drawbacks, such as limited access to COVID-19 data, participants' struggles to manage data, and high costs. The proposed patient-centric framework ensures distributed data access and secure logging of digital transactions and at the same time maintains the security and privacy of patients' data.

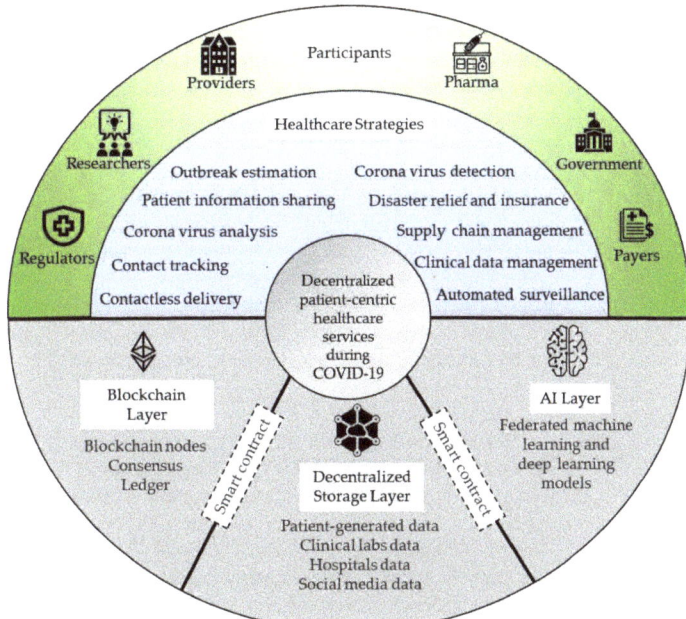

Figure 4. The convergence of blockchain and AI for a decentralized, patient-centric healthcare system to tackle COVID-19.

5.1. Patient-Centric Information Sharing and Clinical Data Management

In COVID-19 research, interoperability among healthcare participants is of predominant importance. However, interoperability mechanisms must avoid violating international and national data-sharing regulations, such as the General Data Protection Regulation (GDPR) compliance and Health Insurance Portability and Accountability Act (HIPAA) [74,75]. These compliances demand that patients be the holder of their data ownership and not organizations, such as hospitals, clinics, or research centers, that generate or create the revenue from data. Therefore, it is necessary to enable individuals to control their COVID-19 data for better communication between healthcare organizations and caregivers to obtain a higher standard of care. The patient's COVID personal health information (PHI), such as scanned medical images, blood oxygen level, heart rates, medication doses, and history of health conditions, are gathered with high privacy through medical IoT (MIoT) and AI-powered decentralized applications (dApps) developed on the blockchain using smart contracts. These gathered data are uploaded directly to the proposed blockchain-based system to eliminate data forging and mutation issues. In addition, the proposed decentralized framework enables patients and physicians to easily participate in telemedicine rather than visiting hospitals during the pandemic. The clinical data are managed using distributed ledger technology and P2P networking features with no centralized management costs, apart from the minimal fees of the Ethereum network [9], thus enhancing patient empowerment.

In general, the actual COVID-19 data are not stored in the blockchain; instead, the metadata of the COVID-19 health information is encrypted and maintained in the blockchain as a pointer. The actual information collected from data sources is stored off-chain in a decentralized storage network, such as IPFS, swarm, and sia. Thus, the blockchain offers security and privacy by storing patients' personal health information in a decentralized storage network. There are several techniques and prototypes that have been recently adopted by researchers to implement permissioned blockchain-based patient information sharing, such as MedChain [76] and MedRec [9]. These healthcare prototypes provide the patient with full control over his or her medical records and enable data sharing and authentication processes. Incorporating such techniques in our proposed architecture eliminates the costly middleman who manages the centralized databases and enables patients to have full control over their data. In addition, a decentralized, patient-centric approach allows data monetization through smart contracts, such as patients retaining their data ownership and remunerating with tokens for their sharing of COVID-19 data with participants, such as researchers. For example, Health Wizz [77] uses blockchain to tokenize data to enable patients to securely aggregate, share, donate, trade, and organize their PHR. Thus, a patient could monetize their COVID data for training an AI model for faster and accurate diagnosis using the patient's X-Ray or CT scans or for predicting the future outbreak [63]. The patient-centric approach helps to protect patients' privacy and maintains trust among participants by providing transparency in storing and sharing data. Smart contracts in the blockchain can serve as security promoters for clinical trial data [78].

5.2. Decentralized Contact Tracing

Contact-tracing applications are among the key digital healthcare services helping to fight the COVID-19 pandemic. There are several technologies that could provide contact tracings, such as mobile phone platforms like quick response (QR) codes, Bluetooth, mobile applications, social graphs, contact details, network-based API, GPS, and wi-fi. However, data privacy and security concerns remain as hurdles that could complicate the process of identifying virus-exposed persons [79]. The decentralized, patient-centric approach based on blockchain and AI can ease those concerns by balancing public health needs with privacy concerns and data analysis [80]. Individuals use blockchain technology to securely share their personal information without revealing their identity to public health agencies, such as a government-aided corporate database or government health authorities. This could help to notify individuals who come into contact with the coronavirus-infected patients without sharing the other personal or medical data of the infected persons [81]. In addition, the gathered data can be used to identify the clusters and hotspots by analyzing the data through an AI model. The outcome of the AI model could be used as a key tool to facilitates a more responsible reopening of the economy without causing a surge in the case. Researchers utilize blockchain technology to issue blockchain-protected digital COVID-19 vaccine passports to immunized citizens. These health certificates can be authenticated easily by public health authorities to verify the status of an individual [82].

5.3. Outbreak Estimation

The general coronavirus data, such as the number of newly infected cases, death cases, recovered cases, and infected regions, are obtained from media platforms to estimate the risks of the infection and its likely spread using AI models. AI enables the identification of the most vulnerable people and countries, and predicts the number of positive cases to take measures accordingly in advance. In addition, AI can combat COVID-19's spread by analyzing people's phone usage patterns to estimate the outbreak size, considering the fact that a COVID-infected patient or a dead person's phone usage patent will change, since the phone might be used by a family member or will be idle. These pattern changes could be detected by analyzing the datasets obtained from wireless operators using AI models [83]. Sarker et al. [84] used ML to model and predict the phone usage records of individuals through learning their personalized diverse mobile activities. Furthermore, J. Shen et al. [85] used DL to accurately estimate the mobile phone application usage, i.e., abnormal calling behaviors and phone service inactivity. Specifically, deploying blockchain-enabled dApps on patients' mobile devices helps to forecast and track the spread of the virus infection globally by anonymously preserving the patient information.

5.4. Coronavirus Detection and Analysis

AI facilitates an automated decision-making system, which helps to develop a new cost-effective diagnosis system for the COVID-19 cases using ML and DL algorithms. For instance, facial recognition [86] using AI helps to detect the temperature on a human face and predict whether the person is wearing a mask or not so that healthcare officials can identify the COVID symptoms and violations related to COVID-19. AI enables computerized diagnosis of the infected cases by analyzing CT, chest X-rays, and MRI scan images. The authors of [87] proposed a detection system using two-dimensional and three-dimensional DL algorithms that were combined with available AI models to identify COVID-19 thoracic CT features with high accuracy. The work in [88] proposed a CT image analysis model to screen COVID-19 by differentiating COVID-19 pneumonia characteristics from influenza A viral pneumonia. The authors used a pulmonary CT image set for feature detection and to differentiate influenza A viral pneumonia, COVID-19 viral pneumonia, and healthy cases. In another study [89], convolutional neural network-based models were used to analyze chest X-ray radiographs to detect patients' viral pneumonia caused by the COVID-19 virus. From the aforementioned examples, we can note that coronavirus data plays a crucial role. However, the healthcare data for training the AI models are fragmented and stored in a private server to maintain privacy. Thus, creating a robust result across populations is a difficult task. The decentralized, patient-centric framework facilitates a federated learning approach to train a shared AI global model within a blockchain network. Meanwhile, keeping all the sensitive patient COVID-19 data in the decentralized storage network, ensures to connect the fragmented healthcare data sources with privacy preservation. This approach increases trust by allowing advanced machine learning to be developed on distributed data with full respect of the confidentiality for the data providers and maintains the property rights of the companies that propose the machine learning models.

5.5. Disaster Relief and Insurance

COVID pandemic situations are often accompanied by significant threats, such as disrupting the healthcare delivery infrastructure and extending the effect of the physical health of individuals living in affected communities for short- and long-term periods due to nationwide lockdowns and social distancing rules. Governments, financial organizations, and healthcare delivery infrastructures are compromised by the loss of facilities; difficulties in providing loans and other financial lifelines; scarcity of health professionals in the impacted area; and disruption of critical supports, such as information sharing and data management technology, pharmaceuticals supplies, supply chain management, and medically necessary social services. The key reasons for such challenges are that the existing healthcare infrastructure is centralized, non-transparent, and relayed on paper-based procedures, which consumes more time and is ineffective.

The blockchain smart contract in the decentralized, patient-centric approach eliminates third-party intermediaries and the inherent processing delays associated with traditional paper-based policies. The smart contract simplifies complicated applications to ease the approval process for providing insurance and loans with reduced operational risk. The policy agreements are created and deployed in blockchain networks by the participants, such as governments, pharma, and regulators, to enable fast, reliable, and scalable solutions in the patient-centric healthcare consortium. Furthermore, patients are now at the center of healthcare operations, such as the revenue cycle [90]. Therefore, patients have choices for the providers they utilize, such as the hospitals, payers, and pharma, and the providers are now expected to deliver retail-like service levels. This patient-centric healthcare model calls for new solutions in infrastructure, technology, and mindset to ensure a transparent financial experience for both the patient and provider. Another application includes managing the medical billing data by AI. The AI model helps to learn about health plans by feeding the sensitive databases into the AI models from different platforms stored on a blockchain. AI would analyze the necessary sensitive information in the blockchain provided by the appropriate entity, disseminate the understandable data, and provide answers related to health plans and medical bills.

5.6. Supply Chain Management

The healthcare provider and the supply chain play a critical role in protecting the patients' safety and treatment. The shockwave of the COVID-19 pandemic created disruptions in the global supply chain due to the abrupt changes in delivery routes, individuals buying patterns, and supply shortages. For example, there was a surge in demand for household essentials due to panic buying. Specifically, COVID-19 exposed the difficulties in managing medical equipment and pharmaceutical supply chains due to the lack of integration and alignments of interest in the healthcare supply chain. Therefore, it is necessary to critically redesign the existing supply chain system to manage the flow of medical supplies and respond to additional challenges presented due to the ongoing global pandemic.

The decentralized, patient-centric approach plays a crucial role in designing a more resilient, fully connected, and trustworthy supply chain environment using blockchain technology. Here, the blockchain anonymously considers various stakeholders with uniting factors, such as delivering a higher quality of care and improved customer service. The patients will be at the center of the healthcare supply chain and integrated with the system data using blockchain-enabled dApps. Thus, immutable recording of data logs supports auditability, transparency, and provenance. By using a blockchain, supply chain organizations achieve a rapid flow of supplies from the origins to the destinations in a reliable and trusted manner. These help to harmonize just-in-time manufacturing with disaster preparedness. Meanwhile, a well-programmed smart contract gives a high level of automation and access restrictions to save billions of dollars and thousands of lives [91]. The patient-centric supply chain management system utilizes AI to increase the system's efficiency for reporting and analyzing the obtained data from medical and logistic teams. The supply chain data are interpreted to derive insights that will enable continued tweaking of the system for even better results.

5.7. Contactless Delivery and Automated Surveillances

Contactless delivery eliminates direct communications among people (e.g., person–person interactions changed to person–machine or person–machine–person) [92] and delivers healthcare services or products between individuals, patients, healthcare professionals, and other providers through digital technologies. Thus, many people and mildly infected patients prefer contactless online treatments and contactless (automated robotic) delivery of essential supplies, such as medicine and food, during a lockdown or quarantine period. The goal is to maintain an individual's safety by avoiding face-to-face interactions and sending a person for doorstep delivery. Accordingly, telemedicine services were naturally contactless and widely practiced in the pre-COVID period. The telemedicine services encompass remote consultation through audio/video calls using a robot with a camera and video features with a tablet, smartphone, or computer. In telemedicine services, patient data are generally stored and managed through a centralized platform [36]. Hence, there is a possibility of security attack, raising questions regarding the patient's privacy of data. In addition, it is necessary to monitor people who violate COVID-19 rules by not wearing facemasks and not maintaining social distancing.

To address challenges, drones and robots are used for contactless delivery and automated surveillance in response to COVID-19, such as monitoring public space; providing guidance during lockdown and quarantine; lab sample pick-up and delivery; transporting medical supplies to minimize the transportation times and infection exposure; and aerial spraying of public areas in order to disinfect potentially contaminated places [29]. Though the utilization of AI technologies facilitates UAVs and robots to precisely operate and execute the task without human interventions, it leads to security attacks, such as device hacking, data theft, and modifications in robot functions. A blockchain- and AI-enabled, patient-centric approach offers a vast range of possibilities to mitigate the issues by integrating with technologies, such as robots and UAVs. The blockchain enables independent drones or robots to reach a consensus in a decentralized way, and shares knowledge to improve the performance of the system [93]. The blockchain, along with smart contracts designed to ensure a high level of security, automates the operations of robots [94] under policies implemented via the government or healthcare organizations' supervision. Blockchain and AI empower personalized care for patients and monitors people using secured and automated UAVs and robots.

6. Discussions

6.1. Challenges and Solutions

Healthcare professionals and medical industries around the globe are urged to fight the pandemic with rapid screening, forecasting, contact tracing, and the development of drugs or vaccines with more accurate and reliable operation. Blockchain- and AI-based, patient-centric approaches enable a personalized healthcare service to patients and healthy people. However, some challenges must be addressed for a patient-centric approach to embrace blockchain and AI technology and to leverage maximum benefit.

The first challenge is related to the increased volume of raw clinical data, and the verification of new transactions can take time on the blockchain, depending on the consensus algorithm. For example, the latency for PoW is higher due to the time taken to approve each transaction by the blockchain infrastructure, which leverages scalability issues. The scalability issues could be overcome by utilizing a permissioned blockchain built to handle large transaction volumes without time-intensive validation. Recently, researchers have been developing novel solutions, such as sharding [95], to achieve network-wide scalability by dividing rapidly growing blockchain networks into groups called shards. Furthermore, designing specific hierarchical blockchain systems and consensus algorithms could help to resolve the scalability issues.

The second challenge is related to privacy and security issues. The blockchain data are distributed to all the nodes which, in turn, leads to non-compliance with privacy laws (e.g., HIPPA and GDPR) and vulnerabilities [96]. Therefore, it is necessary to store data off-chain in order to maintain data privacy and security. The privacy of data can possibly be achieved by new privacy methods, such as homomorphic and attribute-based encryption, secure multiparty computation, zero-knowledge proof, obfuscation, and format-preserving encryption. The different security levels in a system could be accelerated by designing with hybrid privacy methods and using security-enhancing technologies, such as a homomorphic signature [97], which works better than public key certificates. More importantly, COVID-19 data gathered from hospitals, clinical labs, and patients can be altered by any malicious attacker and makes AI learning invalid. Therefore, it is necessary to collect the COVID-19 data without any privacy leakage from different sources using federated learning combined with blockchain technology. Possibly the largest barrier to the adoption of a patient-centric framework based on AI and blockchain relates to legal disputes or regulatory issues. The central entity of each healthcare organization is liable for any legal issues and is responsible for the overall smooth functioning of the centralized healthcare systems. However, a decentralized, patient-centric system leads to difficulties in solving any legal dispute or discrepancies in the public blockchain infrastructure. For example, copyright infringement and defamation problems arise when personal information runs on converged AI and blockchain platforms. In addition, countries are reluctant to share coronavirus-related databases, which creates additional difficulties in performing a large-scale AI operation. Therefore, regulatory approaches would need to be cleverly balanced by developing corresponding administrative processes and a new legal framework among countries and healthcare organizations, such as the WHO, while recognizing the possibility of the technology [98].

6.2. Future Work

In short, the proposed conceptual framework tries to generalize the process of a decentralized, patient-centric healthcare ecosystem to fight the COVID-19 situation with a clearer understanding of possible applications and functionalities. The framework takes full advantage of blockchain and AI technologies to establish better solutions in solving pandemic-related issues. In our future work, we aim to implement the conceptually proposed framework and test our system with the applications related to healthcare strategies. We will focus on conducting experiments by optimizing the blockchain technology to achieve better performance in terms of improved security and increased throughput. In addition, we will deploy a real-time adaptive AI architecture model using a blockchain-based federated learning approach with the potential to manage multimedia healthcare data for predictive modeling, patient monitoring, and emergency department operations in response to critical healthcare situations. Democratizing aspects of healthcare provide personalized care, as well as save time and money for patients. Moreover, this conceptual framework will motivate researchers to pay more attention and explore the combination of other technologies, such as drones, smart MIoT, robots, and digital twin technologies, to help fight future epidemics and pandemics.

7. Conclusions

In this paper, we provided an overview of digital healthcare services in response to COVID-19 pandemic management services. Then, we presented a conceptual framework for a decentralized, patient-centric healthcare system by integrating blockchain and AI technologies to fight against the coronavirus epidemic. The proposed decentralized, patient-centric framework can contribute in four ways. Firstly, it improves the interoperability of different healthcare platform stakeholders, such as providers, payers, pharma, governments, and researchers. Secondly, patients store COVID-19 health records securely on the patient-centric blockchain platforms and own their sensitive data. Thirdly, the blockchain reduces siloed patient datasets and eliminates centralized organizations, thus improving medical research and treatment by using AI models for predictive diagnosis and analysis. Fourthly, the blockchain enables federated learning techniques, where AI models train the COVID-19 data with the patients' permission at the hospital side while preserving their privacy, and aggregates the knowledge from the nodes to learn a global model. Here, only the global AI model parameters are shared with the hospitals, and once the training is performed locally at hospitals, the model parameters are sent back for aggregation. Thus, the machine learning or deep learning models are trained collaboratively in the distributed network while maintaining hospital and patient data privacy. In addition, we explored the possibilities and potential applications of these combined technologies to facilitate the traditional public health strategies for tackling COVID-19, such as contact tracing, outbreak estimation, coronavirus detection, analysis, clinical data management, supply chain management, contactless delivery, automated surveillance, disaster relief, and insurance. The acceptance of a patient-centric healthcare model could transform the centralized healthcare system into a decentralized healthcare system, thus placing the patients at the center of the healthcare ecosystem to control, access, and share their healthcare data, facilitating research and personalized treatment.

Author Contributions: Conceptualization, M.Y.J.; designing the research work, M.Y.J. and H.-N.L.; writing the manuscript, M.Y.J.; performing investigation, revising the manuscript, and supervising the research work, H.-N.L. All authors have read and agreed to the published version of the manuscript.

Funding: This work was supported in part by a National Research Foundation of Korea (NRF) Grant funded by the Korean government (MSIP) (NRF-2021R1A2B5B03002118).

Informed Consent Statement: Not applicable.

Data Availability Statement: Not applicable.

Conflicts of Interest: The authors declare no conflict of interest.

References

1. Wilder-Smith, A.; Osman, S. Public health emergencies of international concern: A historic overview. *J. Travel Med.* **2020**, *27*, 1–13. [CrossRef] [PubMed]
2. Economic Effects of Coronavirus Outbreak (COVID-19) on the World Economy. Available online: https://ssrn.com/abstract=3557504 (accessed on 5 June 2021).
3. Kaye, A.D.; Okeagu, C.N.; Pham, A.D.; Silva, R.A.; Hurley, J.J.; Arron, B.L.; Sarfraz, N.; Lee, H.N.; Ghali, G.E.; Gamble, J.W.; et al. Economic impact of COVID-19 pandemic on healthcare facilities and systems: International perspectives. *Best Pract. Res. Clin. Anesthesiol.* **2020**. [CrossRef]
4. Minor, D. The Democratization of Health Care. Stanford Medicine 2018 Health Trends Report. 2018. Available online: https://med.stanford.edu/content/dam/sm/school/documents/Health-Trends-Report/Stanford-Medicine-Health-Trends-Report-2018.pdf (accessed on 5 June 2021).
5. Morley, J.; Cowls, J.; Taddeo, M.; Floridi, L. Ethical guidelines for COVID-19 tracing apps. *Nature* **2020**, *582*, 29–31. [CrossRef]
6. Ko, H.; Leitner, J.; Kim, E.; Jeong, J. Information technology–based tracing strategy in response to COVID-19 in South Korea—Privacy controversies. *JAMA* **2020**, *323*, 2129–2130.
7. Reddy, S.; Fox, J.; Purohit, M.P. Artificial intelligence-enabled healthcare delivery. *J. R. Soc. Med.* **2019**, *112*, 22–28. [CrossRef]
8. Hölbl, M.; Kompara, M.; Kamišalić, A.; Zlatolas, L.N. A systematic review of the use of blockchain in healthcare. *Symmetry* **2018**, *10*, 470. [CrossRef]
9. Monrat, A.A.; Schelén, O.; Andersson, K. A survey of blockchain from the perspectives of applications, challenges, and opportunities. *IEEE Access* **2019**, *7*, 117134–117151. [CrossRef]
10. Griggs, K.N.; Ossipova, O.; Kohlios, C.P.; Baccarini, A.N.; Howson, E.A.; Hayajneh, T. Healthcare blockchain system using smart contracts for secure automated remote patient monitoring. *J. Med. Syst.* **2018**, *42*, 1–7. [CrossRef]
11. Vaishya, R.; Javaid, M.; Khan, I.H.; Haleem, A. Artificial Intelligence (AI) applications for COVID-19 pandemic. *Diabetes Metab. Syndr. Clin. Res. Rev.* **2020**, *14*, 337–339. [CrossRef]
12. McMahan, H.B.; Moore, E.; Ramage, D.; Hampson, S.; Aguera y Arcas, B. Communication-efficient learning of deep networks from decentralized data. In Proceedings of the 20th International Conference on Artificial Intelligence and Statistics, AISTATS, Lauderdale, FL, USA, 20–22 April 2017; pp. 1273–1282.
13. Lu, X.; Liao, Y.; Lio, P.; Hui, P. Privacy-preserving asynchronous federated learning mechanism for edge network computing. *IEEE Access* **2020**, *8*, 48970–48981. [CrossRef]
14. Sharma, A.; Bahl, S.; Bagha, A.K.; Javaid, M.; Shukla, D.K.; Haleem, A. Blockchain technology and its applications to combat COVID-19 pandemic. *Res. Biomed.* **2020**, 1–8. [CrossRef]
15. Chen, H.S.; Jarrell, J.T.; Carpenter, K.A.; Cohen, D.S.; Huang, X.; Hospital, M.G. Blockchain in healthcare: A patient-centered model. *Biomed. J. Sci. Tech. Res. (BJSTR)* **2019**, *20*, 15017–15022.
16. Jabarulla, M.Y.; Lee, H.-N. Blockchain-based distributed patient-centric image management system. *Appl. Sci.* **2020**, *11*, 196. [CrossRef]
17. Ploug, T.; Holm, S. The four dimensions of contestable AI diagnostics—A patient-centric approach to explainable AI. *Artif. Intell. Med.* **2020**, *107*, 101901. [CrossRef] [PubMed]
18. Nguyen, D.C.; Ding, M.; Pathirana, P.N.; Seneviratne, A. Blockchain and AI-based solutions to combat Coronavirus (COVID-19)-like epidemics: A survey. *Preprints* **2020**, 1–15. [CrossRef]
19. Omar, A.; Bhuiyan, M.; Basu, A.; Kiyomoto, S.; Rahman, M. Privacy-friendly platform for healthcare data in cloud based on blockchain environment. *Future Gener. Comput. Syst.* **2019**, *95*, 511–521. [CrossRef]
20. Ramani, V.; Kumar, T.; Bracken, A.; Liyanage, M.; Ylianttila, M. Secure and efficient data accessibility in blockchain based healthcare systems. In Proceedings of the IEEE Global Communications Conference (GLOBECOM), Abu Dhabi, United Arab Emirates, 9–13 December 2018; pp. 206–212.
21. Abugabah, A.; Nizam, N.; Alzubi, A. Decentralized telemedicine framework for a smart healthcare ecosystem. *IEEE Access* **2020**, *8*, 166575–166588. [CrossRef]
22. Patel, V. A framework for secure and decentralized sharing of medical imaging data via blockchain consensus. *Health Inform. J.* **2019**, *25*, 1398–1411. [CrossRef]
23. Shah, R.; Chircu, A. IoT and AI in healthcare: A systematic literature review. *Issues Inf. Syst.* **2018**, *19*, 33–41. [CrossRef]
24. Passerat-Palmbach, J.; Farnan, T.; Miller, R.; Gross, M.S.; Flannery, H.; Gleim, B. A blockchain-orchestrated Federated Learning architecture for healthcare consortia. *arXiv* **2019**, arXiv:1910.12603.
25. Kasnakova, P.; Ivanova, S. Patient-centered approach to pharmaceutical care in the recovery of patients with post-COVID syndrome. *Pharmacia* **2021**, *68*, 381–385. [CrossRef]
26. James, C.; Barfield, M.; Maass, K.; Patel, S.; Anderson, M. Will patient-centric sampling become the norm for clinical trials after COVID-19? *Nat. Med.* **2020**, *26*, 1810. [CrossRef]
27. Nembaware, V.; Munung, N.; Matimba, A.; Tiffin, N. Patient-centric research in the time of COVID-19: Conducting ethical COVID-19 research in Africa. *BMJ Glob. Health* **2020**, *5*, e003035. [CrossRef]
28. Beaverson, M. HealthTech. July 2020. Available online: https://healthtechmagazine.net/article/2020/12/how-covid-19-has-accelerated-digital-transformation-healthcare (accessed on 16 July 2021).

29. Alsamhi, S.H.; Lee, B.; Guizani, M.; Kumar, N.; Qiao, Y.; Liu, X. Blockchain for decentralized multi-drone to combat COVID-19 and future pandemics: Framework and proposed solutions. *Trans. Emerg. Telecommun. Technol.* **2021**, e4255. [CrossRef]
30. Lalmuanawma, S.; Hussain, J.; Chhakchhuak, L. Applications of machine learning and artificial intelligence for COVID-19 (SARS-CoV-2) pandemic: A review. *Chaos Solitons Fractals* **2020**, *139*, 110059. [CrossRef] [PubMed]
31. Tuckson, R.; Edmunds, M.; Hodgkins, M. Telehealth. *N. Engl. J. Med.* **2017**, *377*, 1585–1592. [CrossRef]
32. Rabah, K. Convergence of AI, IoT, big data and blockchain: A review. *Lake Inst. J.* **2018**, *1*, 1–18.
33. Ye, J. The Role of Health Technology and Informatics in a Global Public Health Emergency: Practices and Implications from the COVID-19 Pandemic. *JMIR Med. Inform.* **2020**, *8*, e19866. [CrossRef]
34. Flannery, D.; Jarrin, R. Building A Regulatory and Payment Framework Flexible Enough to Withstand Technological Progress. *Health Aff.* **2018**, *37*, 2052–2059. [CrossRef] [PubMed]
35. Mahmood, S.; Hasan, K.; Carras, M.C.; Labrique, A. Global Preparedness Against COVID-19: We Must Leverage the Power of Digital Health. *JMIR Public Health Surveill.* **2020**, *6*, e18980. [CrossRef]
36. Bahl, S.; Singh, R.; Javaid, M.; Khan, I.; Vaishya, R.; Suman, R. Telemedicine technologies for confronting COVID-19 pandemic: A review. *J. Ind. Integr. Manag. Innov. Entrep.* **2020**, *5*, 547–561. [CrossRef]
37. Ghosh, A.; Gupta, R.; Misra, A. Telemedicine for diabetes care in India during COVID19 pandemic and national lockdown period: Guidelines for physicians. *Diabetes Metab. Syndr. Clin. Res. Rev.* **2020**, *14*, 273–276. [CrossRef]
38. Bahl, S.; Javaid, M.; Bagha, A.; Singh, R.; Haleem, A.; Vaishya, R.; Suman, R. Biosensors applications in fighting COVID-19 pandemic. *Apollo Med.* **2020**, *17*, 221–223. [CrossRef]
39. Javaid, M.; Haleem, A.; Vaishya, R.; Bahl, S.; Suman, R.; Vaish, A. Industry 4.0 technologies and their applications in fighting COVID-19 pandemic. *Diabetes Metab. Syndr. Clin. Res. Rev.* **2020**, *14*, 419–422. [CrossRef] [PubMed]
40. Whitelaw, S.; Mamas, M.A.; Topol, E.; Van Spall, H.G.C. Applications of digital technology in COVID-19 pandemic planning and response. *Lancet Digit. Health* **2020**, *2*, e435–e440. [CrossRef]
41. Ferretti, L.; Wymant, C.; Kendall, M.; Zhao, L.; Nurtay, A.; Abeler-Dörner, L.; Parker, M.; Bonsall, D.; Fraser, C. Quantifying SARS-CoV-2 transmission suggests epidemic control with digital contact tracing. *Science* **2020**, *368*, eabb6936. [CrossRef]
42. Gagliardi, A.; Lemieux-Charless, L.; Brown, A.; Sullivan, T.; Goel, V. Barriers to patient involvement in health service planning and evaluation: An exploratory study. *Patient Educ. Couns.* **2008**, *70*, 234–241. [CrossRef] [PubMed]
43. Mead, N.; Bower, P. Patient-centredness: A conceptual framework and review of the empirical literature. *Soc. Sci. Med.* **2000**, *51*, 1087–1110. [CrossRef]
44. Crawford, M.; Rutter, D.; Manley, C.; Weaver, T.; Bhui, K.; Fulop, N.; Tyrer, P. Systematic review of involving patients in the planning and development of health care. *BMJ* **2002**, *325*, 1263. [CrossRef] [PubMed]
45. Gordon, W.J.; Catalini, C. Blockchain Technology for Healthcare: Facilitating the Transition to Patient-Driven Interoperability. *Comput. Struct. Biotechnol. J.* **2018**, *16*, 224–230. [CrossRef]
46. Nakamoto, S. Bitcoin: A Peer-to-Peer Electronic Cash System. 2008. Available online: https://bitcoin.org/bitcoin.pdf. (accessed on 5 June 2021).
47. Wood, G. ETHEREUM: A Secure Decentralised Generalised Transaction Ledger. 2014. Available online: https://gavwood.com/paper.pdf (accessed on 5 June 2021).
48. Agboo, C.; Mahmoud, Q.; Eklund, J. Blockchain technology in healthcare: A systematic review. *Healthcare* **2019**, *7*, 56. [CrossRef]
49. Zhang, R.; Xue, R.; Liu, L. Security and Privacy on Blockchain. *ACM Comput. Surv.* **2019**, *52*, 1–34. [CrossRef]
50. Jang, J.; Lee, H.N. Profitable Double-Spending Attacks. *Appl. Sci.* **2020**, *10*, 8477. [CrossRef]
51. Khatoon, A. A Blockchain-Based Smart Contract System for Healthcare Management. *Electronics* **2020**, *9*, 94. [CrossRef]
52. Niya, S.R.; Schüpfer, F.; Bocek, T.; Stiller, B. A Peer-to-Peer Purchase and Rental Smart Contract-based Application. *Inf. Technol.* **2018**, *60*, 307–320.
53. Novikov, S.; Kazakov, O.; Kulagina, N.; Azarenko, N. Blockchain and smart contracts in a decentralized health infrastructure. In Proceedings of the IEEE International Conference Quality Management, Transport and Information Security, Information Technologies (IT&QM&IS), St. Petersburg, Russia, 24 September 2018; pp. 697–703.
54. Nguyen, D.; Pathirana, P.; Ding, M.; Seneviratne, A. Blockchain for secure EHRs sharing of mobile cloud based e-health systems. *IEEE Access* **2019**, *7*, 66792–66806. [CrossRef]
55. Zheng, X.; Mukkamala, R.; Vatrapu, R.; Ordieres-Mere, J. Blockchain-based personal health data sharing system using cloud storage. In Proceedings of the IEEE 20th International Conference on e-Health Networking, Applications and Services (Healthcom), Ostrava, Czech Republic, 17–20 September 2018; pp. 1–6.
56. Hasselgren, A.; Kralevska, K.; Gilgoroski, D.; Pedersen, S.; Faxvaag, A. Blockchain in healthcare and health sciences—A scoping review. *Int. J. Med. Inform.* **2019**, *134*, 104040. [CrossRef]
57. Christiansen, P. Artificial Intelligence: Healthcare's New Nervous System. 2017. Available online: https://www.accenture.com/_acnmedia/PDF-49/Accenture-Health-Artificial-Intelligence.pdf (accessed on 5 June 2021).
58. Erickson, B.J.; Korfiatis, P.; Akkus, Z.; Kline, T.L. Machine learning for medical imaging. *Radiographics* **2017**, *37*, 505–515. [CrossRef] [PubMed]
59. Amin, S.; Hossain, M.; Muhammad, G.; Alhussein, M.; Rahman, M. Cognitive smart healthcare for pathology detection and monitoring. *IEEE Access* **2019**, *7*, 10745–10753. [CrossRef]

60. Pouyanfar, S.; Sadiq, S.; Yan, Y.; Tian, H.; Tao, Y.; Reyes, M.; Shyu, L.; Chen, S.; Iyengar, S. A survey on deep learning: Algorithms, techniques, and applications. *ACM Comput. Surv. (CSUR)* **2018**, *51*, 1–36. [CrossRef]
61. Taulli, T. AI (Artificial Intelligence) Companies That Are Combating the COVID-19 Pandemic. 2020. Available online: https://www.forbes.com/sites/tomtaulli/2020/03/28/ai-artificial-intelligence-companies-that-are-combating-the-covid-19-pandemic/ (accessed on 5 June 2021).
62. Ye, D.; Yu, R.; Pan, M.; Han, Z. Federated learning in vehicular edge computing: A selective model aggregation approach. *IEEE Access* **2020**, *8*, 23920–23935. [CrossRef]
63. Kumar, R.; Khan, A.A.; Zhang, S.; Kumar, J.; Yang, T.; Golilarz, N.A.; Zakria; Ikram, A.; Shafiq, S.; Wang, W. Blockchain-Federated-Learning and Deep Learning Models for COVID-19 detection using CT Imaging. *arXiv* **2020**, arXiv:2007.06537.
64. Lu, Y.; Huang, X.; Zhang, K.; Maharjan, S.; Zhang, Y. Blockchain Empowered Asynchronous Federated Learning for Secure Data Sharing in Internet of Vehicles. *IEEE Trans. Veh. Technol.* **2020**, *69*, 4298–4311. [CrossRef]
65. Hua, G.; Zhu, L.; Wu, J.; Shen, C.; Zhou, L.; Lin, Q. Blockchain-Based Federated Learning for Intelligent Control in Heavy Haul Railway. *IEEE Access* **2020**, *8*, 176830–176839. [CrossRef]
66. Harris, J.D. Analysis of models for decentralized and collaborative AI on blockchain. In Proceedings of the The 2020 International Conference on Blockchain, Rhodes Island, Greece, 2–6 November 2020.
67. Lewko, A.; Waters, B. Decentralizing Attribute-Based Encryption. In Proceedings of the Annual International Conference on the Theory and Applications of Cryptographic Techniques, Tallinn, Estonia, 15–19 May 2011; pp. 568–588.
68. Li, D.; Du, R.; Fu, Y.; Ho Au, M. Meta-Key: A secure data-sharing protocol under blockchain-based decentralized storage architecture. *IEEE Netw. Lett.* **2019**, *1*, 30–33. [CrossRef]
69. Zahed Benisi, N.; Aminian, M.; Javadi, B. Blockchain-based decentralized storage networks: A survey. *J. Netw. Comput. Appl.* **2020**, *162*, 102656. [CrossRef]
70. Benet, J. IPFS—Content Addressed, Versioned, P2P File System. *arXiv* **2014**, arXiv:1407.3561.
71. Miyachi, K.; Mackey, T.K. hOCBS: A privacy-preserving blockchain framework for healthcare data leveraging an on-chain and off-chain system design. *Inf. Process. Manag.* **2021**, *58*, 102535. [CrossRef]
72. Drungilas, V.; Vaičiukynas, E.; Jurgelaitis, M.; Butkiene, R. Towards blockchain-based federated machine learning: Smart contract for model inference. *Appl. Sci.* **2021**, *11*, 1010. [CrossRef]
73. Puri, V.; Kataria, A.; Sharma, V. Artificial intelligence-powered decentralized framework for internet of things in healthcare 4.0. *Trans. Emerg. Telecommun. Technol.* **2021**, e4245. [CrossRef]
74. Edemekong, P.F.; Haydel, M.J. *Health Insurance Portability and Accountability Act (HIPAA)*; StatPearls Publishing: Treasure Island, FL, USA, 2018.
75. Truong, N.; Sun, K.; Lee, G.; Guo, Y. GDPR-compliant personal data management: A BlockchainBased Solution. *IEEE Trans. Inf. Forensics Secur.* **2019**, *15*, 1746–1761. [CrossRef]
76. Shen, B.; Guo, J.; Yang, Y. MedChain: Efficient healthcare data sharing via blockchain. *Appl. Sci.* **2019**, *9*, 1207. [CrossRef]
77. Dietsche, E. Health Wizz Leverages Blockchain Technology to Give Patients Power over Their Data. MedCity News. 2017. Available online: https://medcitynews.com/2017/12/health-wizz/ (accessed on 5 June 2021).
78. Nugent, T.; Upton, D.; Cimpoesu, M. Improving data transparency in clinical trials using blockchain smart contracts. *F1000Research* **2016**, *5*, 2541. [CrossRef] [PubMed]
79. Timberg, C.; Harwell, D. Government Efforts to Track Virus through Phone Location Data Complicated by Privacy Concerns. Washington Post. 2020. Available online: https://www.washingtonpost.com/technology/2020/03/19/privacy-coronavirus-phone-data/ (accessed on 5 June 2021).
80. Jones, M.; Johnson, M.; Shervey, M.; Dudley, J.; Zimmerman, N. Privacy-Preserving Methods for Feature Engineering Using Blockchain: Review, Evaluation, and Proof of Concept. *J. Med. Internet Res.* **2019**, *21*, e13600. [CrossRef]
81. Hylock, R.; Zeng, X. A Blockchain framework for patient-centered health records and exchange (HealthChain): Evaluation and proof-of-concept study. *J. Med. Internet Res.* **2019**, *21*, e13592. [CrossRef] [PubMed]
82. Wistrom, B. How Blockchain and Immunization Passports Could Help Us Re-Open. 2020. Available online: https://www.americaninno.com/austin/inno-insights/how-blockchain-and-immunization-passports-could-help-us-re-open/ (accessed on 5 June 2021).
83. Degrasse, M. The Role of Wireless Tech in Fighting the New Coronavirus. 2020. Available online: https://www.lightreading.com/4g-3g-wifi/the-role-of-wireless-tech-in-fighting-the-new-coronavirus/d/d-id/757634 (accessed on 5 June 2021).
84. Sarker, I.; Kayes, A.; Watters, P. Effectiveness analysis of machine learning classification models for predicting personalized context-aware smartphone usage. *J. Big Data* **2019**, *6*, 1–28. [CrossRef]
85. Shen, J.; Shafiq, M. Learning mobile application usage-a deep learning approach. In Proceedings of the 2019 18th IEEE International Conference on Machine Learning and Applications (ICMLA), Boca Raton, FL, USA, 16–19 December 2019; pp. 287–292.
86. Wang, Z.; Wang, G.; Huang, H.; Xiong, Z.; Hong, Q.; Wu, H.; Yi, P.; Jiang, K.; Wang, N.; Pei, Y.; et al. Masked Face Recognition Dataset and Application. *arXiv* **2020**, arXiv:2003.09093.
87. Gozes, O.; Frid-Adar, M.; Greenspan, H.; Browning, P.; Zhang, H.; Ji, W.; Bernheim, A.; Siegel, E. Rapid AI Development Cycle for The Coronavirus (COVID-19) Pandemic: Initial Results for Automated Detection & Patient Monitoring Using Deep Learning CT Image Analysis. *arXiv* **2020**, arXiv:2003.05037.

88. Xu, X.; Jiang, X.; Ma, C.; Du, P.; Li, X.; Lv, S.; Yu, L.; Chen, Y.; Su, J.; Lang, G.; et al. Deep learning system to screen coronavirus disease 2019 pneumonia. *arXiv* **2020**, arXiv:2002.09334. [CrossRef]
89. Narin, A.; Kaya, C.; Pamuk, Z. Automatic detection of coronavirus disease (COVID-19) using x-ray images and deep convolutional neural networks. *Pattern Anal. Appl.* **2021**, *24*, 1207–1220. [CrossRef]
90. Plunk, A. Patient Consumerism and the Need for a Patient-Centric Revenue Model. 2018. Available online: https://www.beckershospitalreview.com/finance/patient-consumerism-and-the-need-for-a-patient-centric-revenue-model.html (accessed on 5 June 2021).
91. Degnarain, N. Five Ways Blockchain Can Unblock the Coronavirus Medical Supply Chain. Forbes 2020. Available online: Forbes.com/sites/nishandegnarain/2020/03/22/5-ways-blockchaincan-%0Aunblock-the-coronavirus-medical-supply-chain/ (accessed on 5 June 2021).
92. Lee, S.; Lee, D. "Untact": A new customer service strategy in the digital age. *Serv. Bus.* **2020**, *14*, 1–22. [CrossRef]
93. Scarlato, M.; Perra, C.; Jabarulla, M.Y.; Jung, G.; Lee, H.N. A blockchain for the collision avoidance and the recovery of crashed UAVS. In Proceedings of the Korean Institute of Electronics Engineers Conference, Jeju, Korea, 27–31 May 2019; pp. 463–467.
94. Kapitonov, A.; Lonshakov, S.; Berman, I.; Ferrer Castello, E.; Bonsignorio, F.; Bulatov, V.; Svistov, A. Robotic services for new paradigm smartcities based on decentralized technologies. *Ledger* **2019**, 56–66. [CrossRef]
95. Yu, G.; Wang, K.; Ni, W.; Zhang, J.; Liu, R. Survey: Sharding in blockchains. *IEEE Access* **2020**, *8*, 14155–14181. [CrossRef]
96. Bernabe, J.B.; Canovas, J.; Hermandez-Ramos, L.; Moreno, R.; Skarmeta, A. Privacy-preserving solutions for blockchain: Review and challenges. *IEEE Access* **2019**, *7*, 164908–164940. [CrossRef]
97. Line, Q.; Yan, H.; Huang, Z.; Chen, W.; Shen, J.; Tang, Y. An ID-based linearly homomorphic signature scheme and its application in blockchain. *IEEE Access* **2018**, *6*, 20632–20640. [CrossRef]
98. Kakavand, H.; Kost De Sevres, N.; Chilton, B. The Blockchain Revolution: An Analysis of Regulation and Technology Related to Distributed Ledger Technologies. *Soc. Sci. Res. Netw. (SSRN)* **2017**, 1–27. [CrossRef]

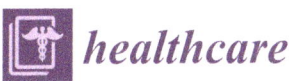

Perspective

Sharing Biomedical Data: Strengthening AI Development in Healthcare

Tania Pereira [1,*], Joana Morgado [1,2], Francisco Silva [1], Michele M. Pelter [3], Vasco Rosa Dias [1], Rita Barros [1], Cláudia Freitas [4,5], Eduardo Negrão [4], Beatriz Flor de Lima [4], Miguel Correia da Silva [4], António J. Madureira [4,5], Isabel Ramos [4,5], Venceslau Hespanhol [4,5], José Luis Costa [5,6,7], António Cunha [1,8] and Hélder P. Oliveira [1,2]

1. INESC TEC—Institute for Systems and Computer Engineering, Technology and Science, 4200-465 Porto, Portugal; joana.p.morgado@inesctec.pt (J.M.); francisco.c.silva@inesctec.pt (F.S.); vasco.r.dias@inesctec.pt (V.R.D.); rita.r.barros@inesctec.pt (R.B.); acunha@utad.pt (A.C.); helder.f.oliveira@inesctec.pt (H.P.O.)
2. FCUP—Faculty of Science, University of Porto, 4169-007 Porto, Portugal
3. Department of Physiological Nursing, School of Nursing, University of California, San Francisco, CA 94143, USA; michele.pelter@ucsf.edu
4. CHUSJ—Centro Hospitalar e Universitário de São João, 4200-319 Porto, Portugal; claudiaasfreitas@gmail.com (C.F.); eduardo.negrao@gmail.com (E.N.); beatrizflordelima@hotmail.com (B.F.d.L.); miguel.ncds@gmail.com (M.C.d.S.); antonio.madureira@chsj.min-saude.pt (A.J.M.); radiologia.hsj@gmail.com (I.R.); hespanholv@gmail.com (V.H.)
5. FMUP—Faculty of Medicine, University of Porto, 4200-319 Porto, Portugal; jcosta@ipatimup.pt
6. i3S—Institute for Research and Innovation in Health of the University of Porto, 4200-135 Porto, Portugal
7. IPATIMUP—Institute of Molecular Pathology and Immunology of the University of Porto, 4200-135 Porto, Portugal
8. UTAD—University of Trás-os-Montes and Alto Douro, 5001-801 Vila Real, Portugal
* Correspondence: tania.pereira@inesctec.pt

Abstract: Artificial intelligence (AI)-based solutions have revolutionized our world, using extensive datasets and computational resources to create automatic tools for complex tasks that, until now, have been performed by humans. Massive data is a fundamental aspect of the most powerful AI-based algorithms. However, for AI-based healthcare solutions, there are several socioeconomic, technical/infrastructural, and most importantly, legal restrictions, which limit the large collection and access of biomedical data, especially medical imaging. To overcome this important limitation, several alternative solutions have been suggested, including transfer learning approaches, generation of artificial data, adoption of blockchain technology, and creation of an infrastructure composed of anonymous and abstract data. However, none of these strategies is currently able to completely solve this challenge. The need to build large datasets that can be used to develop healthcare solutions deserves special attention from the scientific community, clinicians, all the healthcare players, engineers, ethicists, legislators, and society in general. This paper offers an overview of the data limitation in medical predictive models; its impact on the development of healthcare solutions; benefits and barriers of sharing data; and finally, suggests future directions to overcome data limitations in the medical field and enable AI to enhance healthcare. This perspective is dedicated to the technical requirements of the learning models, and it explains the limitation that comes from poor and small datasets in the medical domain and the technical options that try or can solve the problem related to the lack of massive healthcare data.

Keywords: biomedical data; medical imaging; shared data; massive databases; AI-based healthcare solutions

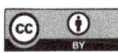

1. Introduction

Artificial intelligence (AI) applications are revolutionizing the way we live, creating automatic solutions for several tasks previously performed by humans with fewer errors [1].

The increase in computational power and the amount of data available has opened up the opportunity to develop novel AI solutions in several areas. Image classification has been one of the most successful AI applications, which has allowed, for example, the creation of a self-driving car or facial recognition on social networks [2]. The great innovation for image classification happened with the creation of the ImageNet [3], which is the most recognizable dataset available with a massive amount of labeled data; thus, allowing a technological breakthrough in image classification. Before the creation of ImageNet, there were only relatively small datasets with tens of thousands of labeled images [4]. These image databases only allow simple recognition tasks [4] since all the variability of the population cannot be covered by these small databases. ImageNet is composed of more than 14 million images with 21,841 synsets and more than 1 million bounding box annotations [5]. However, in order to deal with the variability of data, it was necessary to develop architectures with an automatic feature learning capacity. After the creation of ImageNet, several powerful neural network architectures for image classification were developed, such as AlexNet (2012), ZFNet (2013), VGGNet (2014), Googlenet (2014), Inception (2014), ResNet (2015), ResNeXt (2016), DenseNet (2016), Xception (2017), and SENet (2018) [6,7]. Such progress in a few years was possible due to transparency in the evaluation process. A fair comparison with related works must be done to assess real improvements, and the public availability of ImageNet data allowed this evaluation.

An ideal AI-based model should be robust, reliable, and understandable [8]. To achieve this type of model, it is imperative to have an extremely large amount of data that must be representative of all population features. A massive dataset to cover the population's heterogeneities will only be possible by sharing data collected from multiple institutions. A model trained with this type of representative dataset would then be able to cope with heterogeneities that exist within a population. A robust model should be able to avoid overfitting to generalize well, which would allow the ability to capture the boundaries between classes that will be useful to predict the unseen elements from the test dataset. Generalization is the ability of a classifier to handle new scenarios [9]. One way to test generalization is to evaluate existing models using new independent data that are identically distributed to the original training set [10]. Overfitting occurs when the algorithm, during the learning process, creates a model that performs too well, sometimes by chance, on training data but fails to generalize to new and unseen data (test set) [11]. By allowing the model to achieve an overly specific knowledge of the training examples, it results in a performance decrease on test data [11]. In order to ensure that the model does not rely on the specific elements of the training set, it generally uses strategies such as leave-one-out or splitting a dataset into multiple parts to separate the model training from the validation. With small amounts of data, models will not be able to create a boundary between classes with good accuracy on unseen data and may be biased by some characteristics of the training set [12]. As an alternative way of overcoming the lack of massive training data, Transfer Learning techniques have been explored for several biomedical challenges, allowing to use the knowledge learned with a larger and more generic dataset for a specific application, helping to avoid overfitting by reducing the number of trainable parameters necessary for the learning process of the target task.

Regarding the ideal characteristics of massive data, this has to have five basic dimensions: volume, variety, value, velocity, and veracity, namely the 5 Vs [13]. In fact, the need of large datasets is related with the need to ensure those properties. Only with the extensive collections (high volume of data) is possible to cover the variability of the population using a variety of sources of meaningful data (veracity), which is robust to the noise in the data and labels and allows to capture the statistical relations. The velocity of data generation has an impact on the technological sources available and the protocols, which could change rapidly and influence the acquisition [13]. For example, a novel technological solution can make a traditional clinical exam inadequate and outdated, which makes the previous acquisitions unuseful.

Almost all technological areas have benefited from the combination of powerful AI-based methods, computational resources, and the amount of data available; however, in healthcare, the situation is different. In the exciting era of data-driven and fast growing AI applications, AI-based development in healthcare has been constrained by the lack of access to large datasets [14]. In the healthcare field, AI-based algorithms can aid in the diagnosis, clinical assessment/staging, screening, and/or treatment plan decision making by providing objective and comprehensive information to clinicians that can be taken into consideration for the final decision [15]. Access to large amounts of biomedical data (medical history, medications, allergies, immunization status, laboratory test results (blood and urine), physiologic signals (ECG, PPG, EEG, arterial pressure), medical image (CT, X-ray, MRI, PET), histopathological images, molecular and all "omics" data) will leverage biomedical knowledge, improving the accuracy of diagnosis, allowing early detection of physiological changes and increasing understanding of the clinicopathological events [16–18]. Precision medicine is based on solutions that "provide the right treatments to the right patients at the right time" [19]. Fast and deep characterization of the patient will be aided by AI-based methods that allow the assessment of the main biomarkers that are fundamental for the selection of the most appropriated treatment plan in a short time frame. Massive datasets combined with AI methods allow identifying and inferring meaning of patterns or trends to be directly learned from the data themselves that are not otherwise evident in smaller data sets. Thus, if the hypotheses tested on individual scientific studies were based on a cohort of patients with specific characteristics, chances of lack of generalization for completely different patients are increased. This information will help to develop novel target therapies, innovative biological knowledge, and, as a consequence, personalized medicine. This work gives an overall perspective of the benefits and barriers associated with data sharing (summarized in Figure 1). Current challenges of biomedical data sharing, addressing the impact on the development of healthcare solutions, and major data limitations are discussed.

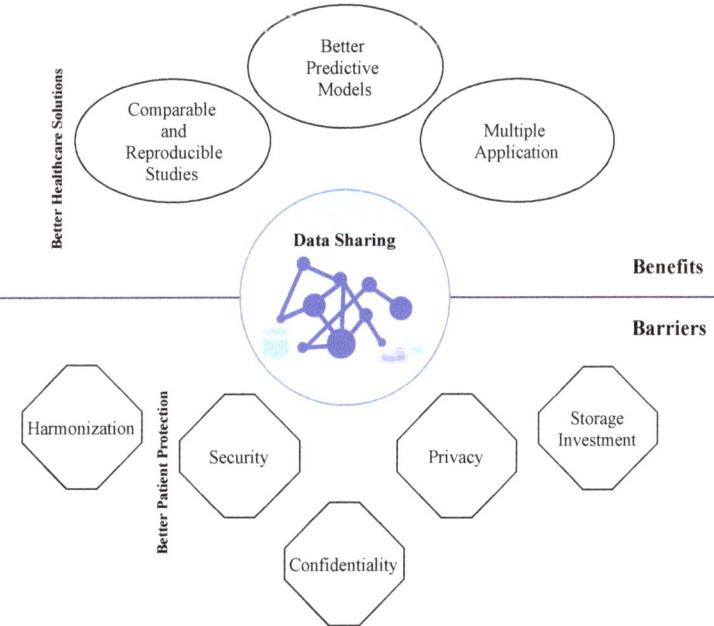

Figure 1. Representation of main benefits and barriers of data sharing. Data sharing has several benefits for healthcare solutions development. Some of the main barriers to data sharing are fundamental for patient data protection.

2. Benefits of Data Sharing

Data sharing, which ensures privacy and security for patients, will enable huge and fast progress in healthcare. Currently, automatic methods, such as computer-aided diagnosis (CAD), have promising results and would lead to improvements in patient care workflow and reduce costs related to examinations, the rate of medical interactions and, as a result, the costs [20]. AI applied to medical diagnosis has been shown to achieve, for the detection of some clinical conditions, better performance than clinicians [21]. Nevertheless, there is still a huge potential to improve CAD performance with large amounts of data in several applications.

On the other hand, scientific studies would be comparable and reproducible, which is only possible with shareable datasets. Usually, each scientific study uses a specific and small dataset that is not representative of all the heterogeneities of the population. Consequently, the performance results depend on the samples used and are not comparable across studies. The use of the same datasets would allow comparison between studies to choose the best solution to be implemented in the clinical decision.

With publicly available datasets, it would be possible to disseminate the use of data collection for multiple projects. Biomedical data have the potential to be used for multiple applications to solve distinct problems, or they can be analyzed from different perspectives to extract relevant clinical information.

From this imperative need of data, institutions promote more synergies with other institutions—companies, universities, R&I organizations and hospitals. The need for data has fostered more collaborations to share this resource, which can be considered as a positive side effect in the biomedical field and, ultimately, benefit patients.

3. Barriers to Access

The barriers to data sharing for health-related research are complex in nature: a combination of economic and social factors intersect with major legal and ethical concerns, to which can be added relevant technical obstacles to overcome.

In the last years, AI-based solutions have created a fundamental shift in business models, and nowadays, data are recognized as a new currency for companies. Data owners will shape the future by creating the new generation of tech solutions [22,23]. From the biggest tech companies to small start-ups, there is a deep and growing commercial interest in healthcare data, since the future and disruptive clinical technological solutions will depend on the data available for use. Biomedical data are even more valuable than other types of data, given the considerable investment required not only in data acquisition, but also in data preservation and storage.

In the healthcare setting, privacy, confidentiality, and security are the fundamental issues that must be addressed [24,25]. The use of health-related information is often strictly regulated, subject to demanding legal requirements regarding information security and organizational measures (anonymization, pseudonymization techniques and encryption), confidentiality, and the respect for data subjects rights. Furthermore, data protection is essentially a fragmented reality worldwide, often mirroring conflicting or, at least, discrepant conceptions with respect to underlying principles and protected social values. The European General Data Protection Regulation (GDPR) represented a major achievement in this regard. It had a global impact, not only as a result of its extraterritorial provisions but also because it was rapidly acknowledged as a relevant international benchmark in the field of data protection, and it was an important source of inspiration for legislation approved shortly after in several states, from Brazil to California, to the UK in the context of Brexit, or to Canada's ongoing reforms. However, and despite its uniformization ambitions, the GDPR abounds in vague clauses and open standards, the application of which often requires balancing competing interests. In the case of AI applications, mostly related to biomedical data, the uncertainties are aggravated by the novelty of the technologies, their complexity, and the wide scope of their individual and social effects. GDPR grants to Member States a significant margin of discretion in several fields, where deviations and specifications are allowed: for example, maintaining or introducing further conditions or limitation regarding the processing of biometric, genetic, or health data. Therefore, lack of harmonization persists in this regard, not only internationally, reflecting different cultures and legal traditions, but, to some extent, even within the EEA. Additionally, the regulation of international data transfers represents another relevant barrier. Following the recent and highly debated case Schrems II, judged by the European Court of Justice, data transfers between EU and US blocks was seriously affected [26], jeopardizing health research collaborations. It should be noted that under EU law, mere (remote) access constitutes a form of data transfer for this purpose.

In the technical realm, harmonization difficulties persist. Biomedical data are usually distributed among several heterogeneous and semantically incompatible health information systems, leading to interoperability problems [27]. The goal of data integration is to create a unique semantic reference to ensure data consistency and reuse and, consequently, improve clinical practice, medical research, and personalized medicine [28]. There has been an increase in the adoption of Semantic Web Technologies in healthcare [29]; however, semantic interoperability is far from being applied across all healthcare organizations. Most of these institutions lack comprehensive semantic definitions of the information they contain and have limitations in extracting parameters to solve semantic service discrepancies [30]. In these cases, a human integrator is required to make final semantic decisions [31]. Furthermore, and since biomedical concepts are constantly evolving, the continuous development of semantic integration is essential [31].

Additionally, the majority of medical solutions have been based on supervised algorithms, which require human annotation of the data. There are several annotation platforms, such as MTurk [32] and Figure Eight (formerly Crowdflower) [33], which are usually based on nonspecialized annotators that follow a very restrict and objective set of rules to define the classes for labeling [34]. However, the annotation of biomedical data needs to be done by experts, usually clinicians, due to the complexity of the physiological knowledge required for annotation. In the end, both data collection and annotation represent a large investment for institutions, due to all the issues related to protecting the large number of samples and the human capital involved in AI-based studies [35]. Because of these large investments and the possible opportunities that data can generate, along with legal barriers, data holders have concerns and economic reasons for not sharing the data collections. While, on the one hand, the sharing of such data, either by hospitals, universities, or other entities for public interest or scientific research purposes, is legally possible under certain conditions and undoubtedly represents a high added value for scientific development, the access and control exerted by companies, especially technological and pharma companies, over such databases raises questions as to their ethical use of health data and the possibility of commercial interests taking precedence over scientific impact and the common good [22].

4. Possible Solution Strategies

Several initiatives have emerged to help healthcare science improve its ability to develop medical tools and overcome the limitation associated with biomedical data access; however, so far none of them can completely overcome the limitation or represent a solution that will solve the problem in the near future.

4.1. Transfer Learning

Recently, TL has been tried as an option to overcome this limitation; however, there is still a lack of large and standardized clinical datasets with potential to be used for multiple biomedical problems [36]. For instance, a dataset from a cohort of patients could be used for several different studies and for the development of multiple AI-based solutions to predict, detect, or assess pathophysiological phenomena, and the multiple associated biological changes. Some studies have attempted to use ImageNet for clinical applications [37,38], using the learning features of a neural network trained on those images; however, due to the dissimilarity between ImageNet and the medical images, its use is limited. Despite the

ImageNet creation and the TL approach, there still remains a need for large and standardized clinical datasets that can be used to train models.

4.2. Blockchain

Blockchain is an extendable database capable of storing large volumes and various types of biomedical data and is an emerging technology with significant potential in the healthcare domain [39]. Compared to traditional databases, blockchain technology offers many advantages for the biomedical field. Besides its decentralized architecture, the key benefits include immutable audit trail, data provenance, availability, and scalability [40]. It has the potential to address interoperability challenges and has so far been proposed to address several security and privacy issues in a number of different applications in the biomedical sector [41], despite the inevitable tension with important data protection principles and individual rights, when considering the current state of the distributed technology [42]. Although this technology is still more associated with the financial area [43], nowadays, there are many pilot projects currently underway, such as FHIRChain [44], Cancer Gene Trust [45], and Zenome [46]. While the implementation of the blockchain technology in clinical routine can address critical issues related to privacy, legal compliance, avoiding fraud, and improving patient care in cases of remote or emergency monitoring, further production developments, detailed proof-of-concept applications, and research articles are crucial for this technology to move forward and be implemented in the biomedical field. In fact, it must be recognized that despite the immense potential of the supporting architecture of blockchain to transform the delivery of healthcare, medical, clinical, and life sciences, challenges still remain, such as standards and interoperability problems, information privacy and security concerns [40], mainly related to the protection of data flows and data retention periods of datasets. A legal obligation established by the GDPR is to ensure that data subjects can invoke their rights and data-protection principles are implemented by means of appropriate technical and organizational measures.

4.3. Synthetic Data

Generative models have recently been applied to generate augmented data for biomedical datasets, thus emerging as a useful tool to increase the number and variability of available examples [47]. Synthetic data are non-reversible, artificially created data that replicate the statistical characteristics and correlations of the original data. This new data overcomes common sharing obstacles, allowing securely access and sharing across institutions, since distributions of real datasets are used to create the synthetic dataset that does not contain identifiable information [48,49], which allows to protect patient privacy while preserving data utility. To build large datasets, synthetic data can be promoted and encouraged, for example, by publishing scientific studies in international journals with the corresponding synthetic data instead of the original datasets. Several studies have been devoted to evaluating synthetic data by analyzing the impact on the performance of learning models compared to the performance obtained with real data. The results showed a small decrease in accuracy for models trained with synthetic data compared to models trained with real data [49]. Synthea™ (MITRE Corporation, Bedford, MA, USA) [50] is one of the most relevant open-source synthetic patient generators due to the massive patient cohort generated; however, the generator showed limited capabilities to model heterogeneous health outcomes [51], and it is still in development. Generating synthetic electronic health records is an enormous challenge because it requires large databases with a combination of linear and nonlinear associations between all medical elements, as well as random associations. Once again, the small databases are the main limitation for data synthesis, restricting the quality of the estimated statistical characteristics of the original data. Furthermore, and since the interactions and correlations are preserved by the synthetic data, the original databases will need to ensure that high-order and complex relationships can be captured. Another limitation is the lack of metrics to evaluate the realism of the generated data. In medical imaging, the validation from clinicians in distinguishing synthetic images from real ones is usually considered the ultimate test, but this evaluation may favor models that concentrate on limited sections of the data (i.e., overfitting, memorizing, or low diversity). Quantitative measures, although less subjective, may not directly correspond to how humans perceive and judge generated images. These, along with other issues such as the variety of probability criteria and the lack of perceptually meaningful image similarity measures, have hindered the evaluation of generative models [52].

4.4. International Strategies

In order to overcome the challenges in accessing biomedical data and facilitate its discovery and use, the set of principles proposed by Wilkison et al. [53] should be fulfilled. These requirements are referred to as the FAIR Data Principles and declare that data should be Findable, Accessible, Interoperable and Reusable [54]. More recently, ten principles for data sharing and commercialization have been proposed, which will help guide healthcare institutions to share clinical data with the aim of improving patient care and fostering innovation [55]. The European Commission (EC) has dedicated special attention to this problem and has adopted strategies to boost actions by the European Union (EU), making the importance of personalized medicine a priority through a shared European data infrastructure [56].

In fact, one of the priorities of the Commission for 2025 is the creation of a European Health Data Space in order to promote a better exchange and access to different types of health data, also for health research and health policy making purposes (not only primary but also secondary use of data). Regarding the entire data system, the EC has announced that will be built on transparent foundations and reinforce the portability of health data, as stated in the GDPR [57]. In addition, it will propose a new data governance model and encourage the creation of common European data spaces in crucial sectors. Fully aware of the problem, the EC is proposing a set of measures to increase data availability in the EU to promote the free flow of non-personal data in the Digital Single Market [58] as part of its new data strategy and the underlying data. Indeed, the White Paper on Artificial Intelligence is another pillar of the new digital strategy of the EC, focusing on the need to put data subjects first in the development of technology, in line with the GDPR goals. European GDPR has been in place since May 2018, and it represents a robust data protection guidelines for better quality healthcare [59]. Some of the key privacy and data protection requirements of the GDPR include consent of subjects for data processing, data anonymization, and secure handling the data transfer across borders [59]. The GDPR outlines a special regime for scientific research, demonstrating that research occupies a privileged position within it. In the healthcare sector there is an ethical and scientific imperative to share personal data for research purposes [60].

The most disruptive solution to this major challenge could be the creation of cloud-based repositories of data abstractions (anonymized and abstracted data). The procedures for data abstraction would be developed for each data format using data abstraction techniques such as data masking, pseudonymization, generalization, data swapping, and other techniques using Neural Networks for feature-based masking. These data abstraction procedures would irreversibly convert patient data into anonymized features, preserving the confidentiality and privacy required for biomedical data and thus fully complying with GDPR and all data protection regulations. This type of platform would enable increased reliability of AI applications in the field and provide more training data for AI systems. The data abstractions extracted from medical data would allow the data to be integrated for several other scientific projects as AI-based solutions to improve diagnosis, treatment, and follow-up and contribute to a more precise and personalized medicine. These infrastructures should also address the issue of harmonization of data storage by designing a standard template to define the roles of data that can be submitted in the platform. Since the objective is to collect data from multiple centers, the infrastructure should allow for the submission of the dataset under an objective protocol. All datasets must be checked after the submission, and if they meet all the requirements related to ethical issues and data protocols, they could be added to the repository.

Data from multiple institutions are generated in numerous formats, frequently without a specific structure and with additional semantic information. Data from multiple sources need to be converted into a unified representation, aggregated, and integrated to extract relevant knowledge that can be used by AI-based models to make predictions, exchange data between different healthcare applications, and enable integration with future data [61]. Clinical annotations, medical reports, lab results, imagiological findings, and expressive description of data using standardized procedures are key elements to maximize the quality and applicability of the next generation of the AI-based models [62]. A common infrastructure with common standards for the integration of multiple data sources into one platform (data integration) is fundamental to allow data sharing [63]. Fast Healthcare Interoperability Resources (FHIR) presents standards and technical specifications to define how the information contained in Electronic Health Records (EHRs) should be structured and semantically described [64]. FHIR ensures the requirements for having patient records in an accessible and available format by providing a comprehensive framework and related standards for the exchange, integration, sharing and retrieval of electronic health information. Despite the extreme importance of standards-based data interoperability and EHR integration, their implementation is not consensual [61].

4.5. Research Resource for Medical Imaging

Despite all the other technical possible options presented, real data remain indispensable. The Cancer Genome Atlas (TCGA) represents the most important source of data for cancer development from thousands of individuals representing over 30 different types of cancers and containing genomic, epigenomic, transcriptomic, and proteomic data, CT images, histopathological images, etc. [65]. The Cancer Imaging Archive (TCIA) hosts a large archive of medical images of cancer accessible for public download, containing MRI, CT, digital histopathology, etc, and supporting image-related data such as patient outcomes, treatment details, genomics, and expert analyses [66]. Database resources of the National Center for Biotechnology Information comprise hundreds of thousands of databases with biological and genomic information for multiple organisms [67]. Those databases have been allowing the most important developments of AI-based solutions on "omics" and cancer; however, the applications based on medical images still suffer from the insufficient number of cases to use the most powerful deep learning methods. *Stanford Center for Artificial Intelligence in Medicine & Imaging* announced the creation of "Medical ImageNet", which would be a searchable repository of annotated de-identified clinical (radiology and pathology) images, linked to other clinical information, for use in computer vision systems [68]. Ideally, these databases should comprise data from multiple centers to cover the heterogeneities of the population. The development of these repositories would be more efficient and reliable if the computer systems in clinics and hospitals had built-in software that automatically integrated the annotations and de-identified images into the databases.

5. Summary

A large amount of data that include population heterogeneities would allow a revolution in the healthcare field. However, current limitations on access to biomedical data are hindering the development of powerful AI-based tools and restricting improvements in healthcare solutions and medical science development. Recognizing that confidentiality and privacy must be fundamental requirements, it is imperative to find a solution to this limitation. This topic deserves special attention from the entire community working in the biomedical engineering field and key healthcare stakeholders. A paradigm shift in the perception of data in society and institutions, regarding its importance and risks, will create novel solutions to share this extremely valuable resource and perhaps even shift perspectives from patient rights to a duty as a citizen [69].

The limitations imposed on data sharing have hindered a wide range of infectious diseases researchers' access to crucial data, even at times like the present, during the COVID-19 pandemic. However, during this pandemic situation, the urgent need allowed for exceptional effort and cooperation to develop rapid knowledge and find solutions [70]. Establishing protocols, regulations, methodologies, and definitions to preserve the confidentiality and privacy of data that permit sharing will enable a faster and better scientific response to a similar situation in the future. In fact, the COVID-19 pandemic exposed the extreme need to cooperate, combine effort and share data and knowledge to enable scientific development at a pace never before experienced.

Author Contributions: T.P., A.C. and H.P.O. conceived the scientific idea. M.M.P., C.F., E.N., B.F.d.L., M.C.d.S., A.J.M., I.R., V.H. and J.L.C. provided the clinical insights. J.M. and F.S. added improvements on the discussion points. V.R.D. and R.B. provided insights on data protection and ownership. All authors contributed to the critical discussion. T.P. drafted the manuscript. All authors provided critical feedback and contributed to the final manuscript. All authors have read and agreed to the published version of the manuscript.

Funding: This work is financed by the ERDF—European Regional Development Fund through the Operational Programme for Competitiveness and Internationalisation—COMPETE 2020 Programme and by National Funds through the Portuguese funding agency, FCT—Fundação para a Ciência e a Tecnologia within project POCI-01-0145-FEDER-030263.

Institutional Review Board Statement: Not applicable.

Informed Consent Statement: Not applicable.

Conflicts of Interest: The authors declare no conflict of interest.

References

1. Makridakis, S. The forthcoming Artificial Intelligence (AI) revolution: Its impact on society and firms. *Futures* **2017**, *90*, 46–60. [CrossRef]
2. Dean, J. The Deep Learning Revolution and Its Implications for Computer Architecture and Chip Design. *arXiv* **2019**, arXiv:1911.05289.
3. Deng, J.; Dong, W.; Socher, R.; Li, L.J.; Li, K.; Li, F.-F. ImageNet: A large-scale hierarchical image database. In Proceedings of the 2009 IEEE Conference on Computer Vision and Pattern Recognition, Miami, FL, USA, 20–25 June 2009. [CrossRef]
4. Krizhevsky, A.; Sutskever, I.; Hinton, G.E. ImageNet classification with deep convolutional neural networks. *Commun. ACM* **2017**, *25*, 1097–1105. [CrossRef]
5. Russakovsky, O.; Deng, J.; Su, H.; Krause, J.; Satheesh, S.; Ma, S.; Huang, Z.; Karpathy, A.; Khosla, A.; Bernstein, M.; et al. ImageNet Large Scale Visual Recognition Challenge. *Int. J. Comput. Vis. (IJCV)* **2015**, *115*, 211–252. [CrossRef]
6. Szegedy, C.; Vanhoucke, V.; Ioffe, S.; Shlens, J.; Wojna, Z. Rethinking the Inception Architecture for Computer Vision. In Proceedings of the IEEE Computer Society Conference on Computer Vision and Pattern Recognition, Las Vegas, NV, USA, 27–30 June 2016. [CrossRef]
7. Alom, M.Z.; Taha, T.M.; Yakopcic, C.; Westberg, S.; Sidike, P.; Nasrin, M.S.; Hasan, M.; Van Essen, B.C.; Awwal, A.A.; Asari, V.K. A state-of-the-art survey on deep learning theory and architectures. *Electronics* **2019**, *8*, 292. [CrossRef]
8. Guidotti, R.; Monreale, A.; Ruggieri, S.; Turini, F.; Giannotti, F.; Pedreschi, D. A survey of methods for explaining black box models. *ACM Comput. Surv.* **2018**, *51*, 1–42. [CrossRef]
9. Urolagin, S.; Prema, K.; Reddy, N.S. Generalization capability of artificial neural network incorporated with pruning method. In Proceedings of the International Conference on Advanced Computing, Networking and Security, Surathkal, India, 16–18 December 2011; pp. 171–178.
10. Chung, Y.; Haas, P.J.; Upfal, E.; Kraska, T. Unknown Examples & Machine Learning Model Generalization. *arXiv* **2018**, arXiv:1808.08294.
11. Mutasa, S.; Sun, S.; Ha, R. Understanding artificial intelligence based radiology studies: What is overfitting? *Clin. Imaging* **2020**, *65*, 96–99. [CrossRef]
12. Ying, X. An Overview of Overfitting and its Solutions. *J. Phys. Conf. Ser.* **2019**, *1168*, 022022. [CrossRef]
13. Hadi, H.J.; Shnain, A.H.; Hadishaheed, S.; Ahmad, A.H. Big Data And Five V's Characteristics. *Int. J. Adv. Electron. Comput. Sci.* **2015**, *2*, 16–23.
14. Kohli, M.; Summers, R.; Geis, J. Medical Image Data and Datasets in the Era of Machine Learning-Whitepaper from the 2016 C-MIMI Meeting Dataset Session. *J. Digit. Imaging* **2017**, *30*, 392–399. [CrossRef]
15. Lysaght, T.; Lim, H.Y.; Xafis, V.; Ngiam, K.Y. AI-Assisted Decision-making in Healthcare. *Asian Bioeth. Rev.* **2019**, *11*, 299–314. [CrossRef]

16. Tobore, I.; Li, J.; Yuhang, L.; Al-Handarish, Y.; Kandwal, A.; Nie, Z.; Wang, L. Deep Learning Intervention for Health Care Challenges: Some Biomedical Domain Considerations. *JMIR mHealth uHealth* **2019**, *7*, e11966. [CrossRef]
17. Hazarika, I. Artificial intelligence: Opportunities and implications for the health workforce. *Int. Health* **2020**, *12*, 241–245. [CrossRef]
18. Kiani, A.; Uyumazturk, B.; Rajpurkar, P.; Wang, A.; Gao, R.; Jones, E.; Yu, Y.; Langlotz, C.P.; Ball, R.L.; Montine, T.J.; et al. Impact of a deep learning assistant on the histopathologic classification of liver cancer. *NPJ Digit. Med.* **2020**, *3*, 23. [CrossRef]
19. Hulsen, T.; Jamuar, S.S.; Moody, A.R.; Karnes, J.H.; Varga, O.; Hedensted, S.; Spreafico, R.; Hafler, D.A.; McKinney, E.F. From big data to precision medicine. *Front. Med.* **2019**, *6*, 34. [CrossRef]
20. Doi, K. Computer-aided diagnosis in medical imaging: Historical review, current status and future potential. *Comput. Med. Imaging Graph.* **2007**, *31*, 198–211. [CrossRef]
21. Liu, X.; Faes, L.; Kale, A.U.; Wagner, S.K.; Fu, D.J.; Bruynseels, A.; Mahendiran, T.; Moraes, G.; Shamdas, M.; Kern, C.; et al. A comparison of deep learning performance against health-care professionals in detecting diseases from medical imaging: A systematic review and meta-analysis. *Lancet Digit. Health* **2019**, *1*, e271–e297. [CrossRef]
22. Campion, E.W.; Jarcho, J.A. Watched by Apple. *N. Engl. J. Med.* **2019**, *381*, 1964–1965. [CrossRef]
23. Perez, M.V.; Mahaffey, K.W.; Hedlin, H.; Rumsfeld, J.S.; Garcia, A.; Ferris, T.; Balasubramanian, V.; Russo, A.M.; Rajmane, A.; Cheung, L.; et al. Large-Scale Assessment of a Smartwatch to Identify Atrial Fibrillation. *N. Engl. J. Med.* **2019**, *381*, 1909–1917. [CrossRef]
24. Abouelmehdi, K.; Beni-Hessane, A.; Khaloufi, H. Big healthcare data: Preserving security and privacy. *J. Big Data* **2018**, *5*, 1. [CrossRef]
25. Cios, K.J.; William Moore, G. Uniqueness of medical data mining. *Artif. Intell. Med.* **2002**, *26*, 1–24. [CrossRef]
26. ALLEA; EASAC; FEAM. *International Sharing of Personal Health Data for Research*; The ALLEA, EASAC and FEAM Joint Initiative on Resolving the Barriers of Transferring Public Sector Data Outside the EU/EEA; 2021; p. 63. Available online: www.doi.org/10.26356/IHDT (accessed on 3 March 2021). [CrossRef]
27. Moner, D.; Maldonado, J.A.; Bosca, D.; Fernández, J.T.; Angulo, C.; Crespo, P.; Vivancos, P.J.; Robles, M. Archetype-based semantic integration and standardization of clinical data. In Proceedings of the 2006 International Conference of the IEEE Engineering in Medicine and Biology Society, New York, NY, USA, 30 August–3 September 2006; pp. 5141–5144.
28. Berlanga, R.; Jimenez-Ruiz, E.; Nebot, V.; Manset, D.; Branson, A.; Hauer, T.; McClatchey, R.; Rogulin, D.; Shamdasani, J.; Zillner, S.; et al. Medical data integration and the semantic annotation of medical protocols. In Proceedings of the 2008 21st IEEE International Symposium on Computer-Based Medical Systems, Jyväskylä, Finland, 17–19 June 2008; pp. 644–649.
29. Cheung, K.H.; Prud'hommeaux, E.; Wang, Y.; Stephens, S. Semantic Web for Health Care and Life Sciences: A review of the state of the art. *Brief. Bioinform.* **2009**, *10*, 111–113. [CrossRef]
30. Sonsilphong, S.; Arch-int, N. Semantic Interoperability for data integration framework using semantic web services and rule-based inference: A case study in healthcare domain. *J. Converg. Inf. Technol. (JCIT)* **2013**, *8*, 150–159.
31. Lenz, R.; Beyer, M.; Kuhn, K.A. Semantic integration in healthcare networks. *Int. J. Med. Inform.* **2007**, *76*, 201–207. [CrossRef] [PubMed]
32. Mortensen, K.; Hughes, T.L. Comparing Amazon's Mechanical Turk platform to conventional data collection methods in the health and medical research literature. *J. Gen. Intern. Med.* **2018**, *33*, 533–538. [CrossRef] [PubMed]
33. Bontcheva, K.; Roberts, I.; Derczynski, L.; Rout, D. The GATE crowdsourcing plugin: Crowdsourcing annotated corpora made easy. In Proceedings of the Demonstrations at the 14th Conference of the European Chapter of the Association for Computational Linguistics, Gothenburg, Sweden, 26–30 April 2014; pp. 97–100.
34. de Herrera, A.G.S.; Foncubierta-Rodríguez, A.; Markonis, D.; Schaer, R.; Müller, H. Crowdsourcing for medical image classification. In Proceedings of the Annual Congress SGMI, 2014; Volume 2014. Available online: https://hesso.tind.io/record/698 (accessed on 3 May 2021).
35. Hannun, A.Y.; Rajpurkar, P.; Haghpanahi, M.; Tison, G.H.; Bourn, C.; Turakhia, M.P.; Ng, A.Y. Cardiologist-level arrhythmia detection and classification in ambulatory electrocardiograms using a deep neural network. *Nat. Med.* **2019**, *25*, 65–69. [CrossRef] [PubMed]
36. Raghu, M.; Zhang, C.; Kleinberg, J.; Bengio, S. Transfusion: Understanding transfer learning for medical imaging. In Proceedings of the Annual Conference on Neural Information Processing Systems 2019, Vancouver, BC, Canada, 8–14 December 2019; pp. 3347–3357.
37. Kim, H.G.; Choi, Y.; Ro, Y.M. Modality-bridge transfer learning for medical image classification. In Proceedings of the 2017 10th International Congress on Image and Signal Processing, BioMedical Engineering and Informatics, Shanghai, China, 14–16 October 2017. [CrossRef]
38. Maqsood, M.; Nazir, F.; Khan, U.; Aadil, F.; Jamal, H.; Mehmood, I.; Song, O.Y. Transfer Learning Assisted Classification and Detection of Alzheimer's Disease Stages Using 3D MRI Scans. *Sensors* **2019**, *19*, 2645. [CrossRef]
39. Drosatos, G.; Kaldoudi, E. Blockchain applications in the biomedical domain: A scoping review. *Comput. Struct. Biotechnol. J.* **2019**, *17*, 229–240. [CrossRef]
40. Justinia, T. Blockchain Technologies: Opportunities for Solving Real-World Problems in Healthcare and Biomedical Sciences. *Acta Inform. Medica* **2019**, *27*, 284–291. [CrossRef]

41. Kuo, T.T.; Kim, H.E.; Ohno-Machado, L. Blockchain distributed ledger technologies for biomedical and health care applications. *J. Am. Med. Inform. Assoc.* **2017**, *24*, 1211–1220. [CrossRef]
42. Finck, M. Blockchains and Data Protection in the European Union. *Eur. Data Prot. Law Rev.* **2018**. [CrossRef]
43. Radanović, I.; Likić, R. Opportunities for use of blockchain technology in medicine. *Appl. Health Econ. Health Policy* **2018**, *16*, 583–590. [CrossRef]
44. Zhang, P.; White, J.; Schmidt, D.C.; Lenz, G.; Rosenbloom, S.T. FHIRChain: Applying blockchain to securely and scalably share clinical data. *Comput. Struct. Biotechnol. J.* **2018**, *16*, 267–278. [CrossRef]
45. Glicksberg, B.S.; Burns, S.; Currie, R.; Griffin, A.; Wang, Z.J.; Haussler, D.; Goldstein, T.; Collisson, E. Blockchain-Authenticated Sharing of Genomic and Clinical Outcomes Data of Patients With Cancer: A Prospective Cohort Study. *J. Med. Internet Res.* **2020**, *22*, e16810. [CrossRef]
46. Kulemin, N.; Popov, S.; Gorbachev, A. The Zenome Project: Whitepaper blockchain-based genomic ecosystem. *Zenome* **2017**. [CrossRef]
47. Lata, K.; Dave, M.; Nishanth, K.N. Data Augmentation Using Generative Adversarial Network. *SSRN Electron. J.* **2019**. [CrossRef]
48. Benaim, A.R.; Almog, R.; Gorelik, Y.; Hochberg, I.; Nassar, L.; Mashiach, T.; Khamaisi, M.; Lurie, Y.; Azzam, Z.S.; Khoury, J.; et al. Analyzing medical research results based on synthetic data and their relation to real data results: Systematic comparison from five observational studies. *JMIR Med. Inform.* **2020**, *8*, e16492. [CrossRef]
49. Rankin, D.; Black, M.; Bond, R.; Wallace, J.; Mulvenna, M.; Epelde, G. Reliability of supervised machine learning using synthetic data in health care: Model to preserve privacy for data sharing. *JMIR Med. Inform.* **2020**, *8*, e18910. [CrossRef]
50. Walonoski, J.; Kramer, M.; Nichols, J.; Quina, A.; Moesel, C.; Hall, D.; Duffett, C.; Dube, K.; Gallagher, T.; McLachlan, S. Synthea: An approach, method, and software mechanism for generating synthetic patients and the synthetic electronic health care record. *J. Am. Med. Inform. Assoc.* **2018**, *25*, 230–238. [CrossRef]
51. Chen, J.; Chun, D.; Patel, M.; Chiang, E.; James, J. The validity of synthetic clinical data: A validation study of a leading synthetic data generator (Synthea) using clinical quality measures. *BMC Med. Inform. Decis. Mak.* **2019**, *19*, 44. [CrossRef]
52. Borji, A. Pros and cons of GAN evaluation measures. *Comput. Vis. Image Underst.* **2019**, *179*, 41–65. [CrossRef]
53. Wilkinson, M.D.; Dumontier, M.; Aalbersberg, I.J.; Appleton, G.; Axton, M.; Baak, A.; Blomberg, N.; Boiten, J.W.; da Silva Santos, L.B.; Bourne, P.E.; et al. The FAIR Guiding Principles for scientific data management and stewardship. *Sci. Data* **2016**, *3*, 160018. [CrossRef]
54. Koehorst, J.J.; van Dam, J.C.; Saccenti, E.; Martins dos Santos, V.A.; Suarez-Diez, M.; Schaap, P.J. SAPP: Functional genome annotation and analysis through a semantic framework using FAIR principles. *Bioinformatics* **2018**, *34*, 1401–1403. [CrossRef] [PubMed]
55. Cole, C.L.; Sengupta, S.; Rossetti, S.; Vawdrey, D.K.; Halaas, M.; Maddox, T.M.; Gordon, G.; Dave, T.; Payne, P.R.O.; Williams, A.E.; et al. Ten principles for data sharing and commercialization. *J. Am. Med Inform. Assoc.* **2020**, *28*, 646–649. [CrossRef] [PubMed]
56. European Commission. *Managing Health Data*; European Commission: Brussels, Belgium, 2019.
57. European Commission. *eHealth: Digital Health and Care*; European Commission: Brussels, Belgium, 2020.
58. European Commission. *Digital Single Market*; European Commission: Brussels, Belgium, 2019.
59. Information Commissioner's Office (ICO). *Guide to the General Data Protection Regulation (GDPR)*; ICO: Wilmslow, UK, 2018.
60. Mostert, M.; Bredenoord, A.L.; Van Der Slootb, B.; Van Delden, J.J. From privacy to data protection in the EU: Implications for big data health research. *Eur. J. Health Law* **2017**, *25*, 43–55. [CrossRef]
61. Dridi, A.; Sassi, S.; Chbeir, R.; Faiz, S. A flexible semantic integration framework for fully-integrated EHR based on FHIR standard. In Proceedings of the 12th International Conference on Agents and Artificial Intelligence (ICAART 2020), Valletta, Malta, 22–24 February 2020. [CrossRef]
62. Weiler, G.; Schwarz, U.; Rauch, J.; Rohm, K.; Lehr, T.; Theobald, S.; Kiefer, S.; Götz, K.; Och, K.; Pfeifer, N.; et al. XplOit: An ontology-based data integration platform supporting the development of predictive models for personalized medicine. *Stud. Health Technol. Inform.* **2018**. [CrossRef]
63. Zillner, S.; Neururer, S. Big data in the health sector. In *New Horizons for a Data-Driven Economy: A Roadmap for Usage and Exploitation of Big Data in Europe*; Springer: Cham, Switzerland, 2016. [CrossRef]
64. Hong, N.; Wen, A.; Shen, F.; Sohn, S.; Wang, C.; Liu, H.; Jiang, G. Developing a scalable FHIR-based clinical data normalization pipeline for standardizing and integrating unstructured and structured electronic health record data. *JAMIA Open* **2019**, *2*, 570–579. [CrossRef]
65. Wang, Z.; Jensen, M.A.; Zenklusen, J.C. A practical guide to The Cancer Genome Atlas (TCGA). In *Methods in Molecular Biology*; Springer: New York, NY, USA, 2016. [CrossRef]
66. Clark, K.; Vendt, B.; Smith, K.; Freymann, J.; Kirby, J.; Koppel, P.; Moore, S.; Phillips, S.; Maffitt, D.; Pringle, M.; et al. The cancer imaging archive (TCIA): Maintaining and operating a public information repository. *J. Digit. Imaging* **2013**, *26*, 1045–1057. [CrossRef]
67. Sayers, E.W.; Beck, J.; Bolton, E.E.; Bourexis, D.; Brister, J.R.; Canese, K.; Comeau, D.C.; Funk, K.; Kim, S.; Klimke, W.; et al. Database resources of the National Center for Biotechnology Information. *Nucleic Acids Res.* **2021**, *36*, D13–D21. [CrossRef]
68. Stanford Center for Artificial Intelligence in Medicine and Imaging. *Medical ImageNet*; Stanford Center for Artificial Intelligence in Medicine and Imaging: Stanford, CA, USA, 2019.

69. Tang, A.; Tam, R.; Cadrin-Chênevert, A.; Guest, W.; Chong, J.; Barfett, J.; Chepelev, L.; Cairns, R.; Mitchell, J.R.; Cicero, M.D.; et al. Canadian Association of Radiologists White Paper on Artificial Intelligence in Radiology. *Can. Assoc. Radiol. J.* **2018**, *69*, 120–135. [CrossRef]
70. National Institutes of Health—Office of Data Science Strategy. *Open-Access Data and Computational Resources to Address COVID-19*; National Institutes of Health: Bethesda, MD, USA, 2020.

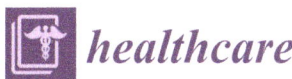

Article

Telemedicine in the Time of the COVID-19 Pandemic: Results from the First Survey among Italian Pediatric Diabetes Centers

Gianluca Tornese [1], Riccardo Schiaffini [2], Enza Mozzillo [3], Roberto Franceschi [4], Anna Paola Frongia [5], Andrea Scaramuzza [6,*], on behalf of HCL Expert Pathway Pediatric Group [†] and the Diabetes Study Group of the Italian Society for Pediatric Endocrinology [‡]

1. Institute for Maternal and Child Health, IRCCS Burlo Garofolo, 34137 Trieste, Italy; gianluca.tornese@burlo.trieste.it
2. Diabetes Unit, Bambino Gesù Children's Hospital, 00165 Rome, Italy; riccardo.schiaffini@opbg.net
3. Regional Center for Pediatric Diabetes, Section of Pediatrics, Department of Translational Medical Science, University of Naples Federico II, 80131 Naples, Italy; mozzilloenza@gmail.com
4. Department of Pediatrics, Santa Chiara Hospital Trento, 38122 Trento, Italy; roberto.franceschi@apss.tn.it
5. Unit of Pediatric Diabetes, Brotzu Hospital, 09134 Cagliari, Italy; annapaolafrongia@aob.it
6. Division of Pediatrics, ASST Cremona, "Ospedale Maggiore di Cremona", Viale Concordia 1, 26100 Cremona, Italy
* Correspondence: a.scaramuzza@gmail.com; Tel.: +39-0372-405375
† Membership of the HCL Expert Pathway Pediatric Group is provided in the Acknowledgments.
‡ Membership of the Diabetes Study Group of the Italian Society for Pediatric Endocrinology is provided in the Acknowledgments.

Citation: Tornese, G.; Schiaffini, R.; Mozzillo, E.; Franceschi, R.; Frongia, A.P.; Scaramuzza, A.; on behalf of HCL Expert Pathway Pediatric Group; the Diabetes Study Group of the Italian Society for Pediatric Endocrinology. Telemedicine in the Time of the COVID-19 Pandemic: Results from the First Survey among Italian Pediatric Diabetes Centers. *Healthcare* **2021**, *9*, 815. https://doi.org/10.3390/healthcare9070815

Academic Editor: Daniele Giansanti

Received: 27 May 2021
Accepted: 23 June 2021
Published: 28 June 2021

Publisher's Note: MDPI stays neutral with regard to jurisdictional claims in published maps and institutional affiliations.

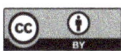

Copyright: © 2021 by the authors. Licensee MDPI, Basel, Switzerland. This article is an open access article distributed under the terms and conditions of the Creative Commons Attribution (CC BY) license (https://creativecommons.org/licenses/by/4.0/).

Abstract: Background: Use of telemedicine for children and adolescents with type 1 diabetes at the beginning of the COVID-19 pandemic was investigated. Method: 68 Italian pediatric diabetes centers were invited to complete a survey about telemedicine usage in their pediatric patients, allocated to the no-tech group (multiple daily injections and self-monitoring blood glucose) and the tech group (insulin pump and/or flash- or continuous-glucose monitoring). Results: 60.3% of the centers completed the survey. In both the no-tech and tech groups, the most used ways of communication were generic download portals, instant messaging with personal physicians' mobiles, working emails, and phone calls to physicians' mobiles, with no difference, except for the use of email being higher in the no-tech group ($p = 0.03$). Seventy-four percent of the centers did not have any systematization and/or reimbursement, with significant differences among regions ($p = 0.03$). Conclusions: Almost all Italian pediatric diabetes centers use telemedicine in a semi-volunteering manner, lacking proper codification, reimbursement system, legal traceability, and accreditation system.

Keywords: telemedicine; continuous glucose monitoring; insulin pump; continuous subcutaneous insulin infusion; pediatric diabetes

1. Introduction

Telemedicine is a term thought up in the 1970s, which literally means "healing at a distance" [1]. It involves the use of information and computer technology to improve patient outcomes by increasing access to care and medical information. Recognizing that there is no definitive description of telemedicine, a 2007 study revealed the existence of 104 peer-reviewed definitions of the word [2] and the World Health Organization adopted a broad delineation of the term: "The delivery of healthcare services, where distance is a critical factor, by all healthcare professionals using information and communication technologies for the exchange of valid information for diagnosis, treatment, prevention of disease and injuries, research, evaluation, and for the continuing education of healthcare providers, all in the interests of advancing the health of individuals and their communities" [3].

Some think that telemedicine differs from telehealth, with the former limited to the service provided only by physicians, and the latter including healthcare professionals in general, such as nurses, pharmacists, and others.

Telemedicine has four key elements: (1) Its purpose is to provide clinical support; (2) it is intended to overcome geographical barriers, connecting users who are not in the same physical location; (3) it involves the use of various types of information and computer technology; (4) its goal is to improve health outcomes [4].

Initially, it was intended to be used, especially in developing countries, to overcome the distances between people and hospitals. However, during these hard times due to COVID-19, where social distancing has become a rule in many countries, including Italy, telemedicine could play a crucial role. In this regard, Hollander and Carr [5] in their recently published perspective on telemedicine stated that "disasters and pandemics pose unique challenges to health care delivery."

Due to the COVID-19 pandemic, on 9 March 2020, Italy was placed under its first national lockdown. A law decree issued by the Prime Minister's Office (called #stayhome, or #iorestoacasa in Italian) ordered people across the entire peninsula, with unprecedented measures, to stay at home, and banned all public meetings and travel, excluding only those for "urgent, verifiable work situations and emergencies or health reasons" [6]. This occurrence led Italy to rediscover smart working in many contexts, including telemedicine.

However, if telemedicine already offers a way to be close to patients even from afar, there is still insufficient evidence to support its use in glycemic control and other clinically relevant outcomes among patients with type 1 diabetes [7]. Moreover, there is still little information available about the use of telemedicine in pediatric diabetes, and so far, no studies have evaluated its extension and modalities in Italy.

This survey aimed to investigate in all Italian pediatric diabetes centers at the beginning of the COVID-19 pandemic: (a) The tools used to provide telemedicine services for children and adolescents with type 1 diabetes, both in patients using or not using technological tools (e.g., insulin pumps and/or flash/continuous glucose monitoring systems); (b) the administrative recognition for telemedicine activities; (c) the reimbursement of telemedicine activities.

2. Materials and Methods

2.1. Participants

All of the 68 Italian pediatric diabetes centers belonging to the Italian Society for Pediatric Endocrinology and Diabetes (ISPED) [8] were invited to complete a survey to collect data about telemedicine usage in their patients.

2.2. Questionnaire Development and Pre-Testing

A survey tool was developed composing questions using distinct and interactive steps [9]. The initial list included ten questions evaluated for face and content validity by two expert pediatric diabetologists (G.T. and E.M.) who worked independently and then agreed on the final list, providing feedback on content accuracy, wording, question order, and survey structure. A preliminary version of the survey composed of ten questions was self-administered and piloted in a convenient sample of six pediatric diabetologists. The sample reported that questions were not ambiguous, the wording was straightforward, and the self-administered experience was successful.

According to insulin treatment and blood glucose monitoring, patients were allocated into two groups to detect any differences in telemedicine use: No-tech group for patients using multiple daily injections and self-monitoring blood glucose, and tech group for patients using insulin pumps and/or flash- or continuous-glucose monitoring.

2.3. Questionnaire Implementation

A self-administered questionnaire divided into two sections (A and B) was used: In section A, the demographic variables of respondents (i.e., sex and age class) and information about the center (i.e., city, number of individuals with T1DM treatment, setting, and staff) were investigated by one open-ended question (i.e., city) and five closed-ended questions; in section B, data on telemedicine were examined by four closed-ended questions (telemedicine ways used for the no-tech and tech groups, codification, and reimbursement of telemedicine activities). The possible answers, which could be selected through a list of checkboxes shown to the respondents, were decided by the study authors, then modified and confirmed by the authors during the survey structuring phases.

2.4. Data Collection Procedure

The survey was web-based, using a commercially available survey host (it.surveymonkey.com, accessed on 10 March 2020). Responses were collected over three weeks, which started on 22 March 2020 up until 12 April 2020. An email reminder was sent two weeks after the initial contact. After ISPED permission, all subscribers of the Diabetes Study Group were contacted by email containing the link to the survey and a brief note outlining the aim of the study, data handling, informed consent statement, invitation to complete the survey, and presentation of the authors. By clicking on the survey link, respondents provided their consent to participate. Participation was voluntary, and no incentives were offered to the participants; all questions were compulsory, although it was possible to quit the questionnaire at any time. The participants were able to review or change their responses using a back button before submitting their answers. Data were downloaded and stored on an encrypted computer, and only the authors had access to the information during all stages of the study. The participants were ensured that their identities would not be disclosed to the investigators: All data were de-identified to maintain confidentiality and data protection [9].

2.5. Data Analysis

The empirical analysis was based on the survey data downloaded from SurveyMonkey into Excel spreadsheets and reviewed for accuracy and missing value. Cities were grouped according to geographical regions (i.e., northern, central, and southern Italy). Statistical analysis was conducted using JMP™ software (version 15.1.0, SAS Institute Inc., Cary, NC, USA). Data are presented as frequencies and percentages or as median and interquartile ranges (IQRs). Mann–Whitney rank-sum and two-tailed Fisher exact tests were performed to evaluate the relationship between variables. The Wilcoxon signed-rank test was carried out to check the differences of paired data. A p-value < 0.05 was considered statistically significant.

3. Results

Among the 68 centers belonging to the Italian Society for Pediatric Endocrinology and Diabetology (ISPED), 41 (60.3%) completed the web-based survey and returned complete data (Table 1). The average time to complete the survey was 3.5 min. In 10 centers, more than one physician completed the survey (two in seven centers and three in three centers) for a total of 54 people who responded to the survey (66.7% female, 45% working in public hospitals, and 55% in academic settings). The percentage of groups divided by age was: 16.4% in the 30–39-year range, 34.6% in the 40–49-year range, 27.3% in the 50–59-years range, and 21.7% in the over 60-year range.

Table 1. Survey center characteristics.

Center Characteristics	Percentage of Centers	Number of Centers
Region		
Northern Italy	43.9%	18
Central Italy	36.6%	15
Southern Italy	19.5%	8
Number of Individuals with T1DM Treated in the Center		
<100 individuals	24.4%	10
100–299 individuals	46.3%	19
≥300 individuals	29.3%	12
Setting		
Hospital	58.5%	24
Academic	41.5%	17
	Median	IQR
Staff		
Pediatric diabetologist	2	(1–2)
Dedicated specialist nurse	1	(1–1)
Dedicated dietician	1	(1–2)
Dedicated psychologist	1	(0–1)

In Table 2, the different methods of using telemedicine have been summarized. The most useful methods to communicate with the diabetes team in the no-tech group were: Generic download portals (e.g., Tidepool, Diasend™, and Glooko™) (80%), instant messaging with personal physicians' mobiles (76%), working emails (71%), and phone calls to physicians' mobiles (59%). In the tech group, the ranking of the tools was as follows: Generic download portals (88%), branded download portals (90%), instant messaging with personal physicians' mobiles (76%), working emails (59%), and phone calls to physicians' mobiles (59%). There was no significant statistical difference between or within groups, except for the use of email, which was higher in the no-tech group than in the tech group ($p = 0.03$). No significant difference was observed when analyzing the data according to country macro-region (northern, central, or southern), size of the center and hospital, or academic setting (Table 2). Only one center declared not using any tool to communicate with its tech group patients. All of the other centers declared using more than one method to communicate, with a statistical difference between the no-tech group, with a median of 4 (IQR 3–5), and the tech group, with a median of 5 (IQR 4–6) ($p = 0.002$).

In Italy, the health sanitary system is free of charge for all citizens, while the health interventions listed in the "International Statistical Classification of Diseases, Injuries and Causes of Death" (ICD10) are fully or partially reimbursed, according to age, health, and economic status. No telemedicine intervention is officially listed; however, the survey asked if any of the telemedicine interventions have been recognized and reimbursed locally? Most of the centers (74%) did not have any systematization for their telemedicine interventions (Table 3).

Table 2. Telemedicine methods used for the no-tech and tech groups according to the region, the number of patients with type 1 diabetes treated in the center, and the setting. "Others" in no-tech group: (1) Dedicated app on a smartphone; (2) paid consultation platform; (3) Skype/Webex. "Others" in the tech group: (1) "Visitami" app/Zoom; (2) dedicated app on a smartphone; (3) paid consultation platform; (4) Skype/Webex.

		Hospital Dedicated Portal	Generic Data Download Portal	Branded Data Download Portal	Working Emails	Personal Emails	Instant Messaging with Hospital Phone	Instant Messaging with Personal Phone	SMS to Hospital Phone	SMS to Personal Phone	Call to Hospital Phone	Call to Personal Phone	None of the Previous	Other
No-Tech Group	Total	12%	80%		71% *	29%	2%	76%	10%	32%	51%	59%	0%	7%
	Northern	17%	83%		83%	17%	6%	72%	22%	33%	61%	56%		11%
	Central	0%	80%		67%	20%	0%	80%	0%	27%	53%	47%		7%
	Southern	25%	75%		50% §	75%	0%	75%	0%	38%	25%	88%		0%
	p				<0.01	<0.01								
	<100 individuals	10%	90%		60% †	30%	0%	90%	20%	20%	50%	50%	0%	0%
	100–299 individuals	5%	79%		84%	11%	5%	79%	11%	42%	58%	63%		0%
	>300 individuals	25%	75%		58%	58%	0%	58%	0%	25%	42%	58%		25%
	p					0.02								0.02
	Hospital	4%	75%		63% ‡	25%	4%	88%	13%	33%	46%	54%		8%
	Academic	24%	88%		82%	35%	0%	59%	6%	29%	59%	65%		6%
	p							0.04						
Tech Group	Total	10%	88%	90%	59% *	32%	5%	76%	7%	32%	51%	59%	2%	10%
	Northern	17%	89%	94%	78%	28%	11%	72%	17%	33%	61%	56%	6%	17%
	Central	0%	93%	93%	60%	13%	0%	80%	0%	27%	53%	47%	0%	7%
	Southern	13%	75%	75%	13% §	75%	0%	75%	0%	38%	25%	88%	0%	0%
	p				<0.01	<0.01								
	<100 individuals	10%	90%	80%	30% †	40%	10%	90%	10%	20%	50%	50%	10%	0%
	100–299 individuals	5%	84%	89%	79%	21%	5%	79%	11%	42%	58%	63%	0%	5%
	>300 individuals	17%	92%	100%	50%	42%	0%	58%	0%	25%	42%	58%	0%	25%
	p				0.03			0.04						
	Hospital	4%	83%	88%	50% ‡	33%	8%	88%	8%	33%	46%	54%	4%	13%
	Academic	18%	94%	94%	71%	29%	0%	59%	6%	29%	59%	65%	0%	6%
	p							0.04						
Differences between No-Tech vs. Tech Groups	p				* 0.03 § 0.04 † 0.04 ‡ 0.04									

Table 3. Codification of telemedicine activities.

Hospital Parameter for Codification	Total	Region			Individuals with T1DM Treated			Practice Setting	
		Northern	Central	Southern	<100	100–299	>300	Hospital	Academic
Methods that should be used	9%	11%	20%	0%	20%	0%	18%	13%	12%
Content of requests from individuals	6%	11%	7%	0%	10%	0%	12%	8%	6%
Time within which the doctor has to reply	2%	6%	0%	0%	0%	0%	6%	0%	6%
Possibility during working hours	7%	11%	7%	0%	0%	7%	12%	4%	12%
Not codified	74%	72%	53%	100%	80%	79%	59%	75%	65%
Other (specify): - Specifying "telemedicine" in the report ($n = 2$) - Codified when using hospital portal ($n = 2$) - With a fee for the individual	12%	6%	27%	0%	0%	11%	25%	8%	18%

The academic centers of central Italy, with less than 100 patients, were those with a higher rate of uncodified service (Table 3). Most centers did not have any reimbursement for telemedicine interventions, with significant differences among regions (100% in southern, 72% in northern, and 47% in central Italy; $p = 0.03$) (Table 4).

Table 4. Reimbursement of telemedicine services.

Hospital Parameter for Reimbursement	Total	Region			Individuals with T1DM Treated			Practice Setting	
		Northern	Central	Southern	<100	100–299	>300	Hospital	Academic
Time spent answering	2%	0%	7%	0%	0%	0%	6%	0%	0%
"Exam overview" service	6%	6%	13%	0%	10%	0%	12%	0%	0%
"Diabetes visit" service	26%	28%	47%	0%	10%	29%	41%	0%	0%
None of the above	70%	72% *	47% *	100% *	80%	71%	59%	0%	0%
Other (specify): - After duty hours	2%	0%	7%	0%	0%	7%	0%	0%	0%

* $p = 0.03$, Fisher's exact test.

4. Discussion

On 20 February 2020, the so-called Italian Patient 1 was admitted to the intensive care unit (ICU) of the local hospital due to a deteriorating clinical condition as a result of COVID-19 infection. After a few days, most Italian hospitals, considering the growing number of people infected by COVID-19, decided to suspend outpatient activities. This decision was extended to all hospitals on 9 March 2020, due to the lockdown, which is still ongoing.

For this reason, most ISPED centers have begun telemedicine activities, even if, in many cases, these have never been officially started. Therefore, this survey was conducted, and, to the best of the authors' knowledge, it is the first to be conducted among the pediatric diabetes centers in Italy and perhaps in Europe.

Telemedicine was originally proposed to facilitate contact between people and healthcare providers in developing countries [1–3]. However, to facilitate the containment of the epidemiological emergency due to COVID-19, telemedicine is now the only way to provide healthcare services for the treatment of chronic diseases that do not need physical proximity (e.g., type 1 diabetes in pediatric patients, among others).

The technological development in recent years in the type 1 diabetes field has led to an increase in the use of technology, with the possibility of remote access to continuous glucose monitoring systems and insulin pump data, downloaded by patients in the comfort of their own homes. This opportunity leads to synergy, the involvement of the patients and families, and a sharing of practices that do not require a physical presence (which also remains fundamental in some situations) and could be implemented to save time, travel, and expenses.

In the present survey, all centers, except one, used at least one telemedicine tool, with an average of four methods for the no-tech group and five for the tech group patients, which resulted significantly higher, probably due to the use of insulin pumps and continuous glucose monitoring systems in the latter group.

The most used methods were data download portals, working emails, instant messaging, or phone calls to personal mobiles with no significant differences between the no-tech and tech groups. For the use of working emails only, the no-tech group showed a significantly higher percentage of centers that used them compared to the tech group. The reason could be that the tech group is more prone to using telemonitoring and connection devices than the no-tech group. Indeed, the tech group used the branded download software to a greater extent, which could be of help in data transfer (e.g., CareLink Personal™ and Dexcom Clarity™).

According to the results of this survey, the application of telemedicine appears to be commonly used by Italian pediatric diabetes centers for assisting patients in managing diabetes, as it facilitates the communication of accurate and reliable data between patients and their healthcare providers. It also empowers patients' attitudes and behavior toward a healthier lifestyle, while providing them with an outlook for better glycemic control. These telemedicine services could be categorized into synchronous (real-time), asynchronous (whereby data are stored and forwarded subsequently), and continuous (remote monitoring).

Nevertheless, it is a shame that only one of four centers reported organization and reimbursement of telemedicine activities. Unfortunately, almost all pediatric diabetes centers in Italy used telemedicine in a semi-volunteering manner because of the lack of proper codification and a reimbursement system. Moreover, most of the methods used (i.e., working emails, text messaging, instant messaging, and phone calls) showed a lack of any legal traceability and are not subject to any accreditation system that might guarantee patients, healthcare providers, and the paying subject [10].

The Italian National Guidelines on Telemedicine published in 2014 [11] state that telemedicine "involves the secure transmission of medical information and data in the form of texts, sounds, images or other forms necessary for the prevention, diagnosis, treatment and subsequent monitoring of patients." Moreover, it adds that "the use of Information and Communication Technology tools for the treatment of health information or the online sharing of data and health information do not in themselves constitute telemedicine services: as an example, telemedicine does not include health information portals, social networks, forums, newsgroups, emails or others."

In Italy, though, these guidelines provide the regulatory framework, and the new basic healthcare levels (what the National Health System reimburse) were approved in 2017 [12], comprising of telemedicine as an "alternative and augmentative communication tools and software." However, the present survey showed that telemedicine in pediatric diabetes is still used in a semi-voluntary way, due to the lack of adequate and uniform platforms, legally accurate traceability of most telemedicine tools, and non-recognition of the work and "televisits" in budgetary terms.

The ability to encrypt emails, thereby ensuring patient confidentiality, is considered difficult when using regular email accounts and none of the respondents reported using certified email accounts. Alternative web-based applications (such as dedicated hospital portals) where the encryption could be implemented would be a good option for security and direct codification, as well as subsequent reimbursement; however, to date, only 11% of centers have had the chance to use this option in Italy.

It is believed that telemedicine must be subjected to an accreditation system that guarantees patients, healthcare providers, and paying subjects, but this system has not yet been implemented.

Although the Italian Health Sanitary System is free of charge (including telemedicine services), the issue of equity problems in telemedicine (similarly to in distance learning programs) should be kept in mind, since poorer families often do not have proper technical devices and a reliable internet connection. Data published in May 2020 by the Italian National Institute of Statistics (ISTAT) revealed that 12.3% of young people aged 6–17 years did not have any personal computer or tablet at home [13].

It is vital to build awareness of these barriers regarding the development of telemedicine and to remove financial barriers (e.g., implementing waivers to purchase essential devices and internet access).

5. Conclusions

Almost all of the surveyed Italian pediatric diabetes centers use telemedicine in a semi-volunteering manner, lacking proper codification, reimbursement system, legal traceability, and accreditation system.

Therefore, the time has come, starting from an extraordinary situation, such as the need to assist our pediatric patients during the COVID-19 pandemic, for the Italian National Health System and our hospitals to carefully examine the advantages of telemedicine to fill this gap [14].

Author Contributions: G.T. and E.M. drafted the survey, collected data, and discussed the results. G.T. ran the statistical analysis. R.S., R.F. and A.P.F. collected data, discussed the results, and revised the manuscript. A.S. collected data, discussed the results, wrote the manuscript, and contributed to the discussion. All authors have read and agreed to the published version of the manuscript.

Funding: This research received no external funding.

Institutional Review Board Statement: This study was conducted according to the guidelines of the Declaration of Helsinki and approved by the Institutional Review Board of Burlo Garolfo Hospital, Trieste.

Informed Consent Statement: Not applicable.

Data Availability Statement: The data are available on request.

Acknowledgments: The authors thank Martina Bradaschia for the English revision of the manuscript. List of the contributing authors [†] of the HCL Expert Pathway Pediatric Group and the [‡] Diabetes Study Group of the Italian Society for Pediatric Endocrinology and Diabetology (ISPED). The following people were actively involved in the collection of data and thus have to be considered as authors of this paper: [†] V. Cherubini (Ancona); [‡] A. Bobbio (Aosta); [‡] E. Schieven (Arzignano); [†] E. Piccinno and [‡] M. Delvecchio (Bari); [‡] S. Zucchini and [†] G. Maltoni (Bologna); [‡] P. Reinstadler (Bolzano); [‡] B. Felappi and [‡] E. Prandi (Brescia); [‡] F. Gallo (Brindisi); [†] A.P. Frongia and [†] C. Ripoli (Cagliari); [‡] R. Maccioni (Carbonia); [‡] D. Lo Presti, [‡] L. Tomaselli, and [‡] T. Timpanaro (Catania); [‡] F. Citriniti (Catanzaro); [‡] V. Graziani, [‡] S.Monti, and [‡] T. Suprani, (Cesena, Ravenna); [†] F. De Berardinis (Cetraro); [†] A. Scaramuzza (Cremona); [‡] V. De Donno (Cuneo); [‡] L. Lenzi and [‡] S.Toni (Florence); [‡] B. Mainetti (Forlì); [‡] M.S. Coccioli (Francavilla Fontana); [†] N. Minuto (Genoa); [‡] R. Maccioni (Iglesias); [‡] P. Macellaro (Legnano); [‡] S. Sordelli (Mantova); [†] F. Lombardo (Messina); [†] R. Bonfanti, [‡] A. Rigamonti, [‡] C. Mameli, and [†] M. Macedoni (Milano), [‡] L. Iughetti (Modena); [‡] A. Franzese, [†] E. Mozzillo, [†] D. Iafusco, and [†] A. Zanfardino (Naples); [†] I: Rabbone and [‡] S. Savastio (Novara); [‡] G. Piredda (Olbia); [‡] B. Iovane (Parma); [‡] V. Calcaterra (Pavia); [‡] M.G. Berioli (Perugia);

‡ E. Randazzo (Pisa); ‡ A. Lasagni (Reggio Emilia); ‡ I. Patera, ‡ M.C. Matteoli, and † R. Schiaffini, (Rome); ‡ I. Rutigliano (San Giovanni Rotondo); ‡ L. De Sanctis, ‡ D. Tinti, and ‡ M. Trada (Turin); ‡ L. Guerraggio and ‡ S. Zonca (Tradate); ‡ V. Cauvin and † R. Franceschi (Trento); † G. Tornese and ‡ E. Faleschini (Trieste); ‡ A.A. Trattene (Varese); † M. Marigliano and ‡ C. Maffeis (Verona); † C. Arnaldi (Viterbo).

Conflicts of Interest: No conflict of interest to disclose exist for any of the authors. All authors and members of the HCL group received travel expenses from Medtronic for the meetings.

References

1. Strehle, E.M.; Shabde, N. One hundred years of telemedicine: Does this new technology have a place in paediatrics? *Arch. Dis. Child.* **2006**, *91*, 956–959. [CrossRef] [PubMed]
2. Sood, S.P.; Negash, S.; Mbarika, V.W.A.; Kifle, M.; Prakash, N. Differences in public and private sector adoption of telemedicine: Indian case study for sectoral adoption. *Stud. Health Technol. Inform.* **2007**, *130*, 257–268. [PubMed]
3. WHO. *A Health Telematics Policy in Support of WHO's Health-For-All Strategy for Global Health Development: Report of the WHO Group Consultation on Health Telematics, 11–16 December, Geneva*; World Health Organization: Geneva, Switzerland, 1997.
4. WHO. *Telemedicine: Opportunities and Developments in Member States. Report on the Second Global Survey on eHealth. Geneva*; World Health Organization: Geneva, Switzerland, 2010.
5. Hollander, J.E.; Carr, B.G. Virtually Perfect? Telemedicine for Covid-19. *New Engl. J. Med.* **2020**, *382*, 1679–1681. [CrossRef] [PubMed]
6. Decree of the Italian Prime Minister of March 9th. Further Measures for the Containment and Contrast of the Spread of the Covid-19 Virus throughout the Entire National Territory. 2020. Available online: https://www.simmons-simmons.com/en/publications/ck7m28wsg1uxf0a60ykkd8fre/the-spread-of-covid-19-in-italy-a-wide-legal-approach- (accessed on 26 June 2020).
7. Lee, S.W.H.; Ooi, L.; Lai, Y.K. Telemedicine for the Management of Glycemic Control and Clinical Outcomes of Type 1 Diabetes Mellitus: A Systematic Review and Meta-Analysis of Randomized Controlled Studies. *Front. Pharm.* **2017**, *8*, 330. [CrossRef] [PubMed]
8. Giorgetti, C.; Ferrito, L.; Zallocco, F.; Iannilli, A.; Cherubini, V. Study group for Diabetes of ISPED. Organization and regional distribution of centers for the management of children and adolescents with diabetes in Italy. *Ital. J. Pediatr.* **2015**, *41*, 74. [PubMed]
9. De Leeuw, D.; Hox, J.; Dillman, D. *International Handbook of Survey Methodology*, 1st ed.; European Association of Methodology Series; Taylor and Francis Group: New York, NY, USA, 2008.
10. Caffery, L.J.; Smith, A.C. A literature review of email-based telemedicine. *Stud. Health Technol. Inform.* **2010**, *161*, 20–34. [PubMed]
11. Italian Ministry of Health. Telemedicine National Guidelines. Available online: http://www.salute.gov.it/imgs/C_17_pubblicazioni_2129_allegato.pdf (accessed on 12 September 2020).
12. Ferorelli, D.; Nardelli, L.; Spagnolo, L.; Corradi, S.; Silvestre, M.; Misceo, F.; Marrone, M.; Zotti, F.; Mandarelli, G.; Solarino, B.; et al. Medical legal aspects of telemedicine in Italy: Application fields, professional liability and focus on care services during the COVID-19 health emergency. *J. Prim. Care Community Health* **2020**, *11*, 2150132720985055. [CrossRef] [PubMed]
13. Italian National Institute of Statistics (ISTAT). Computers and Tablets in the ITALIAN Households—Years 2018/2019. Available online: https://www.istat.it/en/archivio/242572 (accessed on 12 September 2020).
14. Tornese, G.; Scaramuzza, A.; Schiaffini, R. Telemedicine in the time of the Coronavirus. *Med. E Bambino* **2020**, *39*, 142.

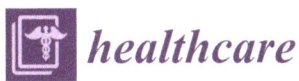

Article

The Impact of Health Information Sharing on Hospital Costs

Na-Eun Cho

College of Business, Hongik University, Seoul 04066, Korea; ncho@hongik.ac.kr

Abstract: Despite substantial progress in the adoption of health information technology (IT), researchers remain uncertain as to whether IT investments benefit hospitals. This study evaluates the effect of health information sharing on the cost of care, and whether the effect varies with context. Our results suggest that information sharing using health IT, specifically the extent (breadth) and level of detail (depth) of information sharing, helps to reduce the cost of care at the hospital level. The results also show that the effects of depth of information sharing on cost savings are salient in poor and less-concentrated regions, but not in wealthier, more-concentrated areas, whereas the the effects of breadth of information sharing on cost savings are equivalent across wealth and concentration. To realize the benefits of using health IT more effectively, policy makers' strategies for encouraging active use of health IT should be informed by market characteristics.

Keywords: health information technology; information sharing; hospital costs; poverty ratio; concentration

1. Introduction

More than 10 years have elapsed since the passage of the Health Information Technology for Economic and Clinical Health (HITECH) act of 2009 designed to spur adoption and promote the use of electronic health records (EHR) for the purposes of improving quality and reducing costs [1]. Putting aside ongoing debate as to whether this policy intervention has helped drive hospital adoption of health IT [2,3], the EHR adoption rate has risen substantially—more than 95% of non-federal acute care hospitals reported to possess certified health IT as of 2017 [4]. The more important question then becomes whether the use of health IT has achieved the predicted benefits.

Research to date examining how adoption of health IT affects hospital outcomes has produced mixed results regarding effects on quality and cost of care [5–9]. Although most studies conclude that effects are generally positive (e.g., lower morality rates, reduced costs, fewer complications, fewer unnecessary tests), some research suggests that health IT implementation does not always generate desired results [5–9]. EHR adoption was found by one study to have no effect on quality and costs [5], and by another to increase costs, especially in non-IT-intensive locations [7].

A number of factors could account for the inconclusive results of prior research. One is that most prior studies have focused simply on the adoption of health IT [5–9]. Since the federal government began emphasizing the prevalence of this new technology, determinants of and barriers to adoption, including financial, technical, psychological, social, legal, organizational, etc., have been the main subjects of the extant literature [10,11]. Although in the early stage of adoption it was difficult to collect data on use patterns, according to the information systems literature, it is use patterns—that is, how information is shared among stakeholders—not adoption, that determine the benefits an organization derives from IT [12–15]. To better understand why some institutions have realized benefits from using health IT and others have not, the present study uses data on use patterns not employed in prior studies. Further, notwithstanding previous scholars' emphasis on the importance of taking into account context when examining the effect of health IT, research examining how the impact of health IT might vary with context remains lacking [8]. The

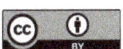

present work addresses the mixed findings of earlier studies by examining the effects of health information sharing, specifically with regard to the extent (breadth) and level of detail (depth) of information shared, and whether the effects vary with context.

Analyzing data variously obtained from the American Hospital Association's (AHA's) annual and IT surveys, the Center for Medicare and Medicaid Services' (CMS') Hospital Compare database, and the Census Bureau's small-area income and poverty estimates, we find that both breadth and depth of information sharing help to reduce the cost of care at the hospital level. We find depth of information sharing to provide cost savings only in poor, less-concentrated regions, not in in wealthier, more-concentrated areas, and breadth of information sharing to yield equivalent cost savings regardless of the wealth and concentration of regions. The results of the current study suggest that policy makers and practitioners carefully modify their strategies for using health IT to reflect market characteristics.

The paper is organized as follows. In Section 2, we describe our data and model, and in Section 3 discuss our empirical tests. The results are discussed in Section 4. We present our conclusions in Section 5.

2. Materials and Methods

2.1. Hypotheses Development

As mentioned in the Introduction, the present study aims to fill a gap in previous research that has produced inconclusive findings [5–9]. The current study examines actual use patterns, specifically, breadth and depth of information sharing, which thus far have received little attention in the literature [12]. The prior literature suggests that hospitals can realize economies of scale and achieve complementarity in operations as information is shared with more external parties [5,6]. Information sharing among multiple stakeholders can also reduce avoidable hospital readmissions and duplicate tests [16,17]. Sharing information at a detailed level reflects a degree of trust between hospitals and external parties that facilitates collaboration across these organizations [12]. This leads to the following hypothesis.

Hypothesis 1 (H1). *Breadth and depth determine the degree to which information sharing decreases hospital costs.*

The current study examines differences in context that might strengthen or weaken the effect of health IT, specifically, how its effect varies with wealth and concentration in the areas in which the hospitals studied operate. We expect health IT to have a greater effect in poor (high poverty ratio) than in rich (low poverty ratio) areas because the need for complementarities from other parties would be greater for those with fewer than for those with abundant resources. Similarly, we expect health IT to have a greater effect in competitive (low HHI) than in concentrated (high HHI) regions. A high concentration level indicates that a market is dominated by a small number of firms. An HHI of 1 implies that there exists only one hospital in our sample. Given only one or a few hospitals in a market, the importance of sharing information about operations decreases, reducing the marginal effect of information sharing. This leads to the following hypothesis.

Hypothesis 2 (H2). *The effects of breadth and depth of information sharing is more salient in poor, less concentrated than in wealthy, highly concentrated regions.*

2.2. Data

We compiled data from the American Hospital Association's annual and IT surveys (https://www.ahadata.com/, accessed on 15 February 2021) and the Census Bureau's small-area income and poverty estimates (https://www.census.gov/, accessed on 1 April 2021) for 2014–2016. We also obtained data on "Medicare Spending Per Beneficiary—National" for 2015–2017 from the Center for Medicare and Medicaid Services' Hospital

Compare database (https://data.cms.gov/provider-data, accessed on 1 April 2021). Note that independent and control variables are lagged by one year. We merged the data from the AHA surveys and CMS database using the respective identification numbers and added the census data using county-level FIPS codes. The AHA's annual surveys provide data on hospital characteristics, including bed size, ownership type, teaching status, system affiliation, physician-hospital integration, revenue models, and total facility admissions. The IT surveys provide information on how broadly a hospital electronically shares patient data with other stakeholders, and the level of detail of the information that is shared. The publicly available CMS data include information on cost of care. The census data provide county-level information on poverty ratios.

2.3. The Model

Our main dependent variable, hospital costs, from Medicare spending per beneficiary (MSPB) at CMS Hospital Compare, is a measure of a specific hospital's expenditure for an episode of care compared to the national median. The measure considers not only patient age and health status, but also geographic payment differences, enabling us to control patient characteristics indirectly. Note that each hospital's expenditure is divided by the median of the national episode-weighted expenditure.

Information sharing, our main independent variable, is measured in terms of breadth and depth of information sharing. AHA IT surveys include the question, "Which of the following patient data does your hospital electronically exchange/share with one or more of the provider types listed below? (check all that apply)" We used the answers to this question to generate the variables of breadth and depth of information sharing [12]. For the breadth variable, we summed the values of the answers to the above question, (1) for hospitals within a system, (2) for hospitals outside a system, (3) for ambulatory providers within a system, and (4) for ambulatory providers outside a system. This implies that the minimum value of breadth is 0 and the maximum value is 4. For the depth variable, we summed the values of the answers to the above question, (1) for patient demographics, (2) for laboratory results, (3) for medication history, (4) for radiology reports, and (5) for clinical/summary care records in any format. This implies that the minimum value of depth is 0 and the maximum value is 5. As theorized above, we expect the coefficients of breadth and depth of information sharing to be negative.

Among several control variables included in our model, bed size, to avoid multicollinearity, is measured with 8 pre-defined codes from the AHA annual survey. Bed size ranges are (1) 6–24 beds, (2) 25–49 beds, (3) 50–99 beds, (4) 100–199 beds, (5) 200–299 beds, (6) 300–399 beds, (7) 400–499 beds, and (8) 500 or more beds. If there exist economies of scale, the ex ante expectation of the effect of bed size on hospital costs is negative; if there exist diseconomies of scale, the ex ante expectation is positive. Thus, our ex ante expectation of the effect of bed size is not predicted. For-profit ownership and government ownership are dummy variables that show differences between for-profit and government-owned hospitals, respectively. When both dummies are equal to zero, a voluntary nonprofit hospital is implied. We expect the for-profit hospital dummy to be positive, for-profit hospitals being likely to offer more profitable services, usually accompanied by expensive equipment and supplies [18]. We expect the government hospital dummy to be negative, with government-run hospitals being supported by limited funds and typically offering unprofitable services [18]. Teaching hospital is a binary variable that takes the value of 1 if the hospital is a member of the Council of Teaching Hospitals (COTH) or Association of American Medical Colleges, and 0 otherwise. We expect teaching hospital to have a negative effect on hospital costs. Contrary to the general perception that teaching hospitals are more expensive than non-teaching hospitals, it has recently been found that despite higher initial hospitalization costs, lower costs of follow-up and fewer readmissions result in overall lower total costs [19]. We also control for system affiliation and physician-hospital integration. System affiliation is a dummy variable that takes the value of 1 if a hospital is part of a system, and 0 otherwise. As with bed size, the sign of which depends on the existence of (dis)economies of scale, the ex ante expectation is not predicted. Physician–hospital integration is a binary variable that takes the value of 1 if a hospital has an arrangement (among many other arrangements) whereby physicians are employed by the hospital under an integrated salary model, and 0 otherwise. Emphasizing the integration costs that arise from changes in the behavior of physicians whose employment status changes [20], we expect the effect of physician–hospital integration on hospital costs to be positive. Capitation revenue ratio is the % of a hospital's net revenue paid on a fixed amount per patient for delivery of healthcare services. We expect the capitation revenue ratio to have a negative effect on hospital costs, as providers with a capitated contract are encouraged to avoid unnecessary tests and procedures in order that overall costs do not exceed the fixed amount.

For market characteristics, we included as controls the poverty ratio and Herfindahl–Hirschman index (HHI). The poverty ratio is the number of people whose income falls below the poverty line divided by the total population at a county-level variable. We expect the effect of poverty ratio to be negative, people in wealthy areas being more likely to be able to afford expensive treatments. The Herfindahl–Hirschman index (HHI) is calculated based on total facility admissions. The lower the Herfindahl index, the more competitive the market. The ex ante expectation of the effect of the Herfindahl index is not predicted for the following reasons. On the one hand, hospitals in highly competitive environments are under greater pressure to strive for efficiency, thereby reducing costs. On the other hand, competition can increase costs as health insurance renders patients insensitive to prices, encouraging hospitals to provide unnecessary services [21].

$$Hosptial\ Costs_{it+1} = \alpha + \beta_1 Information\ Sharing_{it}$$
$$+ \beta_2 Bed\ Size_{it} + \beta_3 For-profit_{it} + \beta_4 Government_{it}$$
$$+ \beta_5 Teaching_{it} + \beta_6 System\ Affiliation_{it}$$
$$+ \beta_7 Physician - Hospital\ Integration_{it}$$
$$+ \beta_8 Capitation\ Revenue\ Ratio_{it} + \beta_9 Poverty\ Ratio_{it}$$
$$+ \beta_{10} HHI_{it} + Year_t + \epsilon_{it}$$

3. Results

Table 1, which presents descriptive statistics for 5291 hospitals, shows the minimum hospital cost for an episode of care compared to the national median to be 0.61 and the maximum to be 1.62. In our sample, 17% are for-profit, 15% are government, and 68% are non-profit hospitals.

Table 1. Descriptive statistics.

Variable	Mean	SD	Min	Max
Hospital costs	0.985	0.074	0.610	1.620
Breadth	3.235	1.138	0	4
Depth	4.709	0.998	0	5
Bed size	4.613	1.845	1	8
For-profit	0.173	0.379	0	1
Government	0.154	0.361	0	1
Teaching	0.096	0.295	0	1
System affiliation	0.710	0.454	0	1
Physician–hospital integration	0.413	0.492	0	1
Capitation revenue ratio	0.450	0.498	0	1
Poverty ratio	15.375	5.409	3.400	46.800
HHI	0.592	0.355	0.027	1.000

Table 2 shows the main results of our OLS regression analyses regarding the effect of breadth (column (1)) and depth (column (2)) of information sharing. As predicted, the coefficients of information sharing are negative and significant for both breadth and depth, supporting H1. The coefficients of for-profit ownership, teaching hospital, and capitation revenue ratio are consistent with our stated ex ante expectations, and thus not discussed further. The coefficient of bed size is positive and statistically significant, supporting the existence of diseconomies of scale. The coefficients of government ownership, system affiliation, and poverty ratio are statistically insignificant, which suggests that they do not affect hospital costs. The coefficient of physician–hospital integration is negative and statistically significant, opposite to our prediction. This result is consistent with transaction cost economics that suggest that opportunistic behavior by physicians can be controlled well within a hierarchy [22]. The coefficient of the Herfindahl index is negative and statistically significant, suggesting that competition can increase overall hospital costs.

Table 2. The impact of health information sharing on spending.

DV: Hospital Costs	(1)	DV: Hospital Costs	(2)
Breadth	−0.003 **	Depth	−0.004 **
	[0.001]		[0.002]
Bed Size	0.010 ***	Bed Size	0.010 ***
	[0.001]		[0.001]
For-profit	0.036 ***	For−profit	0.037 ***
	[0.004]		[0.004]
Government	0.002	Government	0.003
	[0.005]		[0.005]
Teaching	−0.013 ***	Teaching	−0.013 ***
	[0.004]		[0.004]
System Affiliation	−0.000	System Affiliation	−0.001
	[0.003]		[0.003]
Physician-hospital Integration	−0.008 ***	Physician−hospital Integration	−0.009 ***
	[0.003]		[0.003]
Capitation Revenue Ratio	−0.018 ***	Capitation Revenue Ratio	−0.018 ***
	[0.002]		[0.002]
Poverty Ratio	−0.000	Poverty Ratio	−0.000
	[0.000]		[0.000]
HHI	−0.048 ***	HHI	−0.048 ***
	[0.004]		[0.004]
Constant	0.984 ***	Constant	0.991 ***
	[0.009]		[0.011]
Observations	5291	Observations	5291
R-squared	0.180	R-squared	0.180

Standard errors (in brackets) are clustered at the hospital level; *** $p < 0.01$, ** $p < 0.05$.

Noting that market characteristics, the poverty ratio, and the concentration ratio are more or less deterministic from the perspective of policy makers and hospital administrators, we conducted sub-sample analyses to examine whether the effect of breadth and depth of information sharing varies across the variables: county-level poverty ratio and Herfindahl index.

In columns (1) and (2), we divide our sample into wealthy (i.e., low poverty ratio) and poor (i.e., high poverty ratio) regions by median poverty ratio. Results are reported in Table 3. Estimated coefficients of the control variables are the same for the sub-sample (Table 3) as for the full sample (Table 2) analysis. Interestingly, our results suggest that depth of information sharing reduces hospital costs only in poor (i.e., high poverty ratio) areas, as shown in column (4). The effect of depth of information sharing becomes statistically insignificant in relatively wealthy (i.e., low poverty ratio) regions, as shown in column (3). A Wald's test confirmed that the difference in the depth coefficients across the low and high poverty ratio groups (as shown in columns (3) and (4)) is statistically significant (p-value < 0.1), supporting H2. Breadth of information sharing yields cost savings in both poor and wealthy areas, as shown in columns (1) and (2), not supporting H2. Overall, our results partially support H2.

Table 3. The impact of health information sharing on spending by poverty ratio.

DV: Hospital Costs	(1) Low Poverty Ratio	(2) High Poverty Ratio	DV: Hospital Costs	(3) Low Poverty Ratio	(4) High Poverty Ratio
Breadth	−0.003 **	−0.004 ***	Depth	0.000	−0.005 ***
	[0.001]	[0.001]		[0.002]	[0.001]
Bed Size	0.013 ***	0.012 ***	Bed Size	0.000 ***	0.000 ***
	[0.001]	[0.001]		[0.000]	[0.000]
For-profit	0.042 ***	0.038 ***	For−profit	0.040 ***	0.035 ***
	[0.004]	[0.004]		[0.004]	[0.004]
Government	−0.011 ***	0.002	Government	−0.011 ***	−0.001
	[0.004]	[0.004]		[0.004]	[0.004]
Teaching	−0.005	−0.009 **	Teaching	−0.007	−0.004
	[0.005]	[0.005]		[0.006]	[0.005]
System Affiliation	0.003	0.006 *	System Affiliation	0.003	0.009 ***
	[0.003]	[0.003]		[0.003]	[0.003]
Physician-hospital Integration	−0.010 ***	−0.013 ***	Physician−hospital Integration	−0.010 ***	−0.013 ***
	[0.003]	[0.003]		[0.003]	[0.003]
Capitation Revenue Ratio	−0.014 ***	−0.015 ***	Capitation Revenue Ratio	−0.013 ***	−0.013 ***
	[0.003]	[0.003]		[0.003]	[0.003]
Constant	0.934 ***	0.939 ***	Constant	0.961 ***	0.990 ***
	[0.006]	[0.006]		[0.008]	[0.007]
Observations	2692	2599	Observations	2692	2599
R-squared	0.140	0.135	R-squared	0.110	0.101

Standard errors (in brackets) are clustered at the hospital level; *** $p < 0.01$, ** $p < 0.05$, * $p < 0.1$.

We conduct an additional sub-sample analysis by dividing our full sample into more competitive (low HHI) and more concentrated (high HHI) regions by median HHI. The estimated coefficients of the control variables are the same in the sub-sample (Table 4) as in the full sample (Table 2) analysis. Our results suggest that depth of information sharing that reduces cost of care in the full sample analysis does not decrease hospital costs in concentrated areas, as shown in column (4). The coefficient of depth of information sharing is, however, negative and statistically significant in column (3), which suggests that it does decrease hospital costs in competitive regions. A Wald's test confirmed that the difference in the depth coefficients across the low and high HHI groups is statistically significant (p-value < 0.1), supporting H2. Breadth of information sharing consistently decreases hospital costs regardless of concentration ratio, not supporting H2. Overall, the results from Table 4 partially support H2.

Overall, our results suggest that policy makers should consider modifying their strategies for using health IT to account for the finding that benefits are contingent on market characteristics. In countries still in an early stage of health IT investment or with limited resources, poor and competitive regions in which the benefits of health IT can be maximized should be the initial targets of implementation strategy. In countries that have already achieved nationwide adoption of EHR (e.g., the United States), the focus should be on increasing the breadth of information sharing. Policy makers should provide guidelines for increasing the level of detail of information sharing that reflect a consideration of market characteristics.

Table 4. The impact of health information sharing on spending by HHI.

DV: Hospital Costs	(1) Low HHI	(2) High HHI	DV: Hospital Costs	(3) Low HHI	(4) High HHI
Breadth	−0.003 **	−0.004 ***	Depth	−0.006 ***	−0.001
	[0.001]	[0.001]		[0.001]	[0.001]
Bed Size	0.009 ***	0.012 ***	Bed Size	0.009 ***	0.012 ***
	[0.001]	[0.001]		[0.001]	[0.001]
For-profit	0.039 ***	0.035 ***	For−profit	0.038 ***	0.037 ***
	[0.004]	[0.004]		[0.004]	[0.004]
Government	−0.004	0.003	Government	−0.004	0.004
	[0.005]	[0.003]		[0.004]	[0.003]
Teaching	−0.010 **	−0.003	Teaching	−0.011 ***	−0.004
	[0.004]	[0.007]		[0.004]	[0.007]
System Affiliation	0.004	−0.001	System Affiliation	0.004	−0.002
	[0.003]	[0.003]		[0.003]	[0.003]
Physician-hospital Integration	−0.012 ***	−0.008 ***	Physician−hospital Integration	−0.012 ***	−0.008 ***
	[0.003]	[0.003]		[0.003]	[0.003]
Capitation Revenue Ratio	−0.018 ***	−0.015 ***	Capitation Revenue Ratio	−0.017 ***	−0.015 ***
	[0.003]	[0.003]		[0.003]	[0.003]
Constant	0.967 ***	0.929 ***	Constant	0.986 ***	0.925 ***
	[0.006]	[0.006]		[0.008]	[0.007]
Observations	2659	2632	Observations	2659	2632
R-squared	0.096	0.115	R-squared	0.101	0.112

Standard errors (in brackets) are clustered at the hospital level; *** $p < 0.01$, ** $p < 0.05$.

4. Discussion

Despite widespread adoption of EHR systems, not all hospitals seem to benefit from health IT, as evidenced by inconclusive findings regarding its effect [5–9]. Believing the mixed results to be a consequence of an emphasis on adoption and inattention to specific configuration strategies in information sharing, we examine how breadth and depth of information sharing affect hospital costs. There being few studies of how the effects of health IT vary with context [8], we seek to resolve the inconsistency of previous results by specifically examining different contexts (poor vs. wealthy, less concentrated and highly concentrated regions) that may intensify or weaken the effect of health IT. Our finding that depth of information sharing decreases costs in poor and competitive regions, but not in rich and concentrated regions, and that breadth of information sharing decreases overall hospital costs, has implications for both research and practice. Our study enhances the research community's understanding of why some hospitals are successful and others unsuccessful in realizing the benefits of health IT. In the area of practice, our study provides guidance for government in promoting active use of health IT. Our findings regarding positive effects of breadth and depth of information sharing can usefully inform administrators' and providers' monitoring of how adopted IT systems are used. For countries with high health IT adoption to derive greater benefit from using health IT, more incentives should be given to hospitals located in poor and competitive regions. Our findings also have implications for countries that have not yet invested in EHR systems or lack the necessary resources to implement IT systems nationwide. Governments of such countries might purposefully focus on poor or competitive regions in order to maximize the effect of the limited resources they possess, these being the areas that exhibit consistent cost savings when hospitals share information either broadly or in considerable detail.

The present study's limitations present opportunities for future research. For example, we do not have information about precise reductions in duplicate tests or treatment that can result from active information sharing among stakeholders. A future study could examine the number of CT scans or medication changes when patients receive a summary of care record electronically during the process of transitioning to another care setting. Future research could also examine the role specific information (e.g., patient demographics/laboratory results/medication history/radiology reports/clinical/summary care records) plays in reducing tests or treatment. Similarly, whereas our study considers two types of information sharing, breadth and depth, and two contexts that vary by poverty and concentration ratio, a future study might examine other types of information sharing (e.g., volume, diversity) [23] or other contexts, such as patient mix (e.g., Medicare or Medicaid share), race, specific IT vendors, etc.

5. Conclusions

The present research shows an understanding of health information sharing beyond mere adoption of EHR systems to be important to the realization of the benefits of health IT. The study further suggests a significant opportunity to effectively lower healthcare costs by targeting specific areas in which the effect of health IT is maximized. The results of our study can usefully guide efforts to strategically support and tailor policy to enable hospitals to achieve the overarching goal of reducing escalating healthcare costs.

Funding: This work was supported by the National Research Foundation of Korea (NRF) grant funded by the Korea government (MSIT) (No. 2018R1C1B5086201).

Institutional Review Board Statement: Not applicable.

Informed Consent Statement: Not applicable.

Data Availability Statement: American Hospital Association (AHA) IT survey was purchased using the fund provided by the Korea government (MIST). AHA annual survey data were provided by Chang Jongwha. The U.S. Census Bureau's small-area income and poverty estimates that provide information about poverty ratio are publicly available (https://www.census.gov/, accessed on 1 April 2021). Hospital Compare publicly provides data on "Medicare Spending Per Beneficiary—National" where we obtained information about our dependent variable, hospital costs (https://data.cms.gov/provider-data/, accessed on 1 April 2021).

Acknowledgments: The author would like to thank Chang who provided annual AHA surveys.

Conflicts of Interest: The author declares no conflict of interest. The funders had no role in the design of the study, in the collection, analysis, or interpretation of data, in the preparation of the manuscript, or in the decision to publish the results.

References

1. Health Information Technology for Economic and Clinical Health (HITECH). Available online: https://www.cms.gov/ (accessed on 17 May 2021).
2. Adler-Milstein, J.; Jha, A.K. Hitech Act Drove Large Gains in Hospital Electronic Health Record Adoption. *Health Aff.* **2017**, *36*, 1416–1422. [CrossRef]
3. Diana, M.L.; Harle, C.A.; Huerta, T.R.; Ford, E.W.; Menachemi, N. Hospital Characteristics Associated with Achievement of Meaningful Use. *J. Health Manag.* **2014**, *59*, 272–286. [CrossRef] [PubMed]
4. Office of the National Coordinator for Health Information Technology. 'Percent of Hospitals, by Type, that Possess Certified Health IT', Health IT Quick-Stat #52. Available online: https://dash-board.healthit.gov/quickstats/pages/certified-electronic-health-record-technology-in-hospitals.php (accessed on 1 September 2018).
5. Agha, L. The effects of health information technology on the costs and quality of medical care. *J. Health Econ.* **2014**, *34*, 19–30. [CrossRef]
6. Buntin, M.B.; Burke, M.F.; Hoaglin, M.C.; Blumenthal, D. The Benefits of Health Information Technology: A Review of the Recent Literature Shows Predominantly Positive Results. *Health Aff.* **2011**, *30*, 464–471. [CrossRef]
7. Dranove, D.; Forman, C.; Goldfarb, A.; Greenstein, S. The trillion-dollar conundrum: Complementarities and health information technology. *Am. Econ. J. Econ. Policy* **2014**, *6*, 239–270. [CrossRef]
8. Jones, S.S.; Rudin, R.S.; Perry, T.; Shekelle, P.G. Health Information Technology: An Updated Systematic Review with a Focus on Meaningful Use. *Ann. Intern. Med.* **2014**, *160*, 48–54. [CrossRef] [PubMed]
9. Lapointe, L.; Mignerat, M.; Vedel, I. The IT productivity paradox in health: A stakeholder's perspective. *Int. J. Med. Inform.* **2011**, *80*, 102–115. [CrossRef]
10. Kazley, A.S.; Ozcan, Y.A. Organizational and Environmental Determinants of Hospital EMR Adoption: A National Study. *J. Med. Syst.* **2007**, *31*, 375–384. [CrossRef] [PubMed]

11. Miller, R.H.; Sim, I. Physicians' use of electronic medical records: Barriers and solutions. *Health Aff.* **2004**, *23*, 116–126. [CrossRef]
12. Cho, N.; Ke, W.; Atems, B.; Chang, J. How does electronic health information exchange affect hospital performance efficiency? The effects of breadth and depth of information sharing. *J. Healthc. Manag.* **2018**, *63*, 212–228. [CrossRef]
13. Devaraj, S.; Kohli, R. Performance Impacts of Information Technology: Is Actual Usage the Missing Link? *Manag. Sci.* **2003**, *49*, 273–289. [CrossRef]
14. Petter, S.; Delone, W.; McLean, E. Measuring information systems success: Models, dimensions, measures and interrelationships. *Eur. J. Inf. Syst.* **2008**, *17*, 236–263. [CrossRef]
15. Zhu, K.; Kraemer, K.L. Post-Adoption Variations in Usage and Value of E-Business by Organizations: Cross-Country Evidence from the Retail Industry. *Inf. Syst. Res.* **2005**, *16*, 61–84. [CrossRef]
16. Ayabakan, S.; Bardhan, I.; Zheng, Z.; Kirksey, K. The impact of health information sharing on duplicate testing. *MIS Q.* **2017**, *41*, 1083–1103. [CrossRef]
17. Kash, B.A.; Baek, J.; Davis, E.; Champagne-Langabeer, T.; Langabeer, J.R. Review of successful hospital readmission reduction strategies and the role of health information exchange. *Int. J. Med. Inform.* **2017**, *104*, 97–104. [CrossRef] [PubMed]
18. Horwitz, J.R. Making Profits and Providing Care: Comparing Nonprofit, For-Profit and Government Hospitals. *Health Aff.* **2005**, *24*, 790–801. [CrossRef] [PubMed]
19. Burke, L.G.; Khullar, D.; Zheng, J.; Frakt, A.B.; Orav, E.J.; Jha, A.K. Comparison of costs of care for Medicare patients hospitalized in teaching and nonteaching hospitals. *JAMA Netw. Open* **2019**, *2*, e19522. [CrossRef] [PubMed]
20. Cho, N.E. Costs of Physician-Hospital Integration. *Medicine* **2015**, *94*, e1762. [CrossRef] [PubMed]
21. Kessler, D.P.; McClellan, M.B. Is Hospital Competition Socially Wasteful? *Q. J. Econ.* **2000**, *115*, 577–615. [CrossRef]
22. Williamson, O.E. The Economics of Organization: The Transaction Cost Approach. *Am. J. Sociol.* **1981**, *87*, 548–577. [CrossRef]
23. Massetti, B.; Zmud, R.W. Measuring the Extent of EDI Usage in Complex Organizations: Strategies and Illustrative Examples. *MIS Q.* **1996**, *20*, 331. [CrossRef]

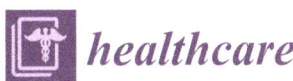

Perspective

The Critical Factors Affecting the Deployment and Scaling of Healthcare AI: Viewpoint from an Experienced Medical Center

Chung-Feng Liu [1,†], Chien-Cheng Huang [2,3,†], Jhi-Joung Wang [4,5], Kuang-Ming Kuo [6] and Chia-Jung Chen [7,*]

1. Department of Medical Research, Chi Mei Medical Center, Tainan 71004, Taiwan; chungfengliu@gmail.com
2. Department of Emergency Medicine, Chi Mei Medical Center, Tainan 71004, Taiwan; jasonhuang0803@gmail.com
3. Department of Environmental and Occupational Health, College of Medicine, National Cheng Kung University, Tainan 701401, Taiwan
4. Department of Anesthesiology, Chi Mei Medical Center, Tainan 71004, Taiwan; 400002@mail.chimei.org.tw
5. Department of Anesthesiology, National Defense Medical Center, Taipei 11490, Taiwan
6. Department of Business Management, National United University, Miaoli 36003, Taiwan; kmkuo@nuu.edu.tw
7. Department of Information Systems, Chi Mei Medical Center, Tainan 71004, Taiwan
* Correspondence: carolchen@mail.chimei.org.tw; Tel.: +886-6-281-2811
† The first two authors contributed equally to this work as first authors.

Abstract: Healthcare Artificial Intelligence (AI) has the greatest opportunity for development. Since healthcare and technology are two of Taiwan's most competitive industries, the development of healthcare AI is an excellent chance for Taiwan to improve its health-related services. From the perspective of economic development, promoting healthcare AI must be a top priority. However, despite having many breakthroughs in research and pilot projects, healthcare AI is still considered rare and is broadly used in the healthcare setting. Based on a medical center in Taiwan that has introduced a variety of healthcare AI into practice, this study discussed and analyzed the issues and concerns in the development and scaling of medical AIs from the perspective of various stakeholders in the healthcare setting, including the government, healthcare institutions, users (healthcare workers), and AI providers. The present study also identified critical influential factors for the deployment and scaling of healthcare AI. It is hoped that this paper can serve as an important reference for the advancement of healthcare AI not only in Taiwan but also in other countries.

Keywords: artificial intelligence; healthcare AI; deployment and scaling; medical center; critical factors; stakeholders

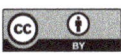

1. Introduction

AI has been given a lot of attention worldwide due to its continued significant scientific and technological advancements. People from all walks of life have gained tremendous interest in AI-related technologies resulting in the development of several amazing AI-related products. For example, the manufacturing industry is now utilizing intelligent solutions through AI in many of its areas, such as defect identification on the production line, automatic process control, predictive maintenance, and raw mix optimization (e.g., [1]). Some industries are using AI for the development of unmanned factories. AI-related research has grown substantially in the past 10 years [2], but most of them only reported the quality of prediction models (such as accuracy, sensitivity, specificity, and Area Under Curve (AUC) values), which makes it difficult to judge their practical feasibility. In terms of the use of AI in healthcare, there is still much space for enhancement, which could overturn the ecology of traditional healthcare. According to Gartner's report [3], 54% of data science projects in most organizations were never deployed or only partially deployed in practice. Indeed, different from other industries, the healthcare industry is strictly limited and restricted by many laws and regulations. Therefore, the experience of using AI in general industries cannot be directly applied to the healthcare industry (an unmanned hospital is obviously impossible).

Two of Taiwan's most competitive industries are healthcare and technology. The development of healthcare AI is an excellent opportunity for Taiwan since it is becoming increasingly popular and could potentially help a lot of people. Therefore, from the perspective of economic development, it is urgent to promote healthcare AI. Two of the four AI Research Centers established in 2018 by the Ministry of Science and Technology in Taiwan are connected with the healthcare industry (one is located at the National Taiwan University and the other at the National Cheng Kung University). The establishment of these centers allows the Taiwanese government to improve the overall quality of the nation's healthcare through AI. The development of healthcare AI also aims to lower the total medical expenditures at a national level. Moreover, as the positive benefits of AI are gradually being recognized and emphasized by healthcare institutions, relevant specialized units have sprung up (e.g., Big data center and AI center) to perform more research and development. Healthcare AI is considered as one of the industries where AI has the most opportunities for development [4,5]. Therefore, many technological manufacturers and start-ups invest heavily in innovative development, hoping to gain an advantage and to initiate the trend in healthcare AI. However, it is important to determine how the biggest consumers of healthcare AI, namely the hospitals and healthcare workers, will react towards such a trend. Whether the hospital obtained AI by developing it or through external purchase, it would require a vast amount of time, special manpower, including AI engineers, and financial resources for building basic infrastructures (GPU servers, data warehouse, and development platform), purchasing various AI products, and storing and transforming big-data. Therefore, calculating the obtainable investment efficiency is the most fundamental and significant concern for hospitals in AI evaluation and development.

The healthcare industry can simplify the calculation of investment efficiency of AI by measuring the income increase, cost reduction, and quality improvement. After this, they could assess the working efficiency improvement, working pressure reduction, and patient satisfaction improvement. In Taiwan, hospital income mainly comes from the national health insurance (NHI) payment under the global budget payment system, which is not directly correlated to the type of equipment and devices used in hospitals (AI could be viewed as a kind of equipment). This means that the introduction of AI in hospitals may not directly generate new sources of income. Additionally, many scholars pointed out that AI performs better than other medical professionals, such as in medical image interpretation (e.g., [6]). Furthermore, many have begun to question whether healthcare workers could be replaced by AI (e.g., [7]). As a response, the government proposed clear regulations to stipulate how the number of healthcare workers should match with the hospital scale. Hence, it may be impractical to say that AI could reduce the volume of healthcare workers in the short term. Additionally, there may be limitations in using AI to reduce the deployment of equipment and devices, and the acceptance of AI by healthcare workers also deserves attention. Since hospitals tend to be busy, many healthcare workers believe that using AI will only consume their time and attention, which they could use in attending to patients instead. Moreover, they believe that they can accurately evaluate some disease outcome changes even without AI; thus, it is safe to assume that some healthcare workers lack the willingness to use AI.

The authors of this paper are affiliated with Chi Mei Hospital, a hospital with three branches in Taiwan. In August 2019, Chi Mei Hospital established the AI Center in its general faculty as the base for developing healthcare AI. Relying on big data accumulated over ten years, the hospital has focused on developing AI-smart clinical outcome prediction. As of March 2021, it has self-developed 15 kinds of AI systems, which are then coordinated with the existing Hospital Information System (HIS) to help healthcare workers in their clinical decision. So far, all of the hospital's branches have installed the AI systems in several departments, including the Emergency, Surgery, Anesthesiology, Intensive Care Unit, and Nursing departments. In addition, as the AI Center is gradually developing and improving the AI systems, it was able to study and observe the use of AI in the healthcare setting and publish them in international journals [8,9]. Based on the experience of Chi Mei Hospital in the implementation of its AI systems, this paper reported the current situation and the challenges being faced by healthcare AI from the perspectives of the government, hospitals, users, and manufacturers. It also determined the key factors affecting the deployment of healthcare AI.

2. Development of AI in Chi Mei Hospital

2.1. AI Computing Infrastructure

Supported by the Board of directors and the Superintendent, Chi Mei Medical Center built the Center for Big Medical Data and AI Computing (hereinafter referred to as AI center) in May 2019. As the base for developing AI in the three branches of the hospital, this center has two main tasks: (1) to establish Big Medical Data (data warehouse) and (2) to develop AI applications. It is hoped that AI will not only be used for academic research but is also expected to produce practical applications for clinical use. The Big Medical Data acts as a retrospective data source for AI development and healthcare researches, and its main source is the online database of HIS. Since the structure of the data warehouse and HIS database are very different from each other, it makes this project enormous and complicated. Therefore, the AI Center usually develops and establishes the topic-specific big database with the most researchers first. To do this, the Department of Information Systems (IS) in hospitals is tasked to help in transferring the needed data from the HIS database. Figure 1 shows the AI Computing Infrastructure of Chi Mei Hospital.

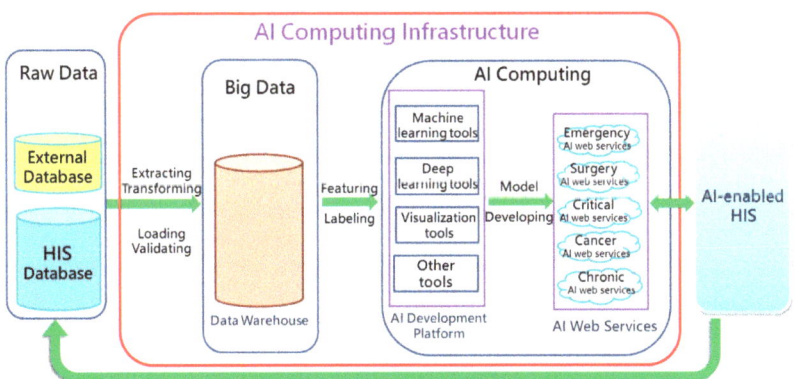

Figure 1. AI Computing Infrastructure of Chi Mei Hospital.

* HIS: Hospital Information System; AI: Artificial Intelligence.

Based on the Service-oriented Architecture (SOA), the IS department designed three types of web service program (WS) that interacts with HIS to process the AI prediction (Figure 2). These are as follows:

i.   HIS interface WS (HWS)
     The HWS receives calls from the existing (HIS) and sends the prediction result (e.g., risk probability) back to the HIS.
ii. Feature extraction WS (FWS)
     The FWS receives calls from HWS, retrieves the patient's characteristic values (such as age, blood pressure, lab data, etc.), and sends them back to HWS. This may include the use of IoT technology to retrieve physiological information at the bedside.
iii. AI prediction WS (AWS)
     The AWS receives calls from HWS, enters the acquired feature values of the patient, performs the AI prediction, and returns the result to HWS.

Six sending/receiving messages are completed while a prediction is triggered by users (healthcare workers). They contain only short messages and only cause minor impacts on the online HIS. So far, 15 healthcare AI predictions (15 AI WSs) are being used on the AI Web Services server (see Figure 1), which is routinely monitored by IS engineers. Because AI is positioned as an assistance role, system failure has little effect on the overall clinical operation.

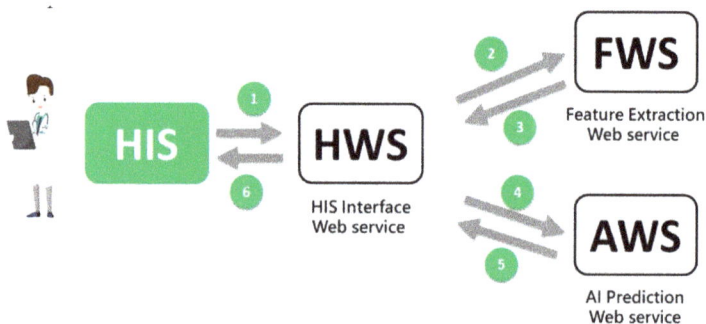

Figure 2. AI Web Service Interaction.

* HIS: Hospital Information System; AI: Artificial Intelligence

2.2. Promotion Strategy

To demonstrate its commitment to developing AI, Chi Mei Hospital has subsidized the training of hundreds of healthcare workers in AI practice. Each training lasts for 4 weeks to 4 months, depending on the complexity of the AI. Moreover, the AI Center has assigned different personnel to give mini-lectures on how to develop AI and create specialized individual roles, evoking wide repercussions among healthcare workers. Because of this, the hospital's workers no longer feel that AI is inaccessible, allowing them to propose various ideas proactively. To determine the plausibility of the staff's ideas, inter-disciplinary meetings with healthcare workers, AI analysts, and IT engineers as participants are being held. The approved ideas are then constructed as AI projects and finally implemented and used in practice. Since the establishment of the AI Center, the emergency department (ED) was the first department to join the AI development and has completed a variety of disease outcome prediction systems (e.g., older patients with influenza, patients with chest pain). Due to the success of the AI systems implementation in the ED, the AI center revised the systems depending on the needs of the other departments and promoted their use (e.g., outcome prediction of burns for surgical treatment, anesthesia risk assessment, mortality prediction and timing prediction for weaning mechanical ventilation in ICU, and fall detection in elderly wards). Figure 3 shows a screenshot of the outcome prediction system in ED patients with chest pain [8]. The system has been integrated with the existing emergency computerized order entry system. Until 30 April 2021, a total of 50 AI projects have been proposed mainly focusing on physicians' clinical requirements; 15 of which have been deployed in the clinical practice (integrated into the existing HIS); 25 are still being completed; 10 have been completed but have not yet been implemented. Among the 10 completed projects, five have not yet been used because the physicians considered their model quality not good enough for clinical use (model AUC < 0.7) and need improvement, while the other five projects are scheduled for further development but are under slow progress due to heavy workload in the IS department.

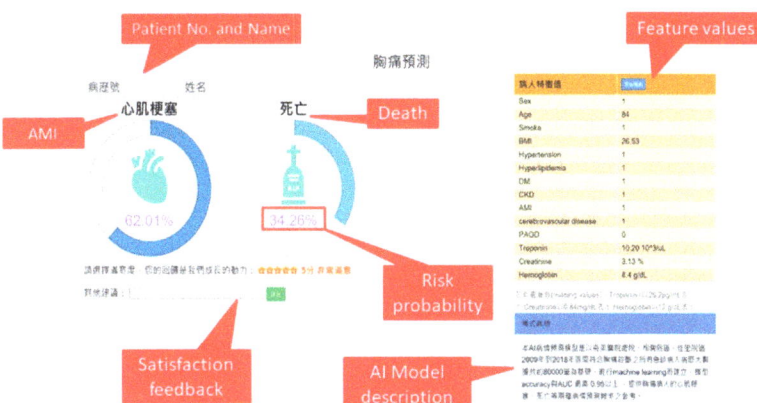

Figure 3. A Screenshot of a Deployed AI System.

* AMI: Acute Myocardial Infarction

Because of previous promotions, the heads of each hospital department are aware of the benefits of AI in healthcare; thus, each gives enough time to discuss AI issues and solve them based on consensus through regular department meetings. Moreover, each department designates specific groups that target specific clinical demands to create AI projects to be submitted to the AI Center. After confirmation and revision, the department can apply the proposed project into practice. In this way, departments are able to carry out subsequent launches of AI systems smoothly and reduce resistance from other healthcare workers. To promote AI, Chi Mei considers it as an assistive tool rather than a substitute for humans' skills and intellect. The hospital also believes that healthcare workers have the right to choose whether they will or will not use AI and shall not suffer any punishment or salary deduction for not using it. Various departments welcomed such policies, which brought out more projects for practical application.

Whether preparing big data or integrating models with HIS, the support of the information department is very much critical. However, the daily workload of the IS department is quite heavy, and understandably, it cannot provide much support on AI development. Therefore, Chi Mei has allotted a data-processing fee in the budget of the in-hospital projects of AI Development every year to encourage IS engineers to support AI development in their free time (off-work time), which has been a feasible and effective approach.

2.3. Emerging Benefits of AI Adoption

AI benefit evaluation is critical but not easy to measure. However, the benefits of Chi Mei's deployment and scaling of AI have gradually emerged. For example, on the basis of no significant differences in gender, age, and disease severity among patients, the periods before and after adopting AI timing prediction for weaning mechanical ventilation in ICU (2019/7–11 vs. 2020/7–11) were compared. It was found that the average time of using a ventilator was reduced by about 22 h while having the same medical quality. This proves that not all the benefits of using AI applications are obvious and may not be recognized in a single AI factor. Therefore, it requires continuous in-depth observation and evaluation.

3. Viewpoint of Stakeholders

The most fundamental consideration for every transaction is the cost-benefit, even for the purchase of information communication technology (ICT) devices. Therefore, the first step to promote healthcare AI is to have careful considerations of the benefits that consumers could obtain by adopting it. These consumers are the most important stakeholders in the development of AI, comprising of the government, healthcare institutions (hospitals), end-users (healthcare workers), and AI providers. Based on the hospital's experience, literature review, and actual observations, this study discussed the viewpoint of AI stakeholders.

3.1. The Government

Using smart technologies to improve healthcare quality has long been one of the government's scientific and technological policies. In the National Healthcare Quality Award (NHQA), an annual competition held by the Joint Commission of Taiwan for hospital accreditation, smart healthcare is always an item of focus. Every year nearly 200 groups attend this competition, and most are from hospitals. Moreover, the truth is, the overall healthcare spending and healthcare insurance expenditure has become increasingly unbalanced. Since technologies could improve public health by both early prevention and intermediary and tertiary care, hospitals could apply AI to different healthcare services on the premise of accurate trend prediction and risk of individual disease outcome change. Thus, through AI, the government could reduce the previously undifferentiated healthcare policies (e.g., nationwide disease screening) and further control the overall healthcare expenditure with guaranteed healthcare quality. After all, national health insurance and healthcare occupy large proportions of the national budget. If AI technologies could accurately predict the public healthcare trend and the epidemiological pattern of diseases and help hospitals plan corresponding strategies with precision, it may create concrete benefits by promoting the government's healthcare and welfare policies. Additionally, from the perspective of detail-oriented healthcare resource management, AI could help avoid healthcare wastes (such as lower examination and medication), meeting the expectations of the government towards smart technology. Therefore, in the short term, the government should be committed to formulating and revising regulations, such as insurance reimbursement policy or specific subsidy programs, to encourage the development and adoption of AI in healthcare institutions.

Another important role of the government is as an industrial promoter. The Taiwan government may pledge AI funding schemes, such as the strategies used in the US and Germany [10,11], for promoting joint efforts in creating breakthroughs in AI. As Taiwan embraces complete big data in national health insurance, it is essential for the government to formulate regulations of data governance [12] and release authorization for the development of the AI industry.

3.2. Healthcare Institutions

Different from other industries, healthcare institutions (e.g., hospitals) are under the strict supervision of various policies and rules regarding their environment, workforce, and medical device deployment. For instance, in Taiwan, the Establishment Standards for Medical Institutions has stipulated the human resource arrangement in hospitals providing minimum requirements on the type and the number of medical professionals in a hospital (to be more specific, a minimum of two physicians for every 10 beds; a minimum of two nurses for every three beds for hospitals over 50 beds; a minimum of one pharmacist for every 40 beds; a minimum of three clinical laboratory technologist for every 50 beds; a minimum of two radiologists for every 35 beds). Even though the introduction of AI into healthcare institutions may bring out promising benefits (e.g., the AI-assisted medical image interpretation), it cannot significantly reduce the actual cost of manpower due to the restrictions of laws and regulations. In fact, the scope of payment under the NHI system is based on the total amount and the Diagnosis Related Groups (DRG), aside from calculating the relative declarations of each healthcare institution and reasonable load for outpatient services in recent years (referring to the Standard Reimbursements for Medical Services and Treatment for the National Health Insurance in Taiwan). As a result, hospitals can barely accumulate surpluses from the NHI system, and some treatments may even operate at a loss, which AI's introduction cannot simply change.

Compared with the control of manpower allocation, the government has relatively no explicit regulations on medical equipment. However, the "arms race" is used as a major promotion topic for the healthcare industry, at least in Taiwan. As can be seen from the popularity of the costly "da Vinci Surgical System" in large hospitals in Taiwan, those hospitals are not reserved in investing in medical equipment. The added value of AI in medical equipment (e.g., the ventilator may be equipped with AI patient risk prediction) could increase the attractiveness of the equipment. AI providers have proposed many innovative diagnostic methods, but hospitals need to confirm first whether these could replace the original ones, especially in terms of practical use. For example, AI could help identify the risk of Obstructive Sleep Apnea Syndrome (OSAS) based on patients' neck CT scans. However, healthcare professionals need to rigorously determine if they could use AI as a reference for diagnosis (traditional diagnosis of OSAS includes nocturnal polysomnography).

The manufacturing industry can establish unmanned factories thanks to smart technologies, but hospitals are different; they cannot run without medical professionals. After the introduction of smart technologies, the manufacturing industry can easily calculate quantitative benefits by measuring production increase, manpower reduction, and yield (healthcare quality) improvement. However, it is difficult for hospitals to reflect the same quantitative benefits because there is lesser variation in production capacity (e.g., the outpatient visit is regulated by Reasonable Load for Outpatient Services Policy), manpower (the healthcare staffing quota is limited by the Establishment Standards for Medical Institutions), and yield (the healthcare quality is in line with hospital accreditation standard). Hence, hospital operators are suspicious about the necessity to invest huge capital in AI development. At present, most hospitals initially use AI for education and research and not for clinical purposes because they believe that AI can be helpful in academic research (research publication is required in teaching hospitals). As for the clinical benefits of AI, hospitals need more time to observe and assess the results.

Other organizational and managerial challenges such as organizational resistance to data sharing and lack of strategy for AI development were pointed out in previous research [13], which could also appear in healthcare institutions and need to be overcome as well.

3.3. End Users (Healthcare Workers)

Based on the user-centered perspectives, understanding the clinical needs of healthcare workers and the difficulties they face in clinical decision-making is the basic principle for the development of healthcare AI. The "coolness" of technology should not be given too much attention as it may generate unnecessary AI, which could neglect the real purpose of AI development, that is, to improve clinical practice.

Furthermore, the cultivation of healthcare workers requires rigorous education and high cost. If technology such as AI could partly replace manpower, it would be called an epoch-making healthcare revolution. However, medical education based on evidence usually emphasizes the accumulation of clinical experience and related skills aside from formal school education. Moreover, practical training is highly significant in medical professionals' practice; this is why many professional units hold regular discussions for clinical cases. In addition, the Objective Structured Clinical Examination (OSCE) provides strict testing of professional skills for healthcare workers. If healthcare professionals rely too much on AI's assistance, they may not develop appropriate professional skills and experience. Therefore, although Chi Mei has introduced AI medical image interpretation, they have discouraged (and even prohibited) medical interns or resident physicians from using it. Nevertheless, the influential factors for medical decisions may be too many; using AI as a tool to assist decision-making and provide an additional layer of gatekeepers may reduce the chance of negligence or even misjudgment, and AI will have its value. However, there is no denying that in the long run, healthcare workers may worry about being replaced by AI, and this still requires careful attention [13].

The black-box problem of AI is another major reason that affects healthcare workers' acceptance of AI. Even though AI is highly accurate, healthcare workers cannot completely trust its suggestions if the reference or logic is unclear. After all, life is above all, and healthcare workers would be to blame if anything untoward happens. Hence, it is very important to guarantee and improve healthcare AI's explainability [14,15].

Since hospitals are always busy and healthcare workers are under great pressure, hospital management should introduce AI gradually without increasing the complexity of the care process. To achieve this goal, the AI functions should be integrated seamlessly with the existing HIS or operate automatically as much as possible (while retaining the final decision to the workers) with utmost convenience. Finally, instead of forcing healthcare workers to follow, they should have the right to choose whether they will use AI's suggestions. As long as the AI can perform well consistently in a long time, healthcare workers would gradually accept and routinely use it.

3.4. AI Providers

"To create an AI physician" is the most dreamlike goal of AI development in health care. Many technology providers such as IBM, Google, Microsoft, and other start-ups have all invested in healthcare AI, creating highly innovative products. However, as the profits seem to be unapparent, many AI providers keep losing money, which prompted them to reduce their investment. The sharp cut-down of personnel in the IBM Watson Health Department is an obvious example [16]. As mentioned previously, the medical industry is very different from other industries, and its development and operation are subject to many strict regulations. It may be far from reality to replace healthcare workers with AI. In other words, the development of healthcare AI shall not follow the same way as that of general industries. According to surveys, even though AI and real physicians have the same diagnostic quality, the public would still prefer real physicians. Moreover, even if the AI provides the judgment result, the patient hopes that a real physician can make the final confirmation [17].

The choice of the user-centered target [18] is key in determining the success or failure of AI. If AI products are innovative but difficult or non-critical to use in the hospitals, the investment of providers will just go to waste. Thus, the providers must design AI products based on actual demands or requirements of the healthcare industry rather than technological innovation. AI providers should assign someone (preferably a healthcare professional) who will be tasked to comprehensively understand the needs of the medical field and propose convenient and flexible AI solutions. Particularly, in recent years, several studies proposed precision and personalized medicine that emphasized the complexity of medical factors requiring personalized care and not a "one-size-fits-all" protocol [19,20]. For instance, although the diagnosis of malignant lesions through X-ray may be the same all over the world, the outcome prediction and treatment may vary with the nationality, race, sex, age, eating habits, and social status of the patient. Therefore, before development, providers must determine whether the AI product is for general or special use. Aside from this, AI development requires thorough considerations in terms of user number, obvious effectiveness, and explainability of results.

High-quality big data is an important prerequisite for AI development, which usually comes from the cooperation between healthcare institutions and providers (developers) rather than from providers alone. Therefore, providers need to select qualified healthcare institutions for long-term cooperation and carefully store big data. Additionally, to avoid interference in healthcare operations, AI products should provide convenient interfaces to combine with the existing HIS of healthcare institutions. Further, an AI with a total solution is more competitive than a single function AI. For example, for patients diagnosed with diabetes mellitus, AI should suggest an ophthalmoscopy test and extract images by IoT. Next, it should evaluate the risk for diabetic retinopathy and provide suggestions (combined with other laboratory data of patients) to confirm the diagnosis (could be sent to mobile phones of attending physicians). Moreover, an AI that integrates Business Intelligence (BI, e.g., digital dashboard), Internet of things (IoT), wearable devices, mobile, and remote technologies in the early and late stages of health care would be great added features.

It is an interesting issue to explore whether AI plays a "leading role" or "supporting role" in the healthcare industry; that is, it is essential to determine whether it is worthwhile to create AI products to attract investments from healthcare institutions. For instance, it would be good to know if hospitals would prefer to purchase an X-ray AI interpretation system alone and integrate it with their existing X-ray machines to assist radiologists or purchase built-in AI interpretation X-ray machines at a higher price. According to our observations, AI providing assistance or supporting role in healthcare equipment and devices may be a promising idea due to a lower obstacle of compatibility and connectivity.

In addition, AI providers could act as an assistant to help hospitals establish their own AI models and application systems using the accumulated healthcare big data. Since the healthcare industry has a geographical distribution, the AI model built on the hospital's data would serve its patient group best. The model quality (e.g., the accuracy of prediction) could be good provided there is enough data in the electronic medical records (EMR).

It is necessary for providers to seize the opportunity to apply for patent protection and verification of equipment concerning healthcare AI products since too many R&D manufacturers, and relevant AI technologies are becoming increasingly simple without differences and advantages. The international community is aware of the rapid development of healthcare AI and has put forward relevant regulations and guidelines for reference, such as "The Software as Medical Device: Clinical Evaluation, Proposed Regulatory Framework for Modifications to Artificial Intelligence/Machine Learning-Based Software as a Medical Device" published by the US Food and Drug Administration (FDA) [21,22] and "The Medical Device of Artificial Intelligence/Machine Learning Technology: Technical Guidelines for Software Inspection and Registration" [23].

As for the target market, AI providers could sell their AI products to healthcare institutions with poor medical service quality (if the use of AI will improve the service quality), to countries with limited healthcare resources (if the domestic government will allow AI to partly replace healthcare workers and medical equipment), or to those with low medical insurance coverage (the cost of medical treatment is high, so people can use AI to properly assist in self-care management).

4. Critical Affecting Factors

Based on the above discussion, the critical factors affecting the deployment and scaling of healthcare AI are summarized below:

4.1. Policies and Regulations Amendment

The government should amend related policies and regulations to encourage the introduction of AI in health care, which could reduce or partially replace manpower. Moreover, the government has to subsidize substantively the development of AI in healthcare institutions to improve the overall healthcare quality and efficiency nationwide.

4.2. Top Executive Support

The introduction of AI into hospitals may require resource expenditure and continuous capital investment. Hence, hospital institutions should exert extra efforts to improve the knowledge of medical professionals on AI and its application even when short-term economic benefits may not seem apparent.

4.3. Clinical Actual Demand

Healthcare institutions should adopt/purchase AI products based on the actual demand of healthcare workers. Furthermore, AI needs to be integrated with existing processes and should not create an additional workload for medical workers.

4.4. User Department Consensus

Since AI is costly, it should not be used by only a few people. A consensus within the entire department should be established, putting forward the needs and expected benefits of AI for it to gain wide recognition and encourage healthcare workers' participation in planning and introducing AI, and eventually, into using it regularly.

4.5. Dedicated AI Analysts

AI development is a complex process across all fields. It is necessary to set up special departments or units and prepare specific AI analysts to effectively and extensively promote the development of AI systems in various medical fields. If the AI analysts are only working part-time, or their work is designated to employees with other existing jobs and responsibilities (maybe statisticians or physicians), the progress may become slow, the subject may be limited, and their AI knowledge may be insufficient.

4.6. IS Department Supports

Whether it is the preparation of big data or the subsequent implementation of integration with HIS, it must be strongly supported by the IS department; otherwise, it will be difficult to complete. However, the IS department may already have a heavy routine and may only provide limited support on AI projects. Providing the IS department additional bonuses to encourage it to assist with AI projects during off-hours is a feasible approach.

4.7. Obvious Concrete Benefits

Since AI users and scientific studies have exaggerated AI's functions, the introduction of AI should target clear aims and measurable benefits such as income increase, cost reduction, and improvement in quality and efficiency. Perceptive benefits such as user satisfaction and acceptance can be considered as well.

4.8. Improve AI's Explainability

Studies have proven that AI performs excellently in prediction and is even better than that of healthcare workers. However, if AI cannot clearly explain the rules or basis of its prediction, the issue of AI being just a "black-box" will remain and continue to doubt the public, resulting in lower acceptance and use.

4.9. Continuous Optimization of Products

Along with environmental changes and technological progress, AI products require continuous optimization and improvement, such as model retraining, self-learning, and federated learning [24].

4.10. Easy to Install and Use

Since clinical work is already complex on its own, AI products should be easy to install and use and should work automatically as much as possible, but the final decision-making should ultimately remain within the healthcare workers. In addition, the AI should not interrupt or impede the clinical care process unnecessarily; otherwise, healthcare workers will avert from it.

4.11. Assistance rather than Replacement

The current AI still needs a lot of improvement. Although it can perform well in healthcare projects, it cannot match the overall judgment of an experienced medical professional. Medical decisions are based on numerous factors, including the emotional level of the patient, the stance of family members, and the socio-economic environment. Hence, hospitals should employ AI as an assistant rather than a replacement for healthcare workers.

4.12. Spontaneous rather than Compulsory

Regarding laws, practice, or even public perception, the use of AI still has a lot of problems, including ownership, accuracy, explainability, reliability, stability, morale affection, etc. Therefore, healthcare workers should have the right to choose whether or not to use AI rather than being imposed to do so.

5. Conclusions

The soft power of healthcare services and the hard power of the ICT industry in Taiwan have laid a strong foundation for developing healthcare AI. Although hospitals, technological manufacturers, and start-ups have launched enormous AI products, the mature economic scale and profit model remain unclear because large-scale cases of successful implementation of healthcare AI in medical institutions are still rare.

Based on the experience of the Chi Mei Hospital group that has deployed multiple AI applications, this research summarized the key influencing factors and possible responses that affected the development and diffusion of AI in medical institutions. This type of research is very important but less reported. We believe that relevant stakeholders or the so-called AI consumers, which include the government, medical institutions, end-users, and AI providers, should openly and fully cooperate to understand each other's niches in AI development and jointly solve the problems in its development. Ideally, machines could be utilized to assist humans in generating higher quality predictions, with the final decisions and optimal actions being left to the latter [25]. This could realize AI-enabled hospitals with confidence.

Since this research is only based on Chi Mei Hospital's view on the development of healthcare AI, it may not be enough to represent all hospitals. Chi Mei Hospital mainly develops AI applications based on its structured big data, which may not represent the experience of other types of healthcare AI (such as medical imaging). In addition, this study suggests that future researchers can explore the attitudes and expectations of more stakeholders thoroughly. Additionally, the differences between the development and introduction of AI in hospitals in different countries are worthy of comparative analysis.

Author Contributions: Conceptualization, C.-F.L. and C.-C.H.; methodology, C.-F.L.; formal analysis, J.-J.W.; investigation, K.-M.K.; resources, J.-J.W.; writing—original draft preparation, C.-F.L.; writing—review and editing, C.-J.C.; visualization, C.-J.C.; supervision, C.-C.H. All authors have read and agreed to the published version of the manuscript.

Funding: This research received no external funding.

Institutional Review Board Statement: Not applicable.

Informed Consent Statement: Not applicable.

Data Availability Statement: Not applicable.

Conflicts of Interest: The authors declare no conflict of interest.

References

1. Thilmany, J. Artificial Intelligence Transforms Manufacturing. The American Society of Mechanical Engineers, 31 May 2018. Available online: https://www.asme.org/topics-resources/content/artificial-intelligence-transforms-manufacturing (accessed on 1 May 2021).
2. Zhang, D.; Mishra, S.; Brynjolfsson, E.; Etchemendy, J.; Ganguli, D.; Grosz, B.; Lyons, T.; Manyika, J.; Niebles, J.C.; Sellitto, M.; et al. *The AI Index 2021 Annual Report*; AI Index Steering Committee, Human-Centered AI Institute, Stanford University: Stanford, CA, USA, 2021.
3. Brethenoux, E.; Ingelbrecht, N.; Shen, S.; Ganly, D. *Five Questions for a Successful AI Project*; Gartner: Stamford, CT, USA, 2019.
4. Smith, T. Where Are the Biggest Opportunities for AI? AI Zone. 31 July 2017. Available online: https://dzone.com/articles/where-are-the-biggest-opportunities-for-ai (accessed on 1 May 2021).
5. Shah, H. 5 Industries that are Using Artificial Intelligence the Most. Datafloq, 2 December 2019. Available online: https://datafloq.com/read/5-industries-using-artificial-intelligence/7242 (accessed on 1 May 2021).
6. Leibowitz, D. AI Now Diagnoses Disease Better Than Your Doctor, Study Finds. Medium, 29 September 2020. Available online: https://towardsdatascience.com/ai-diagnoses-disease-better-than-your-doctor-study-finds-a5cc0ffbf32 (accessed on 1 May 2021).

7. Smith, J. Can Artificial Intelligence Replace the Role of Doctors? Readwrite Daily Newsletter. 23 March 2020. Available online: https://towardsdatascience.com/ai-diagnoses-disease-better-than-your-doctor-study-finds-a5cc0ffbf32 (accessed on 1 May 2021).
8. Zhang, P.-I.; Hsu, C.-C.; Kao, Y.; Chen, C.-J.; Kuo, Y.-W.; Hsu, S.-L.; Liu, T.-L.; Lin, H.-J.; Wang, J.-J.; Liu, C.-F.; et al. Real-time AI prediction for major adverse cardiac events in emergency department patients with chest pain. *Scand. J. Trauma Resusc. Emerg. Med.* **2020**, *28*, 93. [CrossRef] [PubMed]
9. Chang, Y.; Hung, K.; Wang, L.; Yu, C.; Chen, C.; Tay, H.; Wang, J.; Liu, C. A real-time artificial intelligence-assisted system to predict weaning from ventilator immediately after lung resection surgery. *Int. J. Environ. Res. Public Health* **2021**, *18*, 2713. [CrossRef] [PubMed]
10. US While House. The White House Launches the National Artificial Intelligence Initiative Office. 12 January 2021. Available online: https://trumpwhitehouse.archives.gov/briefings-statements/white-house-launches-national-artificial-intelligence-initiative-office/ (accessed on 1 May 2021).
11. Schölkopf, B.; Bethge, M.; Black, M.J.; Kuchenbecker, K.J. A Boost for Artificial Intelligence. Max-Planck-Gesellschaft, 18 December 2020. Available online: https://www.mpg.de/16193056/a-boost-for-artificial-intelligence (accessed on 1 May 2021).
12. Tse, D.; Chow, C.K.; Ly, T.P.; Tong, C.Y.; Tam, K.W. The challenges of big data governance in healthcare. In Proceedings of the 17th IEEE International Conference on Trust, Security and Privacy in Computing and Communications, New York, NY, USA, 1–3 August 2018.
13. Dwivedi, Y.K.; Hughes, L.; Ismagilova, E.; Aarts, G.; Coombs, C.; Crick, T.; Duan, Y.; Dwivedi, R.; Edwards, J.; Eirug, A.; et al. Artificial Intelligence (AI): Multidisciplinary perspectives on emerging challenges, opportunities, and agenda for research, practice and policy. *Int. J. Inf. Manag.* **2021**, *57*, 101994. [CrossRef]
14. Payrovnaziri, S.N.; Chen, Z.; Rengifo-Moreno, P.; Miller, T.; Bian, J.; Chen, J.H.; Liu, X.; He, Z. Explainable artificial intelligence models using real-world electronic health record data: A systematic scoping review. *J. Am. Med. Inform. Assoc.* **2020**, *27*, 1173–1185. [CrossRef] [PubMed]
15. Kokkotis, C.; Moustakidis, S.; Baltzopoulos, V.; Giakas, G.; Tsaopoulos, D. Identifying robust risk factors for knee osteoarthritis progression: An evolutionary machine learning approach. *Healthcare* **2021**, *9*, 260. [CrossRef] [PubMed]
16. Weiss, T.R. IBM Reportedly Looking to Sell its Unprofitable Watson Health Business. EnterpriseAI, 25 February 2021. Available online: https://www.enterpriseai.news/2021/02/25/ibm-reportedly-looking-to-sell-its-unprofitable-watson-health-business/ (accessed on 1 May 2021).
17. Longoni, C.; Morewedge, C.K. AI Can Outperform Doctors. So Why Don't Patients Trust It. Harvard Business Review. 30 October 2019. Available online: https://hbr.org/2019/10/ai-can-outperform-doctors-so-why-dont-patients-trust-it# (accessed on 1 May 2021).
18. Spencer, J.; Poggi, J.; Gheerawo, R. Designing out stereotypes in artificial intelligence: Involving users in the personality design of a digital assistant. In Proceedings of the 4th EAI International Conference on Smart Objects and Technologies for Social Good, Bologna, Italy, 28–30 November 2018; pp. 130–135.
19. König, I.R.; Fuchs, O.; Hansen, G.; von Mutius, E.; Kopp, M.V. What is precision medicine? *Eur. Respir. J.* **2017**, *50*, 1700391. [CrossRef] [PubMed]
20. Prainsack, B. *Personalized Medicine Empowered Patients in the 21st Century?* New York University Press: New York, NY, USA, 2017.
21. US FDA. *Software as a Medical Device (SAMD): Clinical Evaluation*; US Food & Drug Administration: Richmond, VA, USA, 2017.
22. US FDA. *Proposed Regulatory Framework for Modifications to Artificial Intelligence/Machine Learning (AI/ML)-based Software as a Medical Device (SAMD)-Discussion Paper and Request for Feedback*; US Food & Drug Administration: Richmond, VA, USA, 2019.
23. Taiwan FDA. *Medical Device of Artificial Intelligence/Machine Learning Technology-Technical Guidelines for Software Inspection and Registration*; Taiwan Food & Drug Administration: Taipei, Taiwan, 2019.
24. Yang, Q.; Liu, Y.; Chen, T.; Tong, Y. Federated machine learning: Concept and applications. *ACM Trans. Intell. Syst. Technol.* **2019**, *10*, 12. [CrossRef]
25. Verghese, A.V.; Shah, N.H.; Harrington, R.A. What this computer needs is a physician: Humanism and artificial intelligence. *JAMA* **2018**, *319*, 19–20. [CrossRef] [PubMed]

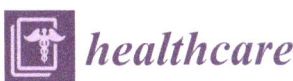 *healthcare*

Project Report

Project Report on Telemedicine: What We Learned about the Administration and Development of a Binational Digital Infrastructure Project

Norbert Hosten [1], Britta Rosenberg [1,*] and Andrzej Kram [2]

[1] Department of Radiology, Universitätsmedizin Greifswald, Fleischmannstraße 8, 17475 Greifswald, Germany; norbert.hosten@med.uni-greifswald.de
[2] Department of Pathology, Westpomeranian Oncology Center, Strzałowska 22, 71-730 Szczecin, Poland; akram@onkologia.szczecin.pl
* Correspondence: britta.rosenberg1@uni-greifswald.de

Abstract: This article describes the development of a German–Polish cross-border telemedicine project. Funded by the European Union Interreg Program, a cooperation between several German and Polish hospitals was developed over the course of 16 years, starting in 2002. Subprojects, governance and outcomes are described, and facilitators and barriers are identified. These points are reviewed with regard to their influence on medical, technical, administrative and medico-legal realisation.

Keywords: telemedicine; telediagnostic; project management; funding; IT infrastructure; cross-border multiprofessional team; European Union; Interreg

Citation: Hosten, N.; Rosenberg, B.; Kram, A. Project Report on Telemedicine: What We Learned about the Administration and Development of a Binational Digital Infrastructure Project. *Healthcare* **2021**, *9*, 400. https://doi.org/10.3390/healthcare9040400

Received: 1 February 2021
Accepted: 25 March 2021
Published: 1 April 2021

Publisher's Note: MDPI stays neutral with regard to jurisdictional claims in published maps and institutional affiliations.

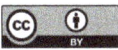

Copyright: © 2021 by the authors. Licensee MDPI, Basel, Switzerland. This article is an open access article distributed under the terms and conditions of the Creative Commons Attribution (CC BY) license (https://creativecommons.org/licenses/by/4.0/).

1. Introduction

This report explores the lessons learnt from a German–Polish telemedicine network funded by the European Union (EU) in Pomerania.

Pomerania is a historic region on the southern shore of the Baltic sea, with a western part located in Germany and an eastern part located in Poland. The area of historic Pomerania was used to create a co-operation structure between Germany and Poland in 1995 ("Euroregion Pomerania"). Ten German cities and districts and 98 Polish municipalities are members of the Euroregion. The purpose of all Euroregions is the promotion of common interests. Euroregions are eligible for funding in the Interreg programs of the European Union. Interreg I started in 1989. The present phase of the program, Interreg V, funded projects until 2020. Interreg was created to promote cross-border cooperation in the EU, thus diminishing the influence of national borders.

The council of the Pomeranian Euroregion is located in (Polish) Szczecin, the historic capital of ancient Pomerania. The council is constituted in equal parts by German and Polish members. Polish members of the Euroregion are members of a Polish association, while German members belong to a "Kommunalgemeinschaft"—an association according to German law.

Eligible projects may apply for funding from current Interreg programs. Only groups that are constituted by both German and Polish members are suitable for application. A lead partner may be either from Germany or Poland. The agency in the lead partner's country of origin will then process the request, aiming to achieve harmonisation between the Polish and the German side.

A complete review of Interreg is beyond the scope of this paper. Perkmann [1] gives an overview of the concept and existing cross-border regions, following Schmitt-Egner's [2] definition of 'cross-border cooperation' as 'cross-border interaction between neighbouring regions for the preservation, governance and development of their common living space, without the involvement of their central authorities" (Perkmann's translation).

The rationale for implementing telemedicine in the Euroregion of Pomerania was twofold: (1) The regions on both sides of the German/Polish border are very thinly populated. The German federal state of "Vorpommern" (Western Pomerania) has a population density of 69 inhabitants/square kilometre, while the Polish voivodeship's (province) "województwo zachodniopomorskie"(Voivodeship Western Pomerania) has 75 inhabitants/square kilometre (mean population density: Germany, 137 inhabitants/square kilometre; Poland, 132 inhabitants/square kilometre). (2) The border in the Pomerania region between Poland and Germany leaves several German and Polish hospitals with small catchment areas (Figure 1). Telemedicine is an accepted means of delivering medical services to people in such areas by enlarging catchment areas [3,4].

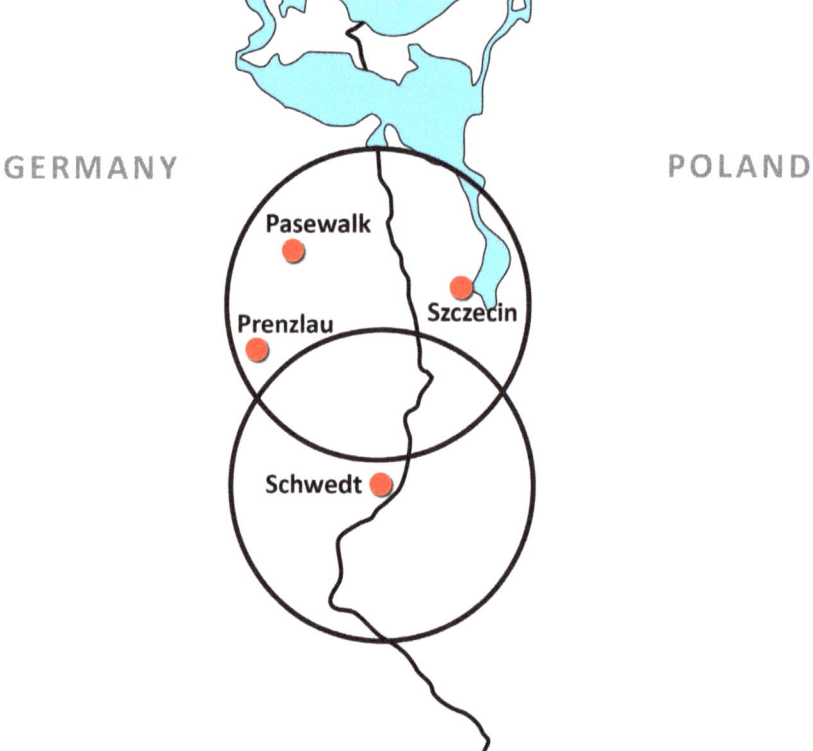

Figure 1. Influence of the boundary between Germany and Poland on the catchment areas of hospitals in the cities of Szczecin, Pasewalk, Prenzlau and Schwedt. It is apparent that the hospitals close to the border have small catchment areas and that there are areas without easily accessible hospitals.

Accordingly, people living in these regions may have reduced access to hospitals. To improve access to specialised medicine, a joint telemedicine project was initiated starting in 2002. With Interreg IVA funding, the most recent phase of this project was initiated with 11 German and 11 Polish hospitals. Specialities taking part were radiology, pathology, ophthalmology, urology and otorhinolaryngology (ear–nose–throat medicine, ENT) as well as radiation therapy, oncology and thoracic surgery in tumour boards. On the German side, an extensive videoconferencing network was laid out, which allowed for the simultaneous transport of x-ray studies, pathology slides, endoscopy images and documents.

As medicine is generally organised nationally, telemedicine tends also to be national. The project described here originated in radiology and pathology, with both of them dealing with physician-to-physician interaction; another focus was videoconferencing. On the German side, an expensive infrastructure had to be bought and installed to support these applications. Management, facilitators and barriers for these parts of the project are described below. We report here on the lessons learned from the implementation of this Interreg IV project.

2. Materials and Methods

2.1. Previous Phases of the Project

The project described here was implemented over the course of four funding periods since 2002. The first author (a university radiologist, chairman of the project's board) has been involved from the beginning; the other two authors (in-house counsel and pathologist) have been involved since 2010. Documentation from the different project phases was used for analysis. Because public funds were used, the written documentation was comprehensive. The work presented here aims to describe facilitators and barriers and thus to provide guidance for colleagues wishing to implement similar international projects. The paper focuses on the last phase of the project which started in 2010. There were three previous project phases, each with six-digit funding (all figures in Euros):

1. A digitisation project focusing on radiology and pathology in Pomerania ("Pommern", Germany) and Poznań.
2. A regional expansion of the digitisation project to North Brandenburg and Poland.
3. Another digitisation phase between Pomerania, northern Brandenburg and Poznań.
4. Beginning in 2010, the current project between Pomerania, northern Brandenburg and the voivodeship of Western Pomerania and Poznań (a fifth phase of the project with cross-border patient treatment has been approved; it is mentioned here as it aims at the cross-border treatment of patients (children with neuroblastoma). Grounded in the first three phases, the project was required to develop a structure that allowed for the implementation of a telemedicine network in a larger state.

The following documents from project phases 1 to 4 were available for analysis:

- From business plans, grant approvals and project applications, we extracted and evaluated objectives and the amount of funding (a low eight-digit amount of funding in the phase described here).
- Accountability reports were available for the project phases between 2002 and 2010. They were evaluated for an overview of newly installed devices.
- Presentation slides.
- For the fourth phase of the project, the following documents were additionally available:
    a. The association's statutes, with descriptions of the organisational structure (Figure 2); protocols of the yearly assembly between 2010 and 2020.
    b. The protocols of the meetings of the Board of Directors between 2010 and 2016.
    c. The business plan for the association from 2010.
    d. The protocols of the technical advisory board's meetings, which had to approve purchases.
    e. Medico-legal and medico-economic analyses as published by the project in specialist journals on the projects: the tele-tumour conference, teleradiology, telepathology, tele-ENT (overview lecture, published), Tele-Glaucoma (technical description) and Tele-Stroke.
    f. Final reports to the sponsor.

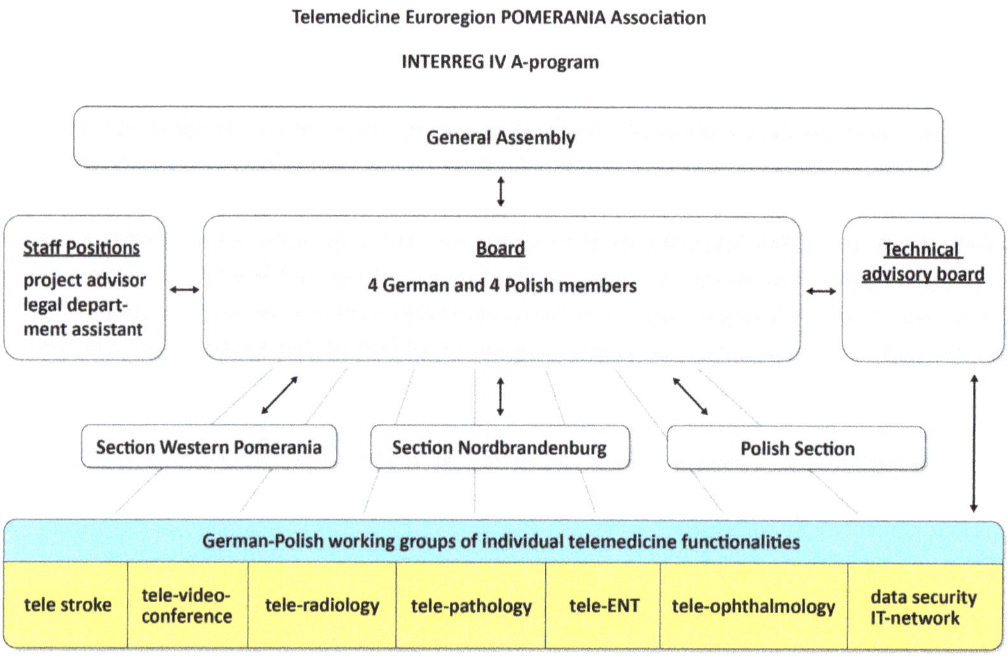

Telemedicine Euroregion POMERANIA Association

INTERREG IV A-program

```
                        ┌─────────────────────────────┐
                        │      General Assembly       │
                        └──────────────┬──────────────┘
                                       ↕
┌──────────────────┐     ┌─────────────────────────────┐     ┌──────────────────┐
│ Staff Positions  │     │           Board             │     │    Technical     │
│ project advisor  │ ↔   │ 4 German and 4 Polish       │ ↔   │ advisory board   │
│ legal depart-    │     │ members                     │     │                  │
│ ment assistant   │     │                             │     │                  │
└──────────────────┘     └─────────────────────────────┘     └──────────────────┘
                         ↙              ↕              ↘
         ┌──────────────────────┐  ┌──────────────────────┐  ┌──────────────┐
         │ Section Western      │  │ Section              │  │ Polish       │
         │ Pomerania            │  │ Nordbrandenburg      │  │ Section      │
         └──────────────────────┘  └──────────────────────┘  └──────────────┘
```

German-Polish working groups of individual telemedicine functionalities						
tele stroke	tele-video-conference	tele-radiology	tele-pathology	tele-ENT	tele-ophthalmology	data security IT-network

Figure 2. Organigram of the association "Telemedicine Euroregion Pomerania". The German project participants organised themselves in an association under German law; three Polish members were co-opted. Their assembly (one representative with voting rights from each of the participating hospitals) approved key decisions and the budget once a year. The assembly elected the association's board. Additional Polish members took part in German–Polish working groups. The German side was the lead partner of the project. It organised the settlement of the funds. The board of directors had several employees for legal, financial and secretarial tasks. A technical advisory board staffed with independent technical experts met twice a year for three years to review the investments.

2.2. Problems Identified in Ihe Scientific Literature on Telemedicine That Were Evaluated

The following text focuses on lessons learned from the Pomerania telemedicine cross-border project. Facilitators and barriers encountered during the implementation of telemedicine in rural regions have been covered in the literature [3–7]. There is, however, hardly any mention of management and organisation matters in such projects. The following barriers are named, among others (they also turned out to be central to our project): high capital expenditure overheads, a lack of motivation and financial benefits for application developers and telehealth service providers, a lack of a strategy to transform telehealth trials into sustainable real-world services, insufficient financial support through government reimbursement (e.g., to buy telehealth equipment) and unmet requirements to train people to deal with cultural differences.

2.3. Participating Hospitals Whose Projects Were Analysed

The participating hospitals on the Polish side were SPSK2 PUM Szczecin, ZCO Szczecin, ZOZ Zdunowo Szczecin, SP Barlinek, SR Kołobrzeg, SZGiChP Koszalin, SW Koszalin, ZOZ Stargard, ZOZ Gryfice, ZOZ Połczyn, and SP Białogard; on the German side, the hospitals were Sana Bergen/Rügen, Asklepios Stralsund, Universitätsmedizin Greifswald, Krankenhaus Wolgast, Asklepios Pasewalk, Dietrich-Bonhoeffer-Klinikum Neubrandenburg, GLG Eberswalde, GLG Prenzlau, Asklepios Schwedt, Sana Templin, and Herzzentrum Bernau (Figure 3).

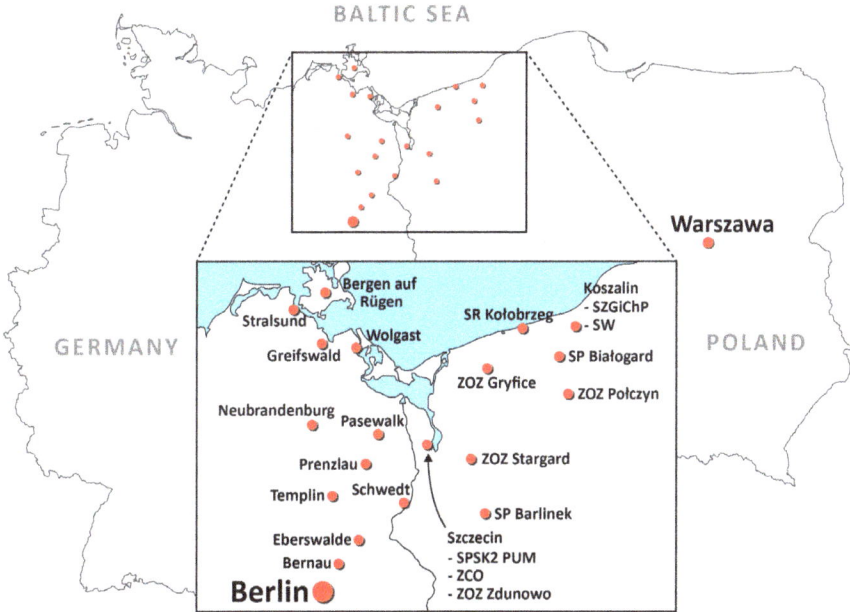

Figure 3. Geographical distribution of hospitals on both sides of the German–Polish border. Berlin, Warsaw and the Baltic Sea are also indicated for the better visualisation of the project.

3. Results

3.1. Results Regarding Organisation of the Project

To develop a structure for a telemedicine network, the Telemedicine Association in the Euroregion of Pomerania was founded in 2008. It was funded in the Interreg program from 2010 onwards. According to German law, an association is not primarily dedicated to generating profits; it receives public funding more easily than a limited company. The association was registered with statutes, and hospitals were invited to a constituent meeting. In the next step, a business plan was drawn up. This budgeted the establishment of an office (see Figure 2) and the financing of staff beyond funding. The association was provided with a low five-digit capital. An IT consultancy (DFC, Munich-Germany) was commissioned to develop a concept for the German side of the funding area. Under the umbrella term "telemedicine", the concept planned the modalities listed in Table 1. They were underlaid with digitised medical devices and equipment for storage, network connection, etc. After several rounds of negotiations with the relevant Ministry of Economics, the concept was accepted and the project was funded.

The EU's outcome parameters differ from the clinical/medical parameters discussed below. Parameters and eligibility requirements for the Interreg program are summarised in manuals. In addition to the basic requirement (beneficiaries from at least two participating countries, at least one of which is a member state of the EU), the following methods of cooperation are also required:

1. Joint conceptualisation, which may for example be achieved by holding regular project development meetings, establishing institutionalised long-term contacts, joint project preparation and/or scheduling.
2. Joint implementation, which may for example be achieved by joint management or partial responsibilities for each of the project partners.
3. Joint staffing.
4. Joint funding.

Table 1. Subprojects. Note, different goals for the German and Polish sides. Outcomes and outcome indicators are given and facilitators and barriers are listed. See details in text.

Subproject	Goal Germany	Goal Poland	Main Outcome Indicator	Outcome	Facilitators	Barriers	Soft Facilitators/Barriers
Tele-tumor conferencing.	To establish a twice-weekly online-only video conference with multiple hospitals and multiple specialties.	-	Economic analysis of working conference.	Established successfully, in permanent full use, economically sound.	Only way to establish tumor conferences in areas with low population density.	-	Implemented by chairman of large hospital in project, prestige project.
Patient's informed consent.	Scientific evaluation.	-	Feasibility.	Feasible.	Obvious advantage of avoiding time and expenses for travel.	Interoperability problems.	Patients remembered content better.
Tele-conference for board meetings.	To avoid travelling to board meetings.	To avoid travelling to board meetings.	-	Established successfully, used when necessary.	Obvious advantage of avoiding time and expenses for monthly travel to board meetings.	Binational meetings too sterile, bonding an important factor for the success of the whole project.	-
Tele-radiology.	To establish 24/7 computed tomography (CT) reporting coverage in German area. Scientific evaluation	To provide digital X-ray equipment.	Establishment of service, equipment delivered, assessment of cost-effectiveness.	Teleradiology established successfully in Germany. Digital X-ray equipment provided to hospitals in Poland. In use.	Teleradiology in off-hours without alternative: no emergency department without computed tomography access (!).	Legal restriction in Germany at time of implementation.	Radiologists in area known to each other from training.
Tele-pathology.	To establish 24/7 pathology coverage in the German area.	To provide digital pathology equipment; tele pathology service.	Establishment of service, equipment delivered.	Telepathology established successfully in Germany and Poland. Also used for teaching.	High cost of digitisation of pathology; funding from project was a very strong incentive.	Low acceptance of telepathology in one provider. Abandoned by one providing hospital as management did not want to support competitors.	Little alternative for providing hospitals, as pathology departments not economically feasible for smaller hospitals.

Table 1. Cont.

Subproject	Goal Germany	Goal Poland	Main Outcome Indicator	Outcome	Facilitators	Barriers	Soft Facilitators/Barriers
Tele-earnose throat (ENT).	To establish 24/7 ENT specialty coverage in the German area.	-	Establishment of service, equipment delivered.	Project was technically implemented, later discontinued.	Technology available, was installed successfully; not enough patients for a university department in this area of low-population density.	Doctors at receiving hospitals not familiar with placement of endoscopic device via nose: legal problems expected.	Smaller hospitals not willing to accept specialty support, prefered to provide for their patients without outside help.
Teleophthalmology.	To establish early diagnoses from retina scans by screening in one hospital.	-	Establishment of service, equipment delivered.	Establishment of tele-screening in hospital, evaluated in university clinic, later discontinued.	Technology was available, was installed successfully.	Program established technically, but no access to financial re-imbursement. Screening.	Started by personally acquainted department heads, stopped when one of them left.
Tele-stroke.	To establish a tele-stroke network.	-	-	-	Pomerania perceived as competitor by neurology. Very strong incentive for neurology to implement own project.	Low-cost of technology employed. No funding necessary. Aspects of organizing services prevailed.	Clinical specialty joined Berlin project, established successful program with minimal funding by Pomerania.

It is important that cross-border cooperation in the specific program context does not have to consist of cross-border patient treatment—a criterion often expected, in particular by the press. The relative freedom in designing the project with the total amount capped at a low eight-digit amount led to the establishment of a technical advisory board on the German side. This independent, national committee of experts had to approve all investments in advance. The State Court of Auditors then reviewed and accepted the entire project financing.

The commitment to fund the office and staff beyond the funding phase was the decisive factor in the project's eligibility. An annual budget was adopted at each of the annual general meetings.

The typical EU outcome parameters are the numbers of persons reached and the amount and quality of the publicity. The facilitator for fulfilling expectations by the EU was the German–Polish structure. This was a definitive advantage for the public perception of the project in Germany. The project was, e.g., visited by the then Federal President Gauck. This generated much publicity. For the organizing IT company, the project was important beyond the level of income due to national visibility. As with the medical community, the IT industry has its own communication channels; the project received also received good press in this context. At the major German trade fairs (Medica, Düsseldorf; conhIT Berlin) there were opportunities to present the project that are not readily available to single-site telemedicine projects. A barrier was the perception of the association as a parallel structure by hospital administrations; the expansion of competencies by physicians was suspected.

3.2. Results by Telemedical Specialty

An overview of subprojects, outcome indicators, outcomes and facilitators/barriers is given in Table 1.

3.2.1. Videoconferencing Network

Telemedical interactions between people benefit from an image transmission that provides facial expressions as well as the other person's spoken language. Naturally, this also applies to interactions between physicians. Common videoconferencing systems, which in the meantime have become widely available to all, can be used for these image transmissions. Data safety has to be ensured when using these devices. Various studies have shown that patients are willing to communicate with their doctors via videoconferencing [8,9]. The prerequisite, however, is that the advantages outweigh the disadvantages. Perhaps the most relevant advantage in particular is saving time due to the elimination of physical transportation from the communication process. In the planning process of the project, we assumed that this would also be the point of view of doctors communicating with colleagues.

Within the project, a videoconferencing system was installed that could connect participants via a "video-bridge" (Figure 4). This system that consisted of 15 sites (14 German and 1 Polish; not all hospitals participated, but some hospitals had more than one site) was the backbone of the entire project. The following situations were covered:

- A tele-tumour conference connected several hospitals and allowed tumour conferences to be held with several specialists.
- Various tumour conferences within a hospital allowed the involvement of specialists (e.g., pathologists) who had only a few points to make for one or two minutes per hour.
- The videoconferencing system could be used experimentally for a doctor–patient project; patient education was simulated here by a two-way-connection.
- Board meetings were organised by videoconferencing.
- In parallel to the videoconferencing, medical image files were transferred. In the projects discussed below, endoscopic images (Tele-ENT), images of the ocular fundus (early diagnosis of diseases), X-ray images (teleradiology) and pathological slides (telepathology) were transmitted.

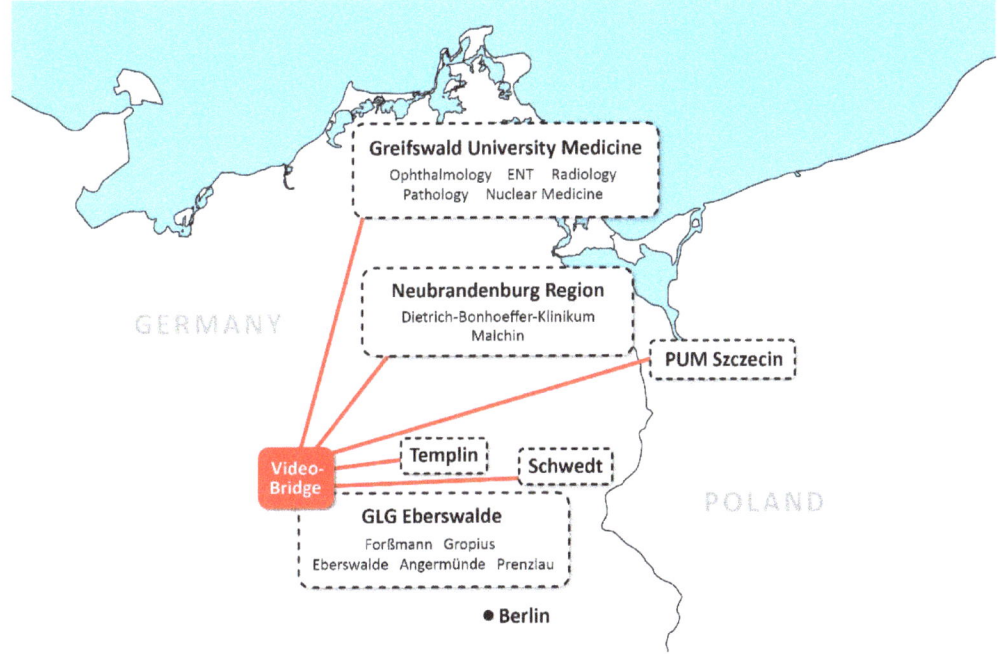

Figure 4. A videoconferencing network was the backbone of the telemedicine project. On the German side, there was a northern (Greifswald), a central (Neubrandenburg) and a southern rail (Eberswalde) with videoconferencing links; in Poland, only Szczecin took part. A "bridge", actually a switch allowing multi-point videoconferencing to be initiated, was located in the south rail. This limited use of the network required three bridges to be installed. The system also allowed for the simultaneous viewing of medical images (x-ray, real-time endoscopy and pathology slides) and various documents on additional monitors. Please note that not all hospitals that participated in the program also participated in the videoconferencing network, explaining the difference in numbers.

In the following, the individual sub-projects are discussed with a focus on facilitators and barriers.

Tele-Tumour Conferencing

Every week, a tumour conference with a regional focus on Eberswalde took place, which connects several hospitals and several modalities (Figure 5). On average, 16.4 patient treatments were discussed in each session. The conferences were attended by an average of 7.9 doctors from various disciplines within the hospital, and 1.4 external specialists from other hospitals were consulted for consultations. The project was scientifically evaluated with business economists. As an example of an objective outcome parameter, the break-even-point for a regional tumour board was calculated at 272 patients discussed per year (main outcome indicator, details in [10]).

The videoconferencing tumour project has been operating without interruption and without external funding since 2012. Facilitators were economic benefits (travelling costs saved) and convenience (travel time saved by doctors). Videoconferencing allows for one physician to be "present" at multiple sites nearly simultaneously. Interoperability was not fully achieved during the installation of the videoconferencing-network: the acquisition of only one "bridge" unnecessarily restricted the initiation of videoconferences to the Eberswalde site and made it difficult to further expand the technology. The acquisition of two additional bridges, costing a middle five-digit amount, would have been easily possible from the generous funding. This was missed by the site planning this subproject (Eberswalde) and resulted in the domination of the network by Eberswalde.

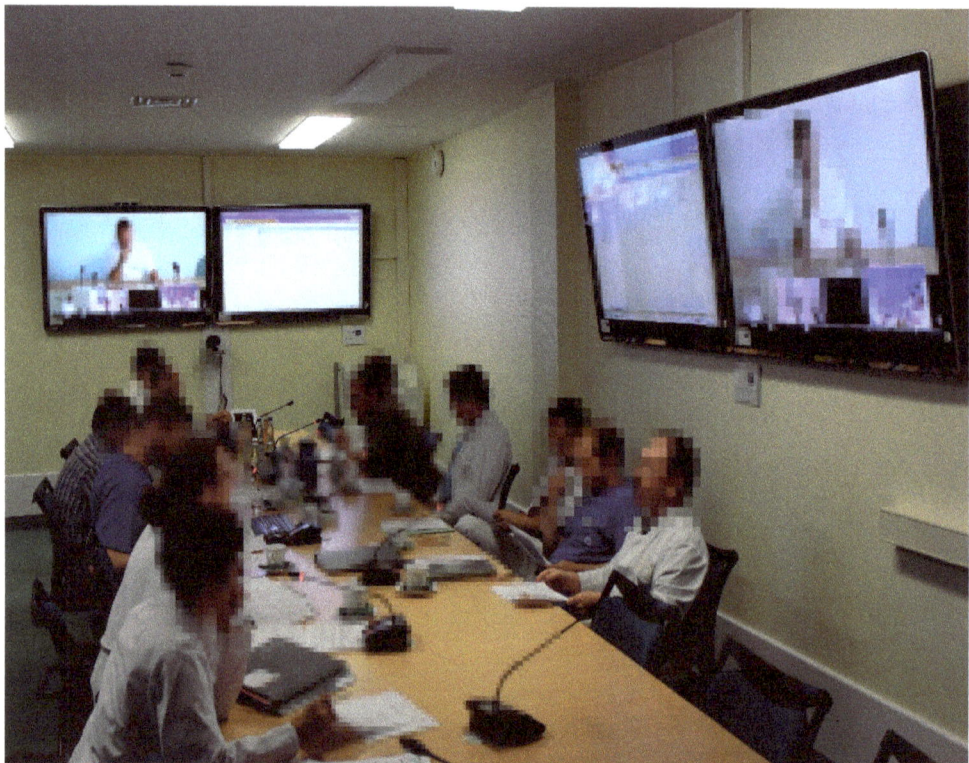

Figure 5. Tele-Tumour Conferencing. A sophisticated subproject included the tumour board of Eberswalde hospital, where smaller hospitals presented their cancer patients to specialists. Seated at the conference table are oncologists, a radiation oncologist and a radiologist. A pathologist in Pasewalk is discussing cases with a referring physician from the Templin hospital, approximately 65 km away. Documents, X-rays and pathology slides can be viewed by all participants simultaneously.

Tumour Videoconferencing within a Hospital

The videoconferencing network on the German side was built around three larger hospitals. Greifswald (videoconferencing units in five clinics and institutes), Neubrandenburg (videoconferencing units in two clinics) and Eberswalde (videoconferencing units in seven affiliated hospitals/locations). Tumour conferences within one hospital are characterised by varying degrees of contribution to the discussion from the participating disciplines. While oncologists and radiotherapists usually provide information on all patients discussed, this is not the case for the diagnostic specialties. Pathologists often have only brief verbal contributions, with short demonstrations of sections. Tumour conferences at Greifswald only call the pathologists' video stream into the conference when they are actually required to make a contribution. This scenario also applied to Eberswalde.

A facilitating factor here is the time saved by the pathologist. This advantage was so obvious that the project was immediately accepted by all involved. One barrier was the need to link different videoconferencing-systems (in-house and inter-hospital). The causes for this were differences in the design of hospitals' in-house meeting-room systems by the hospital administrations and also the inter-hospital purchasing of videoconferencing systems connecting different hospitals from project funds.

Patient Education for Informed Consent via Videoconferencing

In populated regions, patients have to come to a treatment site twice: once to give informed consent and then again for the implementation of the procedure. The reason for this is the often legally required period of consideration of 24 h that must be granted to patients. The acceptance and effectiveness of getting patients' informed consent via videoconferencing was investigated in a prospective study [11].

A facilitating factor was saving patients from a second trip to the hospital by creating the possibility of giving informed consent via a virtual meeting. The benefits—for example, saving sick or vacation days—were so important for patients that they agreed to see their doctor only on-screen. Unexpectedly, a second facilitating factor was the improved concentration of patients on screen, which led to a better memory of the educational contents. Barriers to widespread use were the lack of a uniform technological solution (hospital and at home for patients), difficulties for older patients who were inexperienced with the technology and doubts regarding the security of the video connection.

Board Meetings on Videoconference

The sponsored area has a north–south diameter of about 250 km. In the east–west direction, the diameter is marginally larger, at 280 km. The meetings of the various boards (Figure 6), which took place monthly for years, previously required considerable travel activity. Even short conferences resulted in a significant loss of working days due to travel times (about 20 days per year). In the course of the project, the meetings were converted to a presence-to-videoconferencing-ratio of 1:3. Facilitators and barriers were the same as in the other applications: As might be expected, this changeover was easy due to the installed videoconferencing-network; acceptance was high among all parties involved. However, the acquisition of only one "bridge" unnecessarily restricted the initiation of videoconferences.

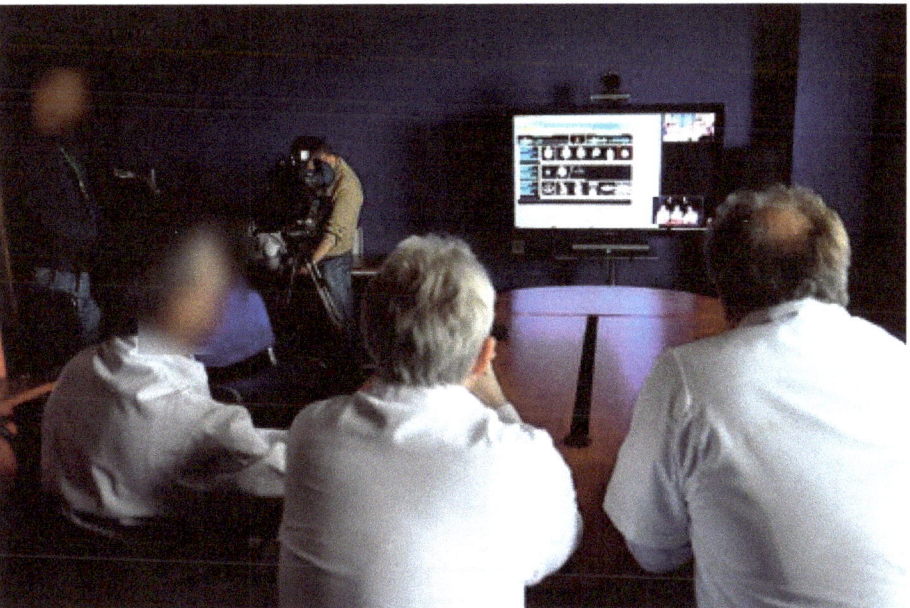

Figure 6. Cross-border meeting (Szczecin/Pasewalk). A working group of the project (in the front of the picture, three participants) and the German members (with modality pictures). From [12].

3.2.2. Teleradiology

In sparsely populated regions, patient care is usually provided by a hospital structure with houses of different sizes. Even in smaller houses, the larger disciplines such as internal medicine and general surgery are often staffed with enough doctors to make 24/7 coverage possible. This does not apply to medical specialties such as radiology, and is even less applicable to pathology. In the studied region, only the hospitals in Greifswald and Neubrandenburg could offer radiological services 24/7. There are two difficulties: if there is a 24/7 radiology service in a sparsely populated region, it is often underutilised; however, in order to operate a German hospital with an emergency department or an intensive care unit, computed tomography diagnostics (CT) must be available 24/7. Teleradiology can compensate for these two situations. This increases the area in which on-call radiologists can provide their medical expertise in the night and on weekends. They are therefore utilised more efficiently by the teleradiological services and the hospitals that use teleradiological services can provide 24/7 CT diagnostics for emergencies. On the German side, the aim in the field of teleradiology was to establish a teleradiological 24/7 network, the development of contracts between supplier and customer and the economic evaluation of the costs that must be reimbursed in order to enable an economic operation, as well as a quality evaluation of the services. A cooperation between the University Radiology Greifswald and seven hospitals was established (Figure 7). On the German side, equipment had been installed in previous phases of the project. On the Polish side, radiological departments were newly equipped with scanners that allowed the digitisation of X-ray images. Several radiology departments in the sponsored houses were given radiological digital workstations consisting of high-resolution monitors and computers. Medical equipment (intraoperative MRI and X-ray workstations) was financed at two hospitals. Computer networks were added to all houses to enable the creation of a digital workflow.

In summary, teleradiology was permanently translated into a sustainable network, and its actual costs were scientifically assessed (main outcome indicator, details in [13,14]). The following figures may give an idea of the scope of services offered permanently; currently, there are approximately 1000 radiological exams per year reported during night and weekend shifts by one institution. A cost analysis of teleradiology from a provider's perspective was performed using Monte Carlo analysis. Costs of reporting head and abdominal CT were calculated in a cooperation with academic economists (with €61.35 as the minimal charge for a head CT report to avoid losses). An increase in the catchment area for radiologists result in the better use of this profession's services during night and weekend shifts.

The facilitating factors for teleradiology were the indispensability of the 24/7 service; the interdisciplinary setup of the project team; the presence of a chair in economics with a focus on medicine, who took over the economic evaluation, as well as the presence of an in-house counsel with a special focus on the legal aspects of teleradiology; and the digitisation of the participating clinics in previous phases with the establishment of a network. Another facilitator was the close cooperation between radiologists all over the area, since a large proportion of the radiologists working in peripheral institutions had been trained in the bigger centres.

There was a chance missed by not supporting the system with weekly videoconferencing between the radiologists in the centres and the surgeons and internists in the area's peripheral regions. This probably will be a barrier to further expanding the service.

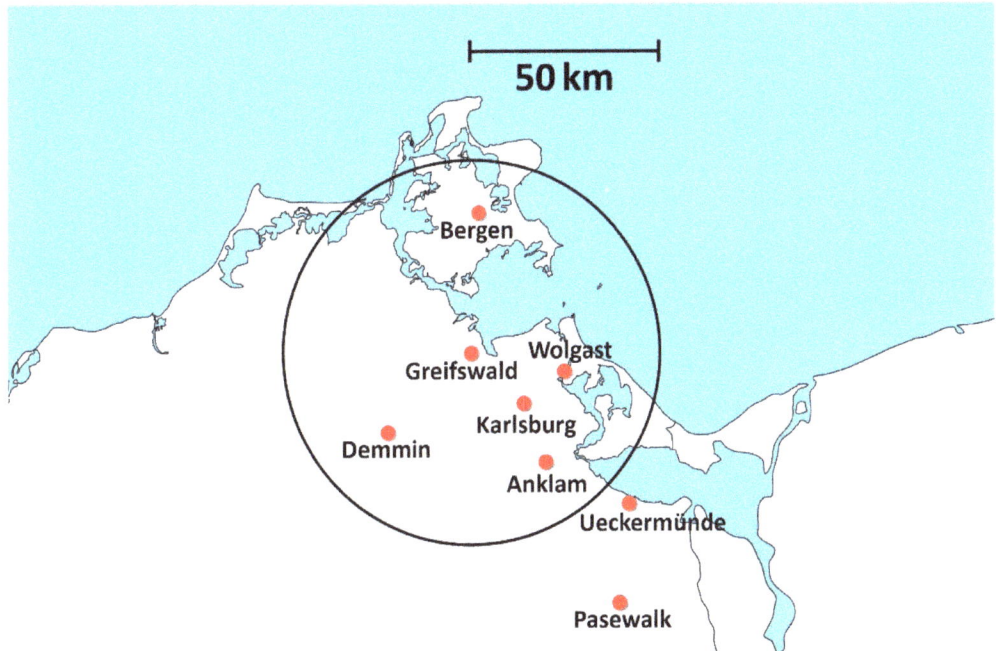

Figure 7. Geographical distribution of the German teleradiology network. The network has been running for more than 15 years. In Greifswald, there is a 24/7 radiological service in the university hospital. The surrounding city names represent the locations of connected houses that are also supplied in the network. According to German law, the backup method for downtime in teleradiology is a radiologist going to the relevant hospital and performing the examination there. Due to this restriction in German law, teleradiology was limited to hospitals that could be reached within an hour (Demmin and Karlsburg were not financed by the project). Conclusion: The loss of catchment areas of the hospitals due to a new territorial delimitation can be increased by the telemedical expansion of catchment areas. Telemedicine thus leads to better access to doctors in territorial states and to the better utilisation of medical services in the same regions (black circle, unbroken: catchment area of Greifswald University Hospital's pathology department with telepathology. Red arrows: pathology connections.).

3.2.3. Telepathology

In sparsely populated regions, most hospitals do not have their own pathologist. The conditions here are even clearer than in radiology. Of the three centres on the German side of our project, only two have a pathology department; none of the smaller houses do. The pathologists provide surgical departments with rapidly processed slides during operations and the reprocessing of surgical material after the operation. The slides are time-critical, as patients remain in anaesthesia until the results are communicated to the surgeon. Telepathological projects create slides cooperatively, using sophisticated technology during surgery (for example, pathologists directing the surgeons regarding from which part of the resectate specimens should be taken). Referring centres can digitally transmit scanned slides and have them evaluated in a pathology department. In our project, providing pathological services for all houses that required them through telepathology was the goal (outcome indicator). Two different approaches (Figure 8) were chosen for this purpose: firstly, Neubrandenburg Hospital's pathology institute permanently provided a pathologist in a branch office in Eberswalde Hospital. Since this pathologist could not work at full capacity due to low case numbers, he was additionally providing telepathology services for the mother institution in Neubrandenburg; secondly, pathologists in Greifswald evaluated rapidly processed slides via telepathology for the hospitals in Bergen, Wolgast, Schwedt and Stralsund (the establishment of the service was the main outcome indicator; for details of the analysis, see [15]).

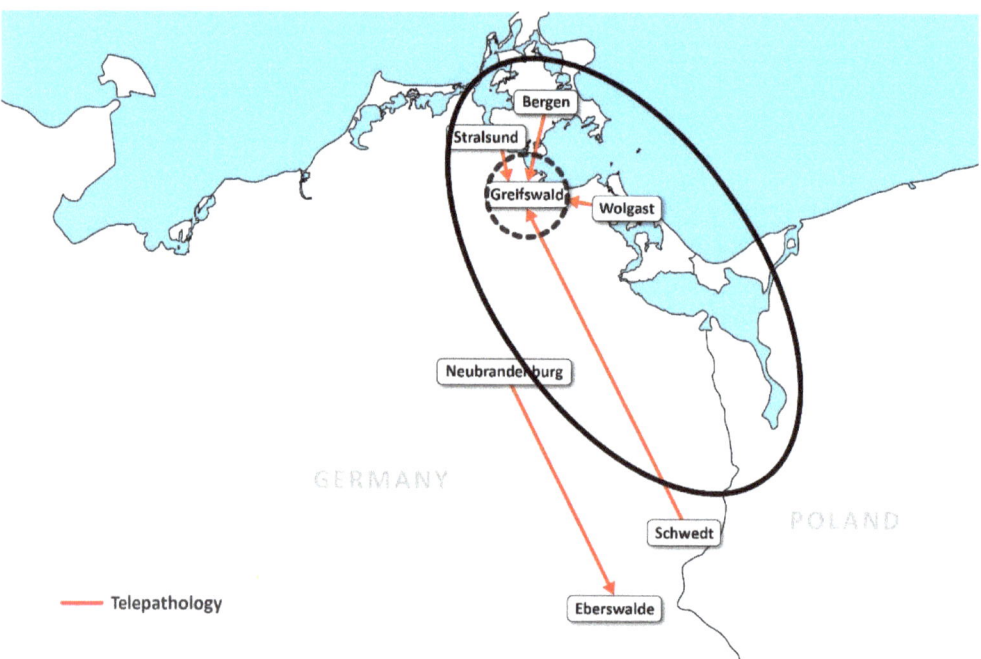

Figure 8. Enlargement of the catchment area of medical facilities through telemedicine. The inner, broken circle shows the direct catchment area of the pathology department at Greifswald University Hospital. Outside working hours, it is limited to the immediate area. Telepathologically, the catchment area is basically unlimited from a purely technical standpoint. The red arrows show telepathology connections in the pathology network.

Equipment on the German side was financed by the project. On the Polish side, the main focus was on funding pathological (and radiological) equipment. In Szczecin, Gryfice and Poznań, scanners for digitising pathological sections were procured and connected for remote consultations.

The Greifswald project has been scientifically evaluated. Retrospectively, the diagnostic accuracy of intraoperative frozen section telepathology was evaluated. It was highly acceptable at 98.95%. The average time for the preparation of virtual slides ranged from 10.58 ± 8.19 min. Investment costs were lower than those of robotic microscopy [15].

A facilitating factor was the fact that a functioning system was already available from the beginning of the project phase. This is not to be taken for granted, because pathology has a very high volume of data; i.e., it requires connections with high bandwidth and a high storage capacity. This barrier is caused by the high number of very thin cuts required for pathological evaluation and the bigger file size (compared to radiology) of the coloured sections (Figure 9).

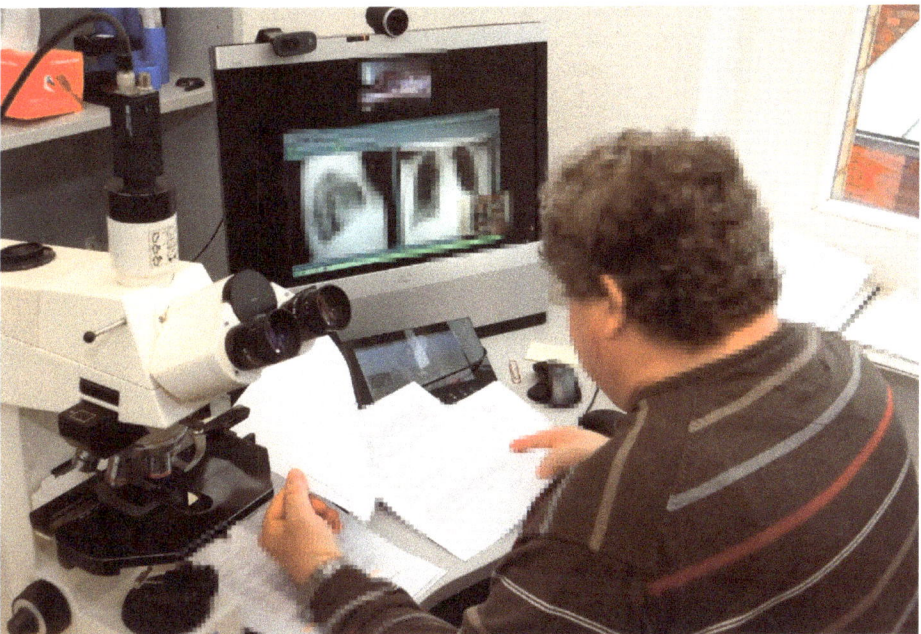

Figure 9. Telepathology. The telepathology workstation of this pathologist shows the pathologist's desk during a tumour conference. He can work on his microscope while following the conference on his monitor. During the few minutes that the pathologist is needed in a typical teleconference, he may be seen and heard and show slides (see Figure 5). The higher productivity that is achieved in this way is particularly important given the few pathologists commonly available.

3.2.4. Tele-Ear-Nose-Throat (ENT)

In the sparsely populated state of Western Pomerania, the economic efficiency before the funding period was poor for the few existing ENT departments. The Tele-ENT subproject consisted of videoconferencing and video endoscopy (Figure 10) between the patient and on-site doctor at the presentation site of the patient in the periphery and the ENT doctor in the centre (Greifswald). Videoconferencing was used to improve communication. The actual tele-ENT diagnostics were carried out with the help of a tele-endoscope. According to the plan [16], the on-site service doctor was able to insert the endoscope into the patient's throat or into the outer ear canal. The endoscopic image was transmitted over the network to the university's ENT department, where the doctor on duty verbally directed the endoscope and used the transmitted images for diagnostics. Specialist medical expertise could therefore be provided to any external location with a primary doctor and appropriate equipment on-site. The outcome indicator was the number of patients assisted with tele-endoscopy for ENT disease, assuming improved quality as a result (the establishment of the service was the main outcome indicator; for details, see [16]).

A facilitating factor was the high quality of the endoscopy devices and the videoconferencing images. Barriers were experienced in two ways: the physicians working on-site used endoscopies—for example, for gastric examinations—and were accustomed to introducing the endoscope through the patient's open mouth, while ENT physicians usually insert the endoscope through the patient's nose. This difference, which seems trivial to the outsider, could not be surmounted in practice. Medical staff feared malpractice claims; the retraining of medical staff in peripheral sites should have been considered. This barrier has been reported in other studies as well [17]. Contractual solutions with external funding should have been worked towards. Another especially crucial barrier was the fact that the treating doctors in the periphery reported feeling devalued by the specialist support. The procedure was evaluated through interviews. A commonly mentioned argument was "We can care for our patients on our own!".

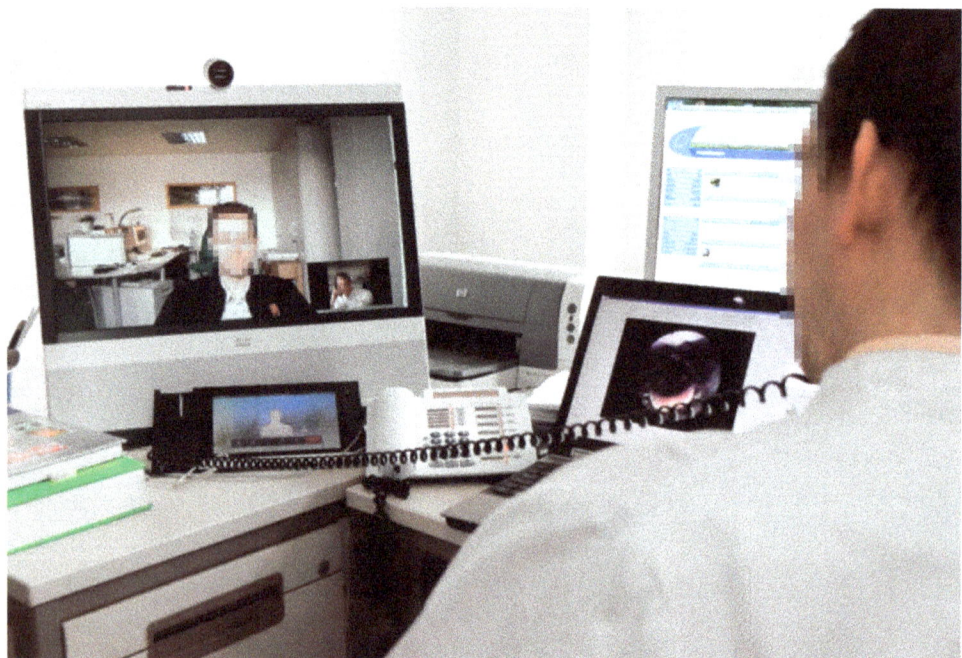

Figure 10. Video endoscopy during an ENT consultation. A non-specialised physician inserted the endoscope and images were automatically transferred to the specialist in a university hospital—in our project, between Templin and Greifswald. The distance between the two cities was roughly 150 km, and the driving time would be nearly 2 h. Specialised diagnosis was thus possible despite the distance, and therapy recommendations could be given. The Greifswald ENT specialist in the image is seen from the back, the general physician in Templin is shown on the monitor of the videoconferencing unit, and the image generated by the endoscope is shown on a smaller monitor to the right.

The difficulties could possibly have been eliminated with help from the medical centre, given sufficient will. The technology appears to be useful, especially in even more sparsely populated locations than our region.

3.2.5. Teleophthalmology Screening

Teleophthalmology screening made apparent another difficulty of telemedical projects. The project planned to use an existing Optical Coherence Tomograph (OTC [18,19])/telefundoscopy system. The system visualises the different retinal layers including blood vessels and the optic nerve head. Images are transferred in automated form to a center, where an experienced clinician can then evaluate the study. Screening for diseases such as increased arterial blood pressure or glaucoma is thus possible. The system was installed for Greifswald University Hospital and a hospital 50 km away without an ophthalmology clinic. The peripheral clinic thus provided its patients with a screening service. The outcome indicator was the statistical recording of a sufficient number of early diagnoses. The reduced number of necessary treatments and follow-up costs should be offset against the costs of maintaining the service. The outcome was not reached.

A facilitating factor was the pre-existing, technically evaluated system that was successfully installed. There was a barrier, however, which could not be overcome: the lack of funding of the prevention project—for example, as a pilot by health insurance companies. The necessary cooperation between the various professional groups (administration, the medical profession and health insurance providers) was not a given, and no contractual arrangement was reached. This should have been required and the possibility to purchase the equipment should have been used as an incentive.

3.2.6. Tele-Stroke Diagnostics

Tele-stroke diagnostics consist of the transmission of clinical findings or a neurological examination of a patient. For the neurological examination, an assistant must be available on-site with the patient. The neurologist communicates and directs necessary examinations and observes the result via the videoconferencing device.

Tele-stroke is a good application of telemedicine. However, it was less suitable in the project presented here, which was based on (and took its influence from) the financing of cost-intensive infrastructure/technology. The cost of equipment for tele-stroke is limited. However, tele-stroke projects must achieve a very well-functioning division of labour between doctors on duty (internists/surgeons), neuroradiologists, neurologists and interventional neuroradiologists. Independent from the project presented here, a Berlin-based tele-stroke project was established and permanently financed in a German innovation project [20]. Greifswald as a location is part of that independent project; the Pomerania telemedicine project only provided equipment in one of the hospitals.

A facilitating factor of this and similar projects is the high treatment pressure: patients who are diagnosed and treated early often have a very good outcome, while not being treated within hours may result in death. The barrier for Pomerania was that, while the initial investment needs are relatively low, telestroke projects have high requirements concerning organisation and long-term-financing. However, Pomerania's interest in tele-stroke possibly motivated neurologists to agree on a project realised by their own profession instead of a radiology-based project. This competition between specialists turned out to be a very potent facilitator.

3.3. Results Regarding Management Issues

3.3.1. Special aspects of a Cross-Border, Binational Project

At the start of the project in 2001, different specialties and regions were unevenly developed with regard to medical services. The project originated between two pathologists located in Pasewalk, Germany (10,000 inhabitants) and Poznań/Poland (536,000 inhabitants); the latter is not even located in an area in which the EU usually funds Interreg projects. Digitisation is a prerequisite of telemedicine in order to provide medical services over a distance. That each side of the project was allowed to start from their own point of development, rather than implementing identical infrastructure in both countries, was an important facilitating factor. Great efforts were made to secure data privacy at this stage. However, the solutions developed later turned out to be unfeasible. Nevertheless, in retrospect, it was crucial to simply start with what was possible.

Facilitating factors were a personal relationship between the founders of the project, the small scope of the initial project and the right timing, with digitisation only beginning in pathology and radiology when the project began. Board meetings by physicians and administrators from different German and Polish hospitals were considered the most rewarding aspect of the project, and this was a facilitator in its own right.

An important barrier at a later stage was binational communication. While German was a common language between the founders of the project, this was not the case for all participants. Law offices, retired diplomats, translators and other organisations exist, which give professional help in cooperation between different countries. However, the leaders of the project, with its public funding, were reluctant to assign the very high fees that specialised law offices commanded. In retrospect, this was incorrect, and a solution should and could have been found by negotiation. For a time, a law office that specialised in German and Polish law provided this service by pointing out basic mistakes which are all but incomprehensible in retrospect; the lack of a Polish translation for the German association's statutes was one such mistake. This probably made it impossible to co-opt Polish members into the association. A translator was present at board meetings, but this was no substitute for a more comprehensive service.

An academic position in psychology, anthropology, etc. financed by the project could have been an important addition to ease integration. Two full-time positions (one in-house counsel, one geographer) were financed for five years by EU project funding, and one, for three more years by the participating hospitals (in-house counsel).

3.3.2. Participation of Multiple Hospitals

An "association" is easily established in Germany, with no capital necessary. It may be tax-exempt, as was the case here. It had serious drawbacks, as associates were not always aware of the financial risks. This led to the telemedicine project being perceived as "not-for-profit" or "pro bono", at least by the participating physicians, while in effect it was a company with considerable financial risk and statutory liability (ranging into an eight-digit sum). It was obviously vital for the project to responsibly handle financial matters and to communicate this to the public. All investments had to be pre-financed by the participating hospitals, with the association later receiving 90% of the funds. The hospitals paid a percentage of the overhead according to the percentage of the EU funding they received. One problem with the accounting was that all of the reimbursements were via the German side and in Euros. Therefore, as this then had to be converted into Polish Złoty, this was a considerable financial risk.

In summary, the formation of an association with a large number of participating hospitals was itself deemed a barrier. While the association is preserved as a mantle under a new board for possible use in the future, the project described here was developed differently. An attending clinician at Greifswald University Hospital (Holger Lode, paediatrician, specialised in neuroblastoma treatment) with a highly specialised area of work and existing referrals from Poland was chosen. His approach received Interreg funding.

3.3.3. Project's Legal Issues

The experiences in telemedicine obtained in the project were partially transferred into the national law of both countries. In the beginning of the project, the legal situation of telemedicine as an innovative medical discipline was—with a few exceptions—unregulated in both Germany and Poland and therefore unclear for the acting hospitals, hospital administrators and physicians. The undefined legal situation was a barrier for all project actors. Legal expertise in the project was a facilitating and essential factor. In connection with the project, telemedical questions that arose were legally processed [21]. During the project´s duration, first regulations for telemedicine were created in Germany and Poland. This circumstance shows that the EU is able to influence, through its projects, national framework and even national health systems, for which the EU has no real legitimisation. Furthermore, the undisputed phrase that law follows the reality of life was confirmed.

Another legal aspect of the project was transporting pilot projects into routine care. Physicians tend to cooperate based on personal trust, and this may help with starting pilot projects. To integrate telemedicine into everyday use, contracts have to be drawn between hospitals (teleradiology, telepathology) or between healthcare providers and hospitals. This last aspect was neglected in the ophthalmology and otorhinolaryngology projects, and these two projects faltered after funding ran out [16,19,20]. In the same way, it does not make sense to give public funding to modalities that are ultimately privately owned. Mammography screening is a multi-million Euro program owned by private practices in Germany, and an attempt to create a comprehensive storage structure for the program was futile [22].

Calling for bids was organised by a specialised law office. Law students were employed to prepare and handle the calls. This worked very well. Procedures were established in this manner, as well as the documentation of bids and contracts awarded.

Associations according to German law were registered. The structures providing this service correspond to parts of local courts. As they were alien to Eastern Germany when the project was first conceived (similar structures did not exist in the German Democratic Republic), they did not function well and were a permanent nuisance to the project. The influence of the project, however, was large enough to achieve improvements with support from local politicians.

Problems arising during the implementation of the project were voiced at binational government meetings by the project's chairman.

4. Discussion

A review of telemedical literature in NIH PubMed does not reveal many multinational, cross-border medical projects. The reasons for this may be the close connection between medical care and a common language between doctor and patient (large price differences between medical services in the border area for lifestyle interventions such as dental care, cosmetic surgery and hair transplants are certainly an exception). The EU considers the goal of cross-border medical care as a building block for the creation of a data network. To this end, it supports projects from neighbouring regional states—in the presented example, Germany and Poland. The prerequisite is the existence of a large city in the development area—in the example, Szczecin, as the historical centre of the region.

Some working groups have named facilitators and barriers for the implementation of telemedicine projects. However, these reports often concern doctor-to-patient telemedicine. A more general recommendation is found in a manual [3] that identified facilitators for the introduction of telemedicine:

1. Existence of a master plan at state level that is well coordinated and financially resourced.
2. Infrastructure data security.
3. The presence of an electronic patient record with interoperability.
4. Adapted legislation.
5. Reimbursement.

Standardised procedures, on the other hand, were not considered necessary.

Brady et al. [4] described in 2021 how publicly available data can be used to prioritize ophthalmic telemedicine. Their work can be understood as the identification of a facilitator. Zanaboni et al. [5] described the early status of Norwegian telemedicine projects and above all identified sparsely populated states as facilitators for the use of telemedicine. This observation can be applied to our project. The same authors [6] later described facilitators for the routine use of telemedicine in Norwegian hospitals. They identified an economy of scale with greater benefits derived from very large telemedicine projects. To this end, the authors reviewed different networks with figures for numbers of per capita consultations. A lack of resources and political guidelines, especially those relating to reimbursement, were described as barriers. A paper from Hawaii [7] proposed three recommendations for improving medical care in unevenly populated areas that suffer from a lack of doctors. As a facilitator, the establishment of a business model to reduce complexity is suggested. A second point concerns the retention of doctors. The approach of the authors is in line with our experience of coaching and training doctors who have remained in the region through telemedical access to specialists on neighbouring islands. This was the rationale of our Tele-ENT project.

The underlying principle of telemedicine is, in short, to expand the catchment areas of medical services. In the Interreg phase described here, which lasted until 2020, this was partially achieved separately on both sides of the border. In Germany, this mainly concerned radiology and pathology as well as tumour conferences, while on the Polish side, pathology and radiology structures were established.

An expansion of the catchment areas of medical offers in the international area makes sense in the case of highly specialised therapy for rare diseases. Accordingly, a paediatric-led, cross-border project for the care of children with neuroblastoma was designed and financed for the next project phase. The EU goal of cross-border care might thus be achieved in a highly specialised and very small, but nevertheless important, field of medicine. A legal framework for cross-border medical services remains desirable.

5. Conclusions

The following recommendations can be given for doctor-to-doctor telemedicine projects with high investments in telemedical infrastructure:

- The establishment of telemedical infrastructure must often be asynchronous in large areas, but always in cross-border projects. The causes are the different stages of development at the beginning of the project.
- Before investing, the financing of future ongoing operations should be secured. An interdisciplinary setup of the project team in EU funded projects is essential.
- Market power in the purchase of expensive technology is an important argument for large infrastructure projects.
- Publicly funded infrastructure projects often require a financial commitment from beneficiaries in the project; in the case shown here, this was 15%. This is ineffective, as 15% of projects that have already been planned by applicants can always be added to applications. Thus, no additional funds in fact have to be raised for the funded projects. It would make more sense to demand from beneficiaries that they add 15% to 25% of the total costs for manpower, supporting the transition into daily practice.
- Cross-border telemedicine projects should have professional counselling from academic institutions or specialised law offices. A law office may also prepare binding contracts, which should be signed before the rolling-out of equipment.
- Projects involving competing hospitals tend to suffer from being labelled as "altruistic", which is not a strategically beneficial term in societies founded on economic success. Input into government decision-making and into regional government authority was a way to resolve this "flaw".

Author Contributions: N.H. and A.K. were members of the board and B.R. was inhouse counsel of the project. B.R. and N.H. wrote the original manuscript, while B.R., N.H. and A.K. revised the manuscript. All authors have read and agreed to the published version of the manuscript.

Funding: The project was supported by Grants INT-08-0001, 2010–2020 and previous grants as well as by FKP-0293-20-C, all of the European Union's Interreg program.

Institutional Review Board Statement: Not applicable.

Informed Consent Statement: Not applicable.

Data Availability Statement: Not applicable.

Acknowledgments: The authors thank Heinz Koehler (1938–2011), Peter Heise, Ursula Brautferger, Andrea Gronwald, Udo Hirschfeld, Janusz Szymas, Andrzej Gajewski, Wenancjusz Domagała, Przemysław Nowacki, Krzysztof Bogusławski, and Denis Feiler.

Conflicts of Interest: N.H. is reimbursed for reporting by teleradiology; the other authors declare no conflict of interest. The funders had no role in the design of the study; in the collection, analyses, or interpretation of data; in the writing of the manuscript; or in the decision to publish the results.

References

1. Perkmann, M. Cross-border regions in Europe: Significance and drivers of regional cross-border co-operation. *Eur. Urban Reg. Stud.* **2019**, *10*, 153–171. [CrossRef]
2. Schmidt-Egner, P. Grenzüberschreitende Zusammenarbeit (GZA) in Europa als Gegenstand wissenschaftlicher Forschung und Strategie transnationaler Praxis. In *Anmerkungen zur Theorie, Empirie und Praxis des Transnationalen Regionalismus*; Brunn, G., Schmitt-Egner, P., Eds.; Nomos: Baden-Baden, Germany, 1998; pp. 27–77.

3. Hartvigsen, G.; Pedersen, S. *Lessons Learned from 25 Years with Telemedicine in Northern Norway*; Norwegian Centre for Integrated Care and Telemedicine, University Hospital of North Norway: Tromsø, Norway, 2015.
4. Brady, C.J.; D'Amico, S.; Withers, N.; Kim, B.Y. Using public datasets to identify priority areas for ocular telehealth. *Telemed. J. eHealth* **2021**. [CrossRef] [PubMed]
5. Zanaboni, P.; Wootton, R. Adoption of telemedicine: From pilot stage to routine delivery. *BMC Med. Inform. Decis. Mak.* **2012**, *12*, 47. [CrossRef] [PubMed]
6. Zanaboni, P.; Wootton, R. Adoption of routine telemedicine in Norwegian hospitals: Progress over 5 years. *BMC Health Serv. Res.* **2016**, *16*, 496. [CrossRef] [PubMed]
7. Scribner, M.N.; Kehoe, K. Establishing successful patient-centered medical homes in rural Hawaii: Three strategies to consider. *Hawaii J. Med. Public Health* **2017**, *76* (Suppl. 1), 18–23. [PubMed]
8. Gilbert, A.W.; Jaggi, A.; May, C.R. What is the acceptability of real time 1:1 videoconferencing between clinicians and patients for a follow-up consultation for multi-directional shoulder instability? *Shoulder Elb.* **2019**, *11*, 53–59. [CrossRef] [PubMed]
9. Viers, B.R.; Pruthi, S.; Rivera, M.E.; O'Neil, D.A.; Gardner, M.R.; Jenkins, S.M.; Lightner, D.J.; Gettman, M.T. Are patients willing to engage in telemedicine for their care: A survey of preuse perceptions and acceptance of remote video visits in a urological patient population. *Urology* **2012**, *85*, 1233–1239. [CrossRef] [PubMed]
10. Spoerl, M.C.; Rosenberg, C.; Kroos, K.; Flessa, S.; Hosten, N. Evaluation of medical teleconference setups. *Health Manag.* **2013**, *13*, 14–18.
11. Guhl, S.; Linngrön, L.; Rosenberg, B.; Hosten, N.; Kirsch, M. Telemedicine: Can in-person pre-treatment communication be expanded by video consultation? *Cardiovasc. Interv. Radiol.* **2019**, *42*, 1812–1813. [CrossRef] [PubMed]
12. Pacjent-Leczony-na-Odleglosc-Ten-Projekt-Robi-fu. Available online: https://radioszczecin.pl/1,99931 (accessed on 25 March 2021).
13. Rosenberg, C.; Langner, S.; Rosenberg, B.; Hosten, N. Medical and legal aspects of teleradiology in Germany. *ROFO* **2011**, *183*, 804–811. [CrossRef] [PubMed]
14. Rosenberg, C.; Kroos, K.; Rosenberg, B.; Hosten, N.; Flessa, S. Teleradiology from the provider's perspective—Cost analysis for a mid-size university hospital. *Eur. Radiol.* **2013**, *23*, 2197–2205. [CrossRef] [PubMed]
15. Ribback, S.; Flessa, S.; Gromoli-Bergmann, K.; Evert, M.; Dombrowski, F. Virtual slide telepathology with scanner systems for intraoperative frozen-section consultation. *Pathol. Res. Pract.* **2014**, *210*, 377–382. [CrossRef] [PubMed]
16. Beule, A.G. Telemedical methods in otorhinolaryngology. *Laryngorhinootologie* **2019**, *98* (Suppl. 1), 129–172. [CrossRef]
17. Jang-Jacard, J.; Nepal, S.; Alem, L.; Li, J. Barriers for delivering telehealth in rural Australia: A review based in Australian trials and studies. *Telemed. eHealth* **2014**. [CrossRef] [PubMed]
18. Swierk, T.; Jurgens, C.; Grossjohann, R.; Flessa, S.; Tost, F. Health economical aspects of telemedical glaucoma monitoring. *Ophthalmologe* **2011**, *108*, 342–350. [CrossRef] [PubMed]
19. Jürgens, C.; Grossjohann, R.; Tost, F. Distribution of mean, systolic and diastolic ocular perfusion pressure in telemedical homemonitoring of glaucoma patients. *Ophthalmic Res.* **2012**, *48*, 208–211. [CrossRef] [PubMed]
20. Weber, J.E.; Angermaier, A.; Bollweg, K.; Erdur, H.; Ernst, S.; Flöel, A.; Gorski, C.; Kandil, F.I.; Kinze, S.; Kleinsteuber, K.; et al. ANNOTeM-consortium. Acute neurological care in north-east Germany with telemedicine support (ANNOTeM): Protocol of a multi-center, controlled, open-label, two-arm intervention study. *BMC Health Serv. Res.* **2020**, *17*, 755. [CrossRef]
21. Rosenberg, B. Legal issues of telemedicine using the example of teleradiology in the context of e-health. *ABW Wiss.* **2019**, *12*, 166.
22. Fröhlich, C.P.; Weigel, C.; Mohr, M.; Schimming, A.; Bick, U.; Hosten, N. Teleradiology and mammography screening: Evaluation of a network with dedicated workstations for reporting. *ROFO* **2007**, *179*, 137–145. [CrossRef]

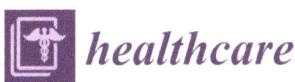

Article

The Accuracy of On-Call CT Reporting in Teleradiology Networks in Comparison to In-House Reporting

Svea Storjohann *, Michael Kirsch, Britta Rosenberg, Christian Rosenberg, Sandra Lange, Annika Syperek, Frank Philipp Schweikhard and Norbert Hosten

Department of Radiology, Universitätsmedizin Greifswald, 17475 Greifswald, Germany; Michael.Kirsch@med.uni-greifswald.de (M.K.); britta.rosenberg1@uni-greifswald.de (B.R.); Christian.Rosenberg@jsd.de (C.R.); sandra.lange@uni-greifswald.de (S.L.); annika.syperek@med.uni-greifswald.de (A.S.); ps143182@uni-greifswald.de (F.P.S.); norbert.hosten@med.uni-greifswald.de (N.H.)
* Correspondence: Svea.Storjohann@uni-greifswald.de; Tel.: +49-383-486-6960

Abstract: (1) Background: We aimed to compare the accuracy of after-hours CT reports created in a traditional in-house setting versus a teleradiology setting by assessing the discrepancy rates between preliminary and final reports. (2) Methods: We conducted a prospective study to determine the number and severity of discrepancies between preliminary and final reports for 7761 consecutive after-hours CT scans collected over a 21-month period. CT exams were performed during on-call hours and were proofread by an attending the next day. Discrepancies between preliminary and gold-standard reports were evaluated by two senior attending radiologists, and differences in rates were assessed for statistical significance. (3) Results: A total of 7209 reports were included in the analysis. Discrepancies occurred in 1215/7209 cases (17%). Among these, 433/7209 reports (6%) showed clinically important differences between the preliminary and final reports. A total of 335/5509 of them were in-house reports (6.1%), and 98/1700 were teleradiology reports (5.8%). The relative frequencies of report changes were not significantly higher in teleradiology. (4) Conclusions: The accuracy of teleradiology reports was not inferior to that of in-house reports, with very similar clinically important differences rates found in both reporting situations.

Keywords: telemedicine; reporting; quality control; resident; diagnostic error

1. Introduction

With the rise of teleradiology, it has become possible to physically separate the sites of image acquisition and interpretation of the resulting scans. Today, radiology reports are not necessarily created at the same facility in which the images are acquired; instead, scans may be read and reported on remotely by physicians in teleradiology networks. Teleradiology networks typically consist of institutions providing 24/7 readings of imaging studies and corresponding requesting institutions, such as smaller hospitals that do not have the financial or personnel means to ensure the around-the-clock presence of radiologists in their imaging departments [1]. The European Society of Radiology (ESR) conducted a survey to obtain the current status of teleradiology [2]. In total, 70.8% out of 25 National societies that responded to the survey answered that in their country, the outsourcing of worklists to teleradiology companies is practiced, i.e., without direct contact between the radiologist and the patient.

In comparison to in-house reporting, "teleradiologists typically do not have access to additional information, including prior studies, plain films, or clinical data, which may assist in-house radiologists in image interpretation" (quoted verbatim from [3]; also [4]). In the teleradiology setting, the reader has to rely on the often-scarce information provided by the referring physician. To protect medical data, prior films and medical files cannot always be accessed remotely when reporting by teleradiology. Direct communication

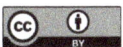

between the radiologist and the patient, which is considered a valuable source of clinical information [5], is rarely possible in this setting. Even if it is not always feasible in the daily routine of in-house diagnostics, it represents another source of information that is lost in teleradiology.

According to German law, teleradiology is intended as an exception to close gaps in care. It is authorized for reporting at night, on weekends, and on bank holidays (24/7 teleradiology as another exception may be approved upon request under certain conditions that must be met). Another requirement based on quality assurance (QA) aspects in the German teleradiology setting is the so-called "regional principle". According to this, the teleradiologist may only work for locations that can be reached within a period of time necessary for emergency care (approx. 45–60 min). In addition, there are strict requirements for the professional experience and qualifications of the radiologists participating in teleradiological reporting [6–10].

A considerable number of existing quality control studies have been conducted in North America. They identified a variety of items which might influence the quality of after-hours reporting. Possible influencing factors were evaluated, such as whether reports were done on a weekend versus a week day, whether reports were done during the hours of a shift or not, and the complexity of a case [11]. There are some studies that reported statistics of a QA program tracking reported disagreements that occurred in observing CT examinations [3,12,13]. In these studies, residents were not involved in the reporting. To the authors' knowledge, no work comparable to the available studies has been reported from Germany to date.

As such, this study was conducted to evaluate the relationship between the imaging setting (teleradiology/network reporting vs. in-house reporting) and the frequency of discrepancies between teleradiology and in-house reports. We evaluated the distribution of neuroradiological examinations, as these are often evaluated separately in quality control studies. We hypothesized that teleradiology reporting would produce more discrepancies—caused, for example, by the lack of contact between the radiologist and the patient, possibly missing preliminary examinations or insufficient clinical information.

2. Materials and Methods

The present study was conducted prospectively. It was reviewed and approved by the local ethics committee and the staff council representing the affected doctors. The teleradiology operation was approved by the local authorities in 2014. In accordance with national laws and regulations, all participating radiologists were informed of the use of their reports in the study. Consent for the necessary diagnostic measure was obtained from all patients involved in the study as far as they were able to give their consent. There was no additional or special risk for the patients from the study. All patient data in the reports were anonymized for evaluation in consideration of the relevant data protection regulations.

CT imaging was chosen as the imaging modality of study since it represents the most frequently requested imaging modality outside core working hours, for the interpretation of which the radiologist is in demand.

2.1. Reporting Process during On-Call Shifts

During nighttime hours (10 p.m. to 7 a.m.) and during the daytime hours on weekends and bank holidays (7 a.m. to 10 p.m.), in accordance with the German teleradiology law rules, on-call radiologists created preliminary reports for CT studies that were either acquired in-house, on our own scanners, or received via the teleradiology network (8 smaller hospitals). The files were sent with point-to-point encryption via a virtual private network (VPN). As is common practice in radiology departments, the on-call radiologist was able to involve an attending radiologist if they decided that the case required a higher level of expertise (for details on the roles of the different readers, see Table 1). During the next regular daytime shift, all of these reports were reviewed by an attending radiologist and corrected if necessary. The resulting proofread final reports were considered to be gold-standard. A correlation of the gold-standard findings with the clinical outcome of patients was not possible, as all data including the patient data and reporting radiologist were required to be deleted in accordance with data protection regulations.

Table 1. Role of the different members of the Department of Radiology involved in the present study. The upper and middle boxes refer to reporting, while the lower box refers to the acquisition of the study data used for assessing discrepancies.

Radiologist on call	First-line reporting.
Attending	Could be consulted by the radiologist taking call; proofread reports the next morning/workday; the resulting final report was considered "gold-standard" for this study.
Senior radiologist	Two attendings specializing in radiology and neuroradiology, respectively; independently, they graded differences as either "clinically unimportant" or "clinically important" and differences as either "in detection" or "in interpretation".

2.2. Availability of Supplementary Information

With in-house imaging, radiologists had full access to all information available on the patient within the Picture Archiving and Communication System (PACS), as well as the hospital and radiological information systems (RIS). This includes prior studies and clinical data such as secondary diagnoses and operative reports. Further information could be acquired by communicating with the referring physician and patients themselves.

For reporting in the teleradiology network, the on-call radiologist could communicate with the referring physician on site and, more importantly, communicate with the technician on site performing the exam, usually focusing on the proposed examination protocol. There was no direct patient–radiologist communication. The written request from the referring colleague communicated clinical information. Prior studies could not be accessed since the requesting and receiving hospitals did not share a PACS or RIS.

2.3. Exclusion Criteria

CT studies which fulfilled one or more of the following criteria were excluded: scans that were not reported the next weekday; scans where the initial report was edited before the next weekday (the initial findings were then overwritten and could no longer be reviewed; any changes made to the report could no longer be traced); scans aborted mid-examination; scans related to an intervention, report created by attending; no verification (in this case, the preliminary report could not be released and a comparison with the gold-standard was impossible at the time of the study).

The contact to an attending was not seen as an exclusion criterion, as it is common practice in both in-house reporting and teleradiology.

2.4. Data Processing

The preliminary on-call reports and the proofread versions were retrieved from our PACS and anonymized by a member of the study group. All data containing the identity of the patient, the reporting radiologist, or the hospital in which the scans were acquired were deleted.

The blinded reports were compiled side-by-side into a single document in order to allow for direct comparisons. In order to evaluate the report quality, both versions (on-call and proofread by a senior attending) were compared, and any apparent differences were highlighted.

2.5. Assessing the Discrepancy Level

If any discrepancies between the on-call report and the proofread final report were identified, the compiled documents were presented to two senior radiologists (>20 years work experience each), who assessed the changes in terms of their clinical and therapeutic consequences. The two readers made their decisions independently. Discrepancies were assigned to five severity levels and subsequently categorized to groups already used in previous publications in the context of studies on second-opinion consultations in radiology (see Table 2) [14,15] (Score 2: addition of a secondary diagnosis such as "maxillary sinus mucocele" when asked about acute ischemia; Score 3: clinically unimportant change in interpretation such as "radiopaque foreign material" to "DD clips"; Score 4: e.g., addition of a missed fracture; Score 5: clinically important change in interpretation such as the age of an ischemic infarction). In case of disagreement, the two readers would discuss this and reach a final consensual decision. One of the readers was also involved in the finalization of on-call reports. There was an interval of several months between the two activities so that no recollection of the circumstances of individual examinations or findings could be assumed.

Table 2. Consensus score [14,15] of final interpretation versus preliminary interpretation in in-house and teleradiology reports. In-house and teleradiology reports were subject to clinically unimportant and clinically important differences at similar rates.

	Discrepancies	Setting		
		In-House [n (%)]	Teleradiology [n (%)]	Sum [n (%)]
1	No difference	4633 (84.1)	1452 (85.4)	6085 (84.4)
2	Clinically unimportant difference in detection	168 (3)	31 (1.8)	199 (2.8)
3	Clinically unimportant difference in interpretation	373 (6.8)	119 (7)	492 (6.8)
4	Clinically important difference in detection	193 (3.5)	51 (3)	244 (3.4)
5	Clinically important difference in interpretation	142 (2.6)	47 (2.8)	189 (2.6)
	sum	5509 (100)	1700 (100)	7209 (100)

2.6. Statistical Analysis

2.6.1. Sample Size

Our aim was to minimize changes in the reporting patterns which might occur if radiologists were aware of an ongoing monitoring process. This is why, instead of determining a certain case number, we instead assigned a period (21 months) over the course of which all CT reports would be evaluated. As a result, because a study duration was assigned rather than a required number of cases, there was a larger number of cases than a pure power calculation would warrant. This was done with the aim of minimizing the on-call radiologists' required attention over time.

2.6.2. Testing

We calculated the absolute and relative frequencies of different severities of report changes and considered the acquisition locations as a risk factor for report changes. Statistical significance of differences in the examined frequencies of discrepancies between comparison groups was tested using the chi-square test. In addition, the chi-square test was used to evaluate the distribution of neuroradiological cases. This aimed at making comparison with other studies easier: Neuroradiological examinations are often evaluated separately in quality control studies. In this study, we intended to investigate emergency imaging of all body regions. Statistical analysis was performed using SPSS for Mac OS (Version 25; IBM, Chicago, IL, USA).

3. Results

3.1. Number of Cases

Within the planned study period, a total of 6037 in-house CT reports and 1724 teleradiology reports were requested outside our hospital's core working hours (nighttime hours: 10 p.m. to 7 a.m.; weekends and bank holidays: 7 a.m. to 10 p.m.) (Figure 1). For 136/6037 (2.3%) and 1/1724 (0.1%) cases, no digital report was created, 234/6037 (3.9%) and 21/1724 (1.2%) reports were edited under unclear circumstances, 5/6037 (0.1%) and 2/1724 (0.1%) scans were aborted mid-procedure, 140/6037 (2.3%) scans were directly related to an intervention (performed by an attending), 6/6037 (0.1%) reports were created by an attending, and in 7/6037 (0.1%) cases, no "gold-standard" report was available at the end of the study period. After excluding these cases, 5509 in-house reports and 1700 teleradiology reports remained for analysis. There were 24 cases excluded from the teleradiology arm (1.4%) and 528 from the in-house arm (8.7%). The higher percentage of in-house cases that were excluded had several reasons: interventional CT, whose reports were excluded because it is performed by attendings, was only performed in-house (without intervention 388 cases were excluded, 6.6%). Immediate clinical feedback led to more reports being changed in-house during the night. Teleradiology reports were reported without additional consultation and therefore more promptly delivered. Unlike in-house reports, they had to be reported; the report could not be delayed till the next morning, e.g., in agreement with the referring physician.

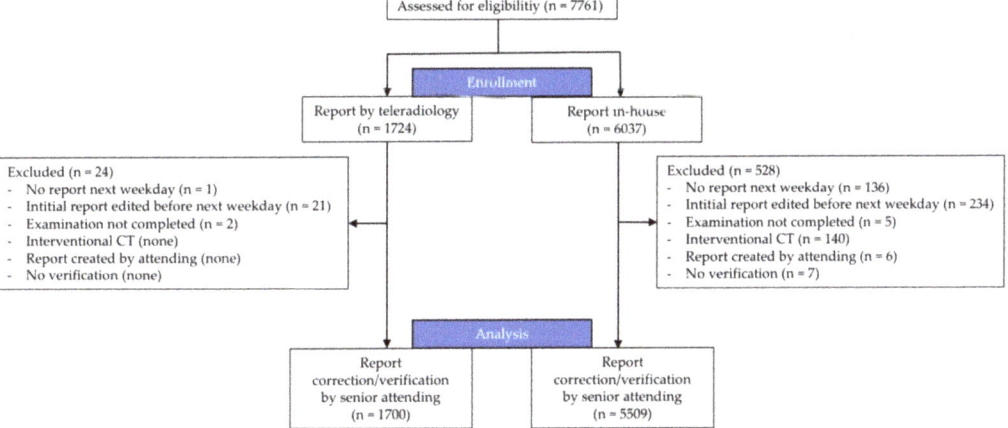

Figure 1. Flowchart of study. During the study period, 7761 consecutive after-hours CT scans were performed. After applying the exclusion criteria, a total of 7209 reports were included in the study.

3.2. Frequency of Report Changes in In-House/Teleradiology Reporting

To investigate the influence of the examination setting on report discrepancies, we calculated error rates and risks in both groups. In the 7209 CT reports which were included in the analysis, discrepancies occurred in 1215 cases (16.9%). A total of 433 clinically important differences between the preliminary report and gold-standard report were identified (6%) (see Table 2).

In the in-house setting, clinically important differences occurred in 335 of 5509 reports (6.1%). Among the 1700 teleradiology reports that were included, 98 underwent clinically important differences (5.8%) (see Figure 2, Table 2).

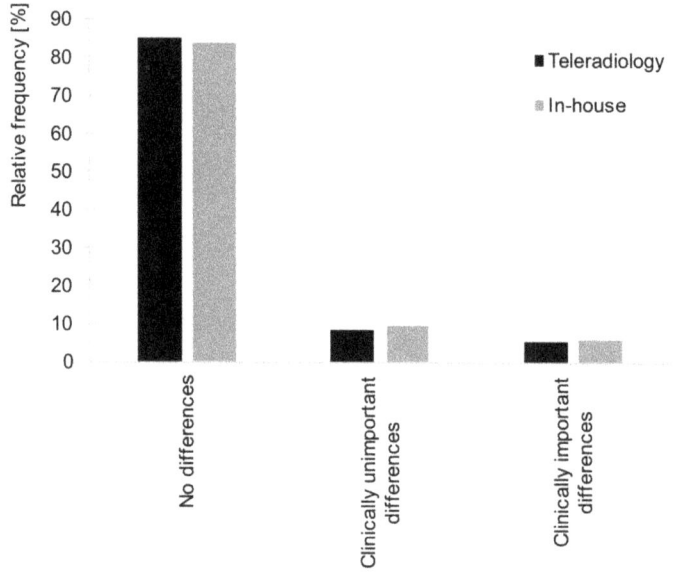

Figure 2. Relative frequencies of no differences, clinically unimportant differences, and clinically important differences for the teleradiology (black bars) versus in-house setting (grey bars). The relative frequencies of reports to which no changes were made; clinically unimportant and clinically important differences did not differ significantly between the teleradiology and the in-house setting ($X^2(2) = 1.828$, $p = 0.401$, $n = 7209$). Found in 5.8% vs. 6.1% of cases, respectively, clinically important differences to CT reports were similarly rare in both teleradiology reporting and in-house.

Overall, the frequency of any kind of report changes was neither significantly higher nor lower for the teleradiology reports compared to in-house imaging ($p > 0.05$). This suggests that in-house reporting and reporting of CT exams transmitted via teleradiology did not differ significantly with regard to reporting errors.

3.3. Scanned Body Regions

To exclude the possible influence of different compositions of the CT reports evaluated in teleradiology and in-house studies, we compared the anatomical regions examined in each arm (see Table 3 for details on the different types of examination). For both in-house imaging and teleradiology, cranial CTs were the most frequently requested examinations, followed by head/neck and abdominal studies. The absolute number of CT images of each body region and their relative frequency in relation to the total number of CT studies in the respective setting type are provided in Table 3 and Figure 3. Results suggest the two types of reporting (network/teleradiology vs. in-house) did not differ in terms of the composition of the exam types.

3.4. Distribution of Reader Groups

Reports were created by 20 different radiologists. All radiologists were equally involved in both in-house and teleradiology reporting. Residents created 5005/7209 (69%) reports. The remaining 2204/7209 cases (31%) were read by board-certified radiologists. The distributions did not differ significantly between in-house and teleradiology reports (residents 69% vs. 71%; board-certified radiologists 31% vs. 29%).

This suggests that the work experience of the reporting radiologists did not differ significantly between in-house reporting and teleradiology.

Table 3. Type of CT examinations included in this study for both settings. The three most frequently examined body regions are highlighted. The proportion of exams from the neuroradiological field, which is often evaluated separately in quality control studies, did not differ between the two groups, as indicated by a low effect size, *Cramers V*. However, there was a statistical difference due to the large number of cases included. (65.4% vs. 69.2%; $X^2(1) = 8.127$, $p = 0.004$, $n = 7209$, *Cramers V* = 0.034).

Scanned Region	Teleradiology		In-House	
	n	[%]	n	[%]
Cranium	1057	62.2	2777	50.4
Head/Neck (incl. Cervical Spine)	119	7.0	828	15.0
Neck	4	0.2	35	0.6
Chest	83	4.9	239	4.3
Abdomen	248	14.6	714	13.0
Chest/Abdomen	48	2.8	124	2.3
Pelvis	11	0.6	23	0.4
Limbs/Joints	35	2.1	266	4.8
Spine (excl. C-Spine)	24	1.4	108	2.0
Multiple Trauma	41	2.4	241	4.4
Other	30	1.8	154	2.8
sum	1700	100.0	5509	100.0

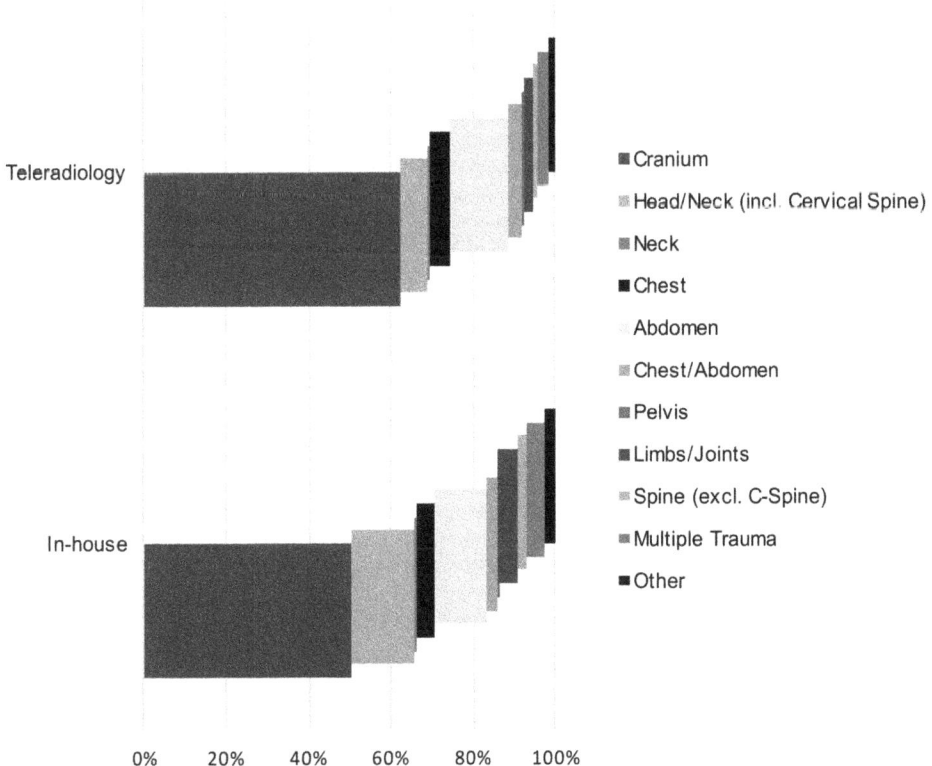

Figure 3. Proportion of examined body regions in the total number of examinations for both settings. A total of 83.8% (teleradiology) and 78.4% (in-house) of all examinations consisted of a cranial CT, a head and neck CT or an abdominal CT. The portions were comparable in both study arms.

4. Discussion

In the present study, report changes did not occur more frequently in the teleradiology setting than in the in-house comparison group. Teleradiology provides affordable full-time access to diagnostic imaging for smaller hospitals [16] by capitalizing on the 24/7 presence of radiologists in larger hospitals. Thrall [17] pointed out that emergency teleradiology has a limited range of indications and does not need results of prior examinations or clinical history; it therefore works well. Nevertheless, adequate report quality should be a top priority in teleradiology: today's teleradiology reporting of emergencies may extend into daytime network reporting [1] and become the new standard. In-house and teleradiology reports did not differ with regard to reporting errors (Figure 2). Clinically important differences to the preliminary reports were made in 6.1% (in-house, n = 335) and 5.8% (teleradiology, n = 98) of cases, respectively.

4.1. Frequency of Report Changes in In-House and Teleradiology Reports

The accuracy of reports generated by teleradiologists is a recurrent concern. According to the authors' knowledge, there is a lack of published QA data from German teleradiology networks. Due to the special legal regulations in Germany, comparability with international studies is limited. Additionally, the QA studies available for teleradiology were conducted without the participation of residents.

The clinically important difference rates observed in this study's teleradiology arm are similar to the 2010 findings by Platt-Mills et al. [3]. Their study, which included head and body CT, revealed that major changes occurred in 6% of reports, while 73% remained entirely unchanged. Teleradiologists there also did not have access to any preliminary images. A study by Hohmann et al. [12] also reported 79% examinations without discrepancies. Previous examinations were provided to the teleradiologists. For both of these studies, teleradiology reports were audited at the department in which the images were acquired rather than at the teleradiology facility itself.

In a 2003 publication by Erly et al. [13], only emergency cranial CT reports were examined. Major discrepancies were found to be less common. In total, 2.0% of the reports created by board-certified general radiologists via teleradiology were subject to significant disagreement. Complete agreement was observed in 95% of cases. However, the examinations were sent as an image file. In this way, only the brightness and contrast of the images could be edited by the radiologists.

4.2. Frequency of Report Changes Depending on Other Factors

Several studies have found that in the context of in-house reporting, the discrepancy rate correlates *inversely* with work experience [18–21]. Meanwhile, Cooper et al. [22] and Mellnick et al. [23] propose that a *positive* correlation between work experience and report discrepancies stems from the increasing responsibility that comes with increased work experience [23]. They found that the risk for report changes was significantly higher when the reader had less than four years of work experience. Lam et al. [24] found that discrepancies were much more likely to occur during the night shift. Developing a protocol for communicating discrepancies between on-call and final reports is essential. The most dreaded consequence of a discrepancy—a change in patient outcome—rarely occurs and only takes place in less than one percent of cases [19,25] but may be necessary and must be addressed. In our institution, difficult cases which gave rise to discrepancies (such as appendicitis, urinary calculus, small-bowel obstruction, diverticulitis) [25] are discussed in the daily morning rounds. Residents may thus familiarize themselves with typical off-hour problems before they start taking calls.

4.3. Does a Lack of Clinical Information and Access to Prior Studies Affect Report Quality?

If it is too costly and time-consuming for the teleradiologist to obtain clinical information, there is a risk that examinations will be interpreted with incomplete preliminary information [17]. So far, there are few data on whether a relative lack of clinical information affects the quality of teleradiology reports. Millet et al. [26] found that the absence of clinical information did not negatively influence diagnostic accuracy in abdominal CT. Mullins et al. [27] saw reports for stroke CTs improve when clinical data were available; MR results did not change, however. A review by Loy and Irwig [28] cited several papers focused on the bias inherent to clinical information, which may inadvertently direct the radiologist's attention toward evidence of the clinically suspected diagnosis. Interestingly, in light of this, sufficient clinical information was found to help to establish a rational examination protocol in a study by Dang et al. [29].

The limitations of this study result from the strict requirements regarding the anonymization of the collected data. It was not possible to calculate the influence of individual radiologists on the group performance. In addition, it was not possible to follow up on patients whose examination underwent a change. Thus, only the final report could be used as a gold standard. The influence of changes on the outcome of patients could not be determined.

5. Conclusions

In conclusion, teleradiologists need to work with the lack of personal contact with patients, technical staff, and referring physicians. This did not compromise the accuracy of CT reports compared to a traditional in-house setting. The frequency of reports to which changes were made did not differ significantly between the teleradiology and the in-house setting. Clinically important differences to CT reports were similarly rare in both settings. Our study, as such, establishes teleradiology as a realizable way of providing after-hours radiology services.

Author Contributions: Conceptualization, S.S., M.K., B.R., and N.H.; methodology, S.S., M.K., B.R., S.L., and N.H.; software, S.S. and S.L.; validation, S.S., S.L., and N.H.; formal analysis, S.S. and S.L.; investigation, S.S., M.K., B.R., and N.H.; resources, M.K., C.R., and N.H.; data curation, S.S. and S.L.; writing—original draft preparation, S.S., S.L., and N.H.; writing—review and editing, M.K., B.R., C.R., A.S., and F.P.S.; visualization, S.S. and S.L.; supervision, M.K., B.R., and N.H.; project administration, S.S., M.K., B.R., and N.H.; funding acquisition, C.R. and N.H. All authors have read and agreed to the published version of the manuscript.

Funding: The project was supported by EU Grants INT-08-0001, 2010–2018 and FKP-0293-20-C.

Institutional Review Board Statement: The study was reviewed and approved by the Institutional Ethics Committee of Universitätsmedizin Greifswald (28 June 2016) and the staff council representing the affected doctors.

Informed Consent Statement: Informed consent was obtained from all participating radiologists involved in the study. Patient consent was waived due to anonymization of reports for evaluation.

Data Availability Statement: Not applicable.

Acknowledgments: Martina Plaehsmann supported the collection of raw data.

Conflicts of Interest: N.H. is reimbursed for reporting by teleradiology; the other authors declare no conflict of interest. The funders had no role in the design of the study; in the collection, analyses, or interpretation of data; in the writing of the manuscript; or in the decision to publish the results.

References

1. Thrall, J.H. Teleradiology. Part I. History and clinical applications. *Radiology* **2007**, *243*, 613–617. [CrossRef] [PubMed]
2. European Society of Radiology. ESR Teleradiology Survey: Results. *Insights Imaging* **2016**, *7*, 463–479. [CrossRef]
3. Platts-Mills, T.F.; Hendey, G.W.; Ferguson, B. Teleradiology interpretations of emergency department computed tomography scans. *J. Emerg. Med.* **2010**, *38*, 188–195. [CrossRef]
4. Rosenkrantz, A.B.; Hanna, T.N.; Steenburg, S.D.; Tarrant, M.J.; Pyatt, R.S.; Friedberg, E.B. The current state of teleradiology across the united states: A national survey of radiologists' habits, attitudes, and perceptions on teleradiology practice. *J. Am. Coll. Radiol.* **2019**, *16*, 1677–1687. [CrossRef] [PubMed]
5. Cohen, M.D. Accuracy of information on imaging requisitions: Does it matter? *J. Am. Coll. Radiol.* **2007**, *4*, 617–621. [CrossRef] [PubMed]

6. Rosenberg, C.; Langner, S.; Rosenberg, B.; Hosten, N. Medizinische und rechtliche Aspekte der Teleradiologie in Deutschland. [Medical and legal aspects of teleradiology in Germany]. *RoFo* **2011**, *183*, 804–811. [CrossRef]
7. Hosten, N.; Rosenberg, B.; Feiler, D. Teleradiologie nimmt weiter Fahrt auf. [Teleradiology continues to gain momentum]. *Radiol. Tech. IT-Syst. (RT)* **2016**, *15*, 16–20.
8. Bundesministerium der Justiz. *Röntgenverordnung in der Fassung der Bekanntmachung vom 30. April 2003 (BGBl. I S. 604), die Zuletzt Durch Artikel 6 der Verordnung vom 11. Dezember 2014 (BGBl. I S. 2010) GeäNdert Worden Ist. [X-ray Regulations in the Version of the Announcement of April 30, 2003 (BGBl. I p. 604), Which Was Last Updated by Article 6 of the Regulation of December 11, 2014 (BGBl. I p. 2010)]*; BGBl. I. Germany; Justiz Bd (Hrsg): Berlin, Germany, 2003.
9. Bundesministerium der Justiz. *Strahlenschutzgesetz vom 27. Juni 2017 (BGBl. I S. 1966), das Durch Artikel 2 des Gesetzes vom 27. Juni 2017 (BGBl. I S. 1966) GeäNdert Worden Ist. [Radiation Protection Law of June 27, 2017 (BGBl. I p. 1966), as Modified by Article 2 of the Law of June 27, 2017 (BGBl. I p. 1966)]*; BGBl. I. Germany; Justiz Bd (Hrsg): Berlin, Germany, 2017.
10. Bohrer, E.; Schäfer, S.B.; Krombach, G.A. Die neue Strahlenschutzgesetzgebung–Teil 2: Änderungen in der Radiologie bezüglich Vorabkontrolle und Sonderbereiche, einschließlich Teleradiologie. [The new radiation protection legislation-part 2: Modifications in radiology regarding approval procedure and special fields including teleradiology]. *Der Radiol.* **2020**, *60*, 959–965. [CrossRef]
11. Bruni, S.G.; Bartlett, E.; Yu, E. Factors involved in discrepant preliminary radiology resident interpretations of neuroradiological imaging studies: A retrospective analysis. *AJR. Am. J. Roentgenol.* **2012**, *198*, 1367–1374. [CrossRef]
12. Hohmann, J.; de Villiers, P.; Urigo, C.; Sarpi, D.; Newerla, C.; Brookes, J. Quality assessment of out sourced after-hours computed tomography teleradiology reports in a Central London University Hospital. *Eur. J. Radiol.* **2012**, *81*, e875–e879. [CrossRef]
13. Erly, W.K.; Ashdown, B.C.; Lucio, R.W., 2nd; Carmody, R.F.; Seeger, J.F.; Alcala, J.N. Evaluation of emergency CT scans of the head: Is there a community standard? *AJR Am. J. Roentgenol.* **2003**, *180*, 1727–1730. [CrossRef] [PubMed]
14. Zan, E.; Yousem, D.M.; Carone, M.; Lewin, J.S. Second-opinion consultations in neuroradiology. *Radiology* **2010**, *255*, 135–141. [CrossRef] [PubMed]
15. Chalian, M.; Del Grande, F.; Thakkar, R.S.; Jalali, S.F.; Chhabra, A.; Carrino, J.A. Second-Opinion Subspecialty Consultations in Musculoskeletal Radiology. *AJR Am. J. Roentgenol.* **2016**, *206*, 1217–1221. [CrossRef]
16. Ebbert, T.L.; Meghea, C.; Iturbe, S.; Forman, H.P.; Bhargavan, M.; Sunshine, J.H. The state of teleradiology in 2003 and changes since 1999. *Am. J. Roentgenol.* **2007**, *188*, W103–W112. [CrossRef] [PubMed]
17. Thrall, J.H. Teleradiology. Part II. Limitations, risks, and opportunities. *Radiology* **2007**, *244*, 325–328. [CrossRef]
18. Davenport, M.S.; Ellis, J.H.; Khalatbari, S.H.; Myles, J.D.; Klein, K.A. Effect of work hours, caseload, shift type, and experience on resident call performance. *Acad. Radiol.* **2010**, *17*, 921–927. [CrossRef]
19. Erly, W.K.; Berger, W.G.; Krupinski, E.; Seeger, J.F.; Guisto, J.A. Radiology resident evaluation of head CT scan orders in the emergency department. *AJNR Am. J. Neuroradiol.* **2002**, *23*, 103–107.
20. Ruutiainen, A.T.; Scanlon, M.H.; Itri, J.N. Identifying benchmarks for discrepancy rates in preliminary interpretations provided by radiology trainees at an academic institution. *J. Am. Coll. Radiol.* **2011**, *8*, 644–648. [CrossRef] [PubMed]
21. Weinberg, B.D.; Richter, M.D.; Champine, J.G.; Morriss, M.C.; Browning, T. Radiology resident preliminary reporting in an independent call environment: Multiyear assessment of volume, timeliness, and accuracy. *J. Am. Coll. Radiol.* **2015**, *12*, 95–100. [CrossRef]
22. Cooper, V.F.; Goodhartz, L.A.; Nemcek, A.A., Jr.; Ryu, R.K. Radiology resident interpretations of on-call imaging studies: The incidence of major discrepancies. *Acad. Radiol.* **2008**, *15*, 1198–1204. [CrossRef]
23. Mellnick, V.; Raptis, C.; McWilliams, S.; Picus, D.; Wahl, R. On-call radiology resident discrepancies: Categorization by patient location and severity. *J. Am. Coll. Radiol.* **2016**, *13*, 1233–1238. [CrossRef]
24. Lam, V.; Stephenson, J. A retrospective review of registrar out-of-hours reporting in a university hospital: The effect of time and seniority on discrepancy rates. *Clin. Radiol.* **2018**, *73*, 590.e9–590.e12. [CrossRef]
25. Ruchman, R.B.; Jaeger, J.; Wiggins, E.F., III; Seinfeld, S.; Thakral, V.; Bolla, S.; Wallach, S. Preliminary radiology resident interpretations versus final attending radiologist interpretations and the impact on patient care in a community hospital. *AJR. Am. J. Roentgenol.* **2007**, *189*, 523–526. [CrossRef]
26. Millet, I.; Alili, C.; Bouic-Pages, E.; Curros-Doyon, F.; Nagot, N.; Taourel, P. Journal club: Acute abdominal pain in elderly patients: Effect of radiologist awareness of clinicobiologic information on CT accuracy. *AJR. Am. J. Roentgenol.* **2013**, *201*, 1171–1179. [CrossRef] [PubMed]
27. Mullins, M.E.; Lev, M.H.; Schellingerhout, D.; Koroshetz, W.J.; Gonzalez, R.G. Influence of availability of clinical history on detection of early stroke using unenhanced CT and diffusion-weighted MR imaging. *AJR. Am. J. Roentgenol.* **2002**, *179*, 223–228. [CrossRef] [PubMed]
28. Loy, C.T.; Irwig, L. Accuracy of diagnostic tests read with and without clinical information: A systematic review. *JAMA* **2004**, *292*, 1602–1609. [CrossRef] [PubMed]
29. Dang, W.; Stefanski, P.D.; Kielar, A.Z.; El-Khodary, M.; van der Pol, C.; Thornhill, R.; Jaberi, A.; Fu, A.Y.; McInnes, M.D. Impact of clinical history on choice of abdominal/pelvic CT protocol in the Emergency Department. *PLoS ONE* **2018**, *13*, e0201694. [CrossRef]

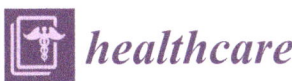

Article

A Study of eHealth from the Perspective of Social Sciences

Juan Uribe-Toril [1], José Luis Ruiz-Real [1,*] and Bruno José Nievas-Soriano [2]

1. Faculty of Economics and Business, University of Almería, 04120 Almería, Spain; juribe@ual.es
2. Nursing, Physiotherapy and Medicine Department, University of Almería, 04120 Almería, Spain; brunonievas73@gmail.com
* Correspondence: jlruizreal@ual.es; Tel.: +34-950-015742

Abstract: The field of social sciences has become increasingly important in eHealth. Patients currently engage more proactively with health services. This means that eHealth is linked to many different areas of Social Sciences. The main purpose of this research is to analyze the state-of-the-art research on eHealth from the perspective of social sciences. To this end, a bibliometric analysis was conducted using the Web of Science database. The main findings show the evolution of publications, the most influential countries, the most relevant journals and papers, and the importance of the different areas of knowledge. Although there are some studies on eHealth within social sciences, most of them focus on very specific aspects and do not develop a holistic analysis. Thus, this paper contributes to academia by analyzing the state-of-the-art of research, as well as identifying the most relevant trends and proposing future lines of research such as the potential of eHealth as a professional training instrument, development of predictive models in eHealth, analysis of the eHealth technology acceptance model (TAM), efficient integration of eHealth within public systems, efficient budget management, or improvement in the quality of service for patients.

Keywords: eHealth; mHealth; telemedicine; telehealth; social sciences; bibliometrics

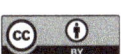

1. Introduction

The Internet is a phenomenon that no one could have predicted [1]. It has changed the way we access and use the information [2]. A few years ago, textbooks were the only source of medical information. Nowadays, anyone can find medical information by accessing the Internet from almost anywhere in the world [3]. As a consequence, people have changed the way they search for information and make decisions about their health [4]. The interest of people in the Internet as a tool for searching for health information is rising rapidly and online searches about health have increased in recent years [5]. Therefore, the way people deal with health issues is changing [1]. For example, it has been found that for pediatric consultations, mothers tend to use Internet resources frequently [6,7].

The delivery of health services using information and communication technologies (ICT), particularly the Internet, has been named eHealth, a concept that first appeared in 2000 [8]. Gunther Eysenbach published one of the most used definitions in 2001. This author defined eHealth as an emerging field at the intersection of medical informatics, public health, and business referring to the health services and information delivered or enhanced through the Internet and related technologies [9].

While Eysenbach's eHealth definition seems to be the most accepted one, universal consensus does not exist [10]. There are essential eHealth aspects such as ICT [1], delivery of healthcare services [11], the Internet [10], and that it is user-centered [12], so eHealth can be understood to be the delivery of user-centered healthcare services through ICT, mainly the Internet.

Some distinctly important advantages are offered by eHealth. Numerous authors highlight its accessibility as one of its most relevant features [13,14]. It is important for users to access health information quickly and easily so they can resolve their queries [2,15,16].

A high degree of accessibility helps to overcome social and geographical barriers, allowing people with fewer resources to access health information and healthcare services [15,17,18]. Another important advantage is the possibility of tailoring interventions via eHealth [19], as personalized medical treatment can be more effective [20,21].

Users can be empowered by eHealth with regard to health issues [22]. This could help them make better informed health decisions [14,18] and aid in improving communication between people and healthcare providers [1], as eHealth is often used to supplement physicians' recommendations [14,15]. Another advantage mentioned in the scientific literature is that eHealth allows people to access community support by facilitating participation in online support forums or in peer-support forums on social media [15,23].

The above notwithstanding, there are also some disadvantages to eHealth. For example, there are some serious concerns within the scientific community about the quality of the health information available online [24,25] as health-related web contents are not always trustworthy or validated [26–28]. Furthermore, information is not always easily understandable or suited to the needs of people [15,24,29]. Some authors have also described differences concerning the access to electronic health information as it relates to the digital divide, a concept that implies that socioeconomically disadvantaged subpopulations are less likely to have access to technologies, including eHealth interventions or health information available on the Internet [30,31]. Socioeconomically disadvantaged families also experience difficulty accessing technology or the Internet [32]. Some authors have described that the appearance of new medical technologies has often increased health disparities [33]. Technical issues could also become a barrier that can contribute to the digital divide [34].

The lack of education or training in the use of eHealth interventions could also generate personal barriers that can limit the access to health information [25]. Some authors state that eHealth can generate distrust among ordinary people. Numerous users are fearful of eHealth interventions and are reluctant to perform online health searches [24]. Parents in particular can feel unsafe and wary when searching health information [35]. Another disadvantage mentioned in the literature are the risk of adverse effects [2,27], especially in children [16]; concerns about privacy and security [34,36]; stress or anxiety of the users when performing health searches [37]; interference in the doctor–patient relationship [30]; or ethical and legal concerns [36].

Numerous authors propose some guiding principles for the future of eHealth. The principles most frequently mentioned in the literature are user empowerment and the improvement of their health and eHealth literacy [34,38]. In addition, healthcare providers should get involved in eHealth development and delivery [28]. It is also important to search for ways to minimize the digital divide [39] such as improving the usability of the eHealth interventions [25] and to investigate methods to ensure eHealth quality [10] and to develop ethical aspects [32].

The world of medicine and health cannot be understood without taking into account the social sciences. Social sciences cover such disciplines as psychology, education, management, public administration, communication, biomedical social sciences, social work, sociology, demography, information and documentation, legislation, etc. The strong focus on the detection and treatment of diseases has given way to a more holistic understanding of the patient, considering both purely medical and social aspects and placing the patient at the center of everything. Patienthood is a social state rather than simply a biological one. Thus, "psychosocial variables influence, not only the social and personal meanings of illness, but also the risk of becoming ill, the nature of the response to illness and its prognosis" [40].

The joint analysis of the social sciences and health allows professionals to understand not only medicine, but also the socioeconomic and political approach to disease and health. This interdisciplinary research facilitates different levels of analysis in the health sciences between social, psychological, behavioral, and biomedical scientists [41]. Thus, interdisciplinary efforts provide researchers new opportunities to refine theories and methods. Specifically, social scientists play different roles in health services, such as framing the issues, intelligence, monitoring, evaluation and assessment, and implementation, contributing to a better understanding of complex organizational arrangements, structures, cultures, management approaches, financial arrangements, and regulatory processes [42].

Social sciences have become an important approach in eHealth studies in the 21st century, and even more significantly in the last decade, a period in which the number of publications and citations has increased notably, as well as the number of areas of knowledge involved in these topics. The rapid and continuous development of new ICT has substantially changed the way in which people interact with healthcare systems [43]. Scholars have moved from debating what eHealth is to examining the technical, human, organizational, and social factors that influence eHealth practices [44–46]. Nowadays, eHealth research is an interdisciplinary field where information science and technology, biomedical science, and social sciences collaborate and create synergies [47].

To all of the above, the abrupt appearance of the coronavirus (COVID-19) pandemic during 2020 must also be added. As this pandemic requires quarantine and isolation, face-to-face visits in medical care have been considerably reduced. This situation calls for rapid and creative changes to the way healthcare is delivered and the development and adoption of new approaches to eHealth resources [48], which should be developed from a global vision, a vision which obviously must include the social sciences.

Despite the importance of this issue, there is a scarcity of systematic literature on what aspects of eHealth have been investigated from the perspective of social sciences. Although the existing bibliometric research addresses specific issues, it does not offer a holistic analysis of eHealth from the perspective of the social sciences. Along these lines there are some interesting papers to be found on topics such as health information systems [49]; Internet studies as a field of social science research around four primary research themes, including eHealth [50]; health informatics competences [51]; physical activity, sedentary behavior, and diet-related eHealth and mHealth [52]; international mobile health research [53]; or the most cited authors in a specific journal [54]. The two papers that carry out a more general analysis of these topics were written by Jiang et al. [41] who performed a systematic review of eHealth literature in the mainstream social science journals by testing the applicability of the 5A categorization (i.e., access, availability, appropriateness, acceptability, and applicability) and Son et al. [55] who reviewed the main research topics and trends of international eHealth through social network analysis.

The main objective of this research was to analyze the research on eHealth from the perspective of the social science areas of knowledge. To contextualize analysis of the relevant areas of knowledge of the documents analyzed, essential aspects like the number of publications per year, the most influential countries, and the most influential journals and papers are studied.

Therefore, this research contributes to academia by analyzing the state-of-the-art research on eHealth from the perspective of various social science areas of knowledge. It also identifies the main trends and proposes future lines of research and topics. To achieve this objective, a bibliometric analysis was developed. This paper has the following structure. First, the methodology is explained. Second, findings are presented to know the annual evolution of publications and citations, the most influential countries on these topics, the most relevant journals and papers, the most important areas of knowledge involved in this field, and significant trends. Finally, in conclusion, future lines of research are proposed.

2. Materials and Methods

For this study, a bibliometric analysis of the scientific literature in the Web of Science (WoS) Core Collection and a cluster analysis of the co-citation and keyword variables were carried out. The bibliometric analysis was based on the qualification and parameterization of scientific production as well as the influence of authors, publications, and institutions on a certain topic. The origin of this type of analysis is found in the article by Garfield [56] and his attempts to evaluate and quantify the importance of scientific articles. In 1960, he created the Institute for Scientific Information, which later became the WoS database.

Bibliometry, as defined by Pritchard [57], is the application of mathematical and statistical methods to books and other communication methods. Therefore, and from this perspective, bibliometric analysis is a meta-analytic systematic review. The success of this methodology lies in the possibility of measuring scientific activity to quickly and concisely study the antecedents, evolution, trends, and future lines of research of a topic, measuring scientific activity around a given topic.

The impact or influence is measured by the number of citations an article receives. In an attempt to unify both positions, Hirsch [58] created an index that provides a balance between the number of articles and citations (h-index).

The procedure used for data collection and subsequent information analysis has been described by Moed [59] or Brereton et al. [60], although there are multiple variants to these procedures. The first stage consisted of selecting the WoS Core Collection database, a source that has been commonly used in bibliometric analysis. It was the first compiler of indexes and a precursor in measuring the impact of journals and covers more research fields compared to other databases. In addition, WoS allows filtering the indicators, prioritization by number of citations, and its journal impact index guarantees the quality of articles.

Five search terms were chosen based on the prevailing literature on the topic: eHealth; mHealth; Telemedicine; Mobile Health; and Telehealth. The documents published in 2020 were eliminated, as the year had not finished at the time of this study and their inclusion could distort the analysis. Furthermore, other documents such as grey literature, books, or proceedings were excluded, limiting the search to the articles published in indexed journals.

The documents in the WoS database are classified into five broad categories: Arts and Humanities; Life Sciences and Biomedicine; Physical Sciences; Social Sciences; and Technology, with all the journals assigned to at least one research area. The final research criterion used was to refine the search by the research related to social sciences (Figure 1).

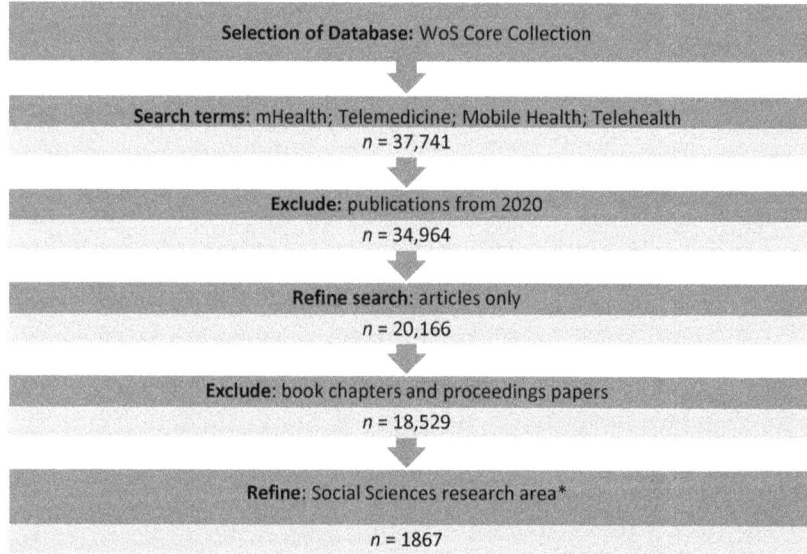

Figure 1. Methodology wtages used in the bibliometric analysis. * Archaeology; Area Studies; Biomedical Social Sciences; Business & Economics; Communication; Criminology & Penology; Cultural Studies; Demography; Development Studies; Education & Educational Research; Ethnic Studies; Family Studies; Geography; Government & Law; International Relations; Linguistics; Mathematical Methods In Social Sciences; Psychology; Public Administration; Social Issues; Social Sciences—Other Topics; Social Work; Sociology; Urban Studies; Women's Studies.

Once the data had been cleaned, the results were exported to files compatible with statistical analysis tools, performing a cluster analysis through the VOSviewer [61]. The text mining functionality of this tool supports the generation of keyword term maps based on a corpus of documents [62]. A term map is a two-dimensional map in which words are located in such a way that the distance between them can be taken as an indication of the affinity of the terms. The relatedness of terms is determined by their cooccurrence in documents [63].

The analysis was limited to the terms that were repeated a minimum of 25 times (111 keywords) with the keywords used for the search eliminated from the count. In this analysis, keywords from authors, journals, as well as the most repeated words in titles and abstracts were selected.

This study also used fractional counting at the network level since it can normalize the relative weights of links and thereby clarify structures in the network [64].

3. Results and Discussion

3.1. Publications Per Year

The first article to focus on the eHealth topic included in the WoS database in the Social Sciences research area is "Some implications of Telemedicine" by Ben Park and Rashid Bashshur published in 1975 in *Journal of Communication* [65]. This paper, published before the existence of the Internet, prophesied that healthcare delivery by two-way television might change roles, authority, and distribution of healthcare professionals.

The number of scientific publications on eHealth during the 20th century is small, even in the late 1990s when mobile phones and the Internet were in common use. It was not until the decade of 2010 when there was an important increase with the number of publications doubling from 199 to 433 (Table 1). Since 2005, there has been a continuous annual growing of manuscripts, with 2019 having the largest number of publications (317).

Table 1. Number of articles per year.

Years	Articles	Citations	h-Index	Mean	≥ 100	≥ 50	≥ 25	≥ 10
2015–19	1103	8475	35	7.68	6	19	70	256
2010–14	433	11,096	53	25.63	15	60	140	279
2005–09	199	5962	44	29.96	7	39	85	125
2000–04	109	4735	33	43.44	6	20	45	72
1995–99	29	1575	16	54.31	3	6	11	16
1990–94	0	0	0	0.00	0	0	0	0
1985–89	1	10	1	10.00	0	0	0	1
1980–84	1	6	1	6.00	0	0	0	0
1975–79	6	59	4	9.83	0	0	1	2
Total	1881	31,918	73	16.97	37	144	352	751

The comparison between articles including all research areas and those limited to the Social Sciences (Figure 2) shows a similar evolution. The lack of differences confirm that the topic is developing in the same way across the whole scientific community. This parallel evolution does not happen when the field does not generate significant scientific interest.

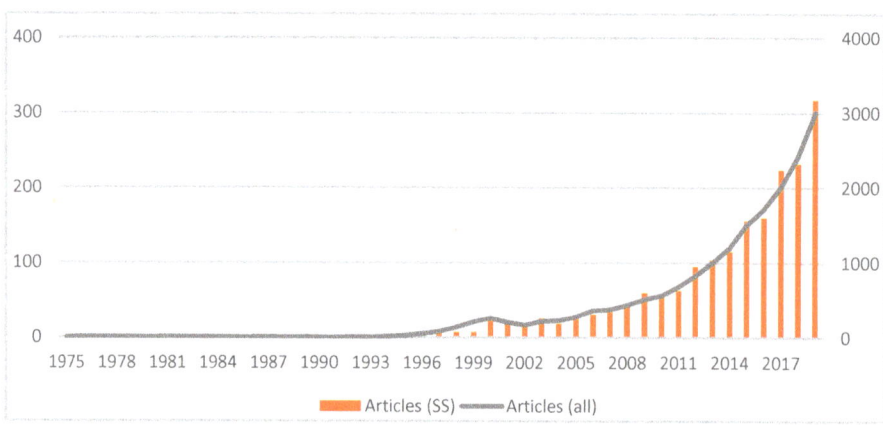

Figure 2. Evolution in the number of articles (Social Sciences (SS) and all areas).

3.2. Most Influential Countries

The ten countries with the largest number of articles published related to eHealth in Social Sciences are shown in Table 2. The USA is the country with the largest number of articles published and citations, with 7.38 times more articles than the second-ranking country, Australia. Among the rest of the countries shown in the table, two groups can be distinguished: Australia, the UK, and Canada have a similar number or articles, between 104 and 150, while the remaining countries (Netherlands, Germany, Spain, China, Italy, South Africa) have a smaller number of publications, between 36 and 71.

Table 2. Number of articles and citations by country.

Country	A	C	h	Mean	≥250 C	≥100 C	≥50 C	≥25 C	≥10 C	≥5 C	≥1 C
USA	1107	20,229	59	18.27	6	22	92	228	485	687	1026
Australia	150	2913	29	19.42	0	5	17	35	65	87	136
UK	148	3038	30	20.53	1	5	16	36	64	82	132
Canada	104	1475	20	14.18	0	1	4	17	44	61	91
Netherlands	71	1347	22	18.97	0	1	7	20	34	45	61
Germany	50	557	11	11.14	0	1	2	6	13	23	42
Spain	41	448	10	10.93	0	1	3	5	11	15	30
China	37	2636	14	71.24	4	6	7	10	16	21	32
Italy	36	370	10	10,28	0	0	1	5	10	20	32
South Africa	36	186	8	5,17	0	0	0	1	5	12	28

A: articles; C: citations; h: h-index.

When analyzing the number of citations, the USA is once again the highest-ranking country, 6.65 times higher than the second country, the UK. Nevertheless, the h-index of the USA is only 1.96 times higher than that of the UK. If we consider mean citations per article, the largest number corresponds to China, with a mean of 71.24 citations per article. This figure seems very high, as it is 3.47 times higher than mean citations of the second most cited country, the UK, considering that China has only 37 articles compared to the 3038 articles published in the UK.

Only three of the ten countries (USA, China, and UK) have eleven articles with more than 250 citations. It is important to highlight that although the USA and China have a similar number of articles in this category, the number of articles published in the USA (1107) far outnumbers the 37 articles published in China. In addition, when considering the categories with more than 100, 50, and 25 citations, China has larger figures than expected when considering the number of articles published and the h-index of each country. Perhaps, this particular finding could benefit from a more detailed analysis of the Chinese articles to find how they are cited and interconnected. If Chinese articles are not taken in account, the rest of the figures of these rankings are in the same order as the list of countries with more published articles.

Another aspect to consider when analyzing the most influential countries is the number of citations in relation to the population of each country (Table 3). In this case, the country with the largest number of citations per population is Australia, followed by the Netherlands, the USA, the UK, and Canada. Despite the large number of absolute citations and the large number of citations per article, China is in the last place due to its large population.

Table 3. Mean citations per population.

Country	Population *	Citations	Mean
Australia	25,499,884	2913	0.114236
Netherlands	17,134,872	1347	0.000079
USA	331,002,651	20,229	0.000061
UK	56,286,961	3038	0.000054
Canada	37,742,154	1475	0.000039
Spain	46,754,778	448	0.000010
Germany	83,783,942	557	0.000007
Italy	60,461,826	370	0.000006
South Africa	59,308,690	186	0.000003
China	1,439,323,776	2636	0.000002

* Source of population data: United Nations 2020 [66].

It seems understandable that a country like the USA has the largest number of publications due to its large population, but surprisingly this is not the case for China, perhaps because their literature production about eHealth is less focused on social sciences. Analyzing the rest of the list, we can find countries like Australia, the UK, Canada, the Netherlands, or Germany, which seem to be more concerned with the development of the social sciences literature.

3.3. Most Influential Journals and Papers

When analyzing the most influential journals related to eHealth in the social sciences, the number of articles published on these topics and the number of citations have been taken into account. The results of the said analysis can be seen in Table 4 in the ranking of the most influential journals. The ranking is led by the journal *Professional Psychology Research and Practice* with 54 articles and 1768 citations in addition to having the highest h-index (23). This journal is followed by *Patient Education and Counseling* (a medical journal covering patient education and health communication) with 44 articles and 880 citations and by *Journal of Health Communication* (focused on information and library science), 42 articles and 1026 citations. However, the high impact of the journal *Social Science & Medicine* is very striking since, with 24 articles on this topic, it has received 1043 citations, which makes it the journal with the largest number of citations per article (43.46).

When focusing the analysis on the articles published in the 21st century, which represent 96.52% of the total articles on these topics, it can be observed (Figure 3) that the most relevant journals are *Social Science & Medicine* (43.26), *Professional Psychology Research and Practice* (28.53), *Journal of Health Communication* (24.43), *Patient Education and Counseling* (19.33), and *AIDS and Behavior* (13.71).

Table 4. Most relevant journals on the eHealth and Social Sciences.

Journal	Articles	Citations	h-Index	Cit/Paper	IF-5 Years	Q
Professional Psychology Research and Practice	54	1768	23	32.74	2.077	Q2
Patient Education and Counseling	44	880	18	20	3.408	Q1
Journal of Health Communication	42	1026	17	24.26	2.358	Q2
Digital Health	39	106	5	2.72	-	-
AIDS and Behavior	38	520	14	13.68	3.298	Q1
Psychological Services	33	335	10	10.15	2.201	Q2
Psycho-Oncology	31	215	7	6.94	3.581	Q1
Frontiers in Psychology	24	147	7	5.92	2.723	Q2
Social Science & Medicine	24	1043	15	43.46	4.241	Q1
Journal of Pediatric Psychology	23	384	11	16.7	3.505	Q3

Cit/paper: citations per paper; IF-5 years: impact factor in the last five years; Q: quartile in WoS.

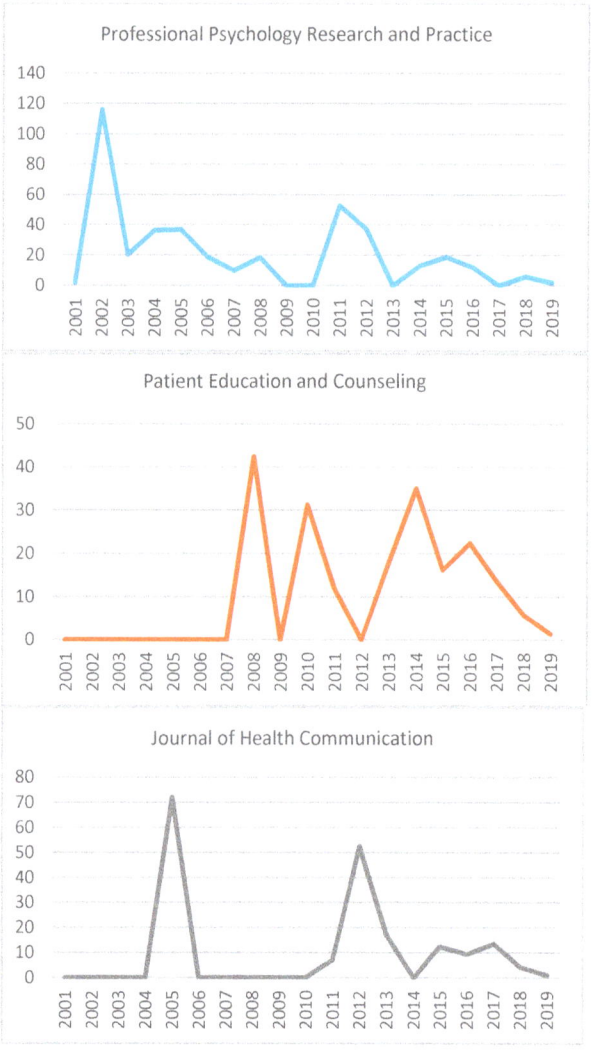

Figure 3. *Cont.*

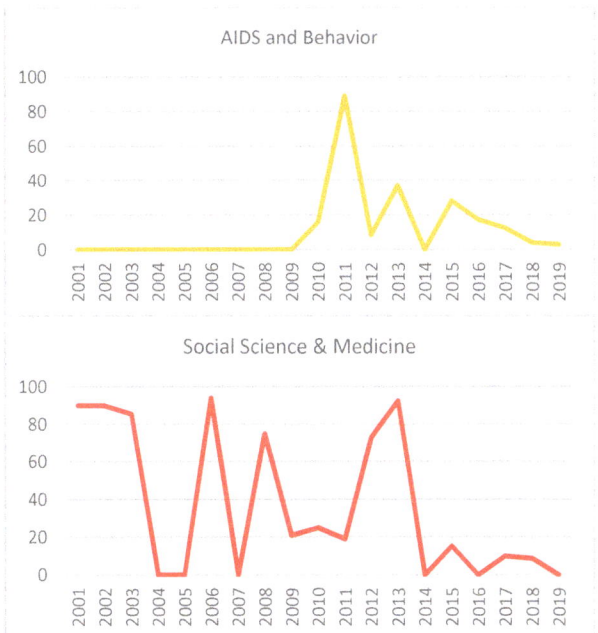

Figure 3. Citations per article of journals in the 21st century.

It is noteworthy that, of the top ten journals that publish articles about eHealth in the field of Social Sciences, 50% of them have psychology applied to various fields as their main field of research. This is the case for *Professional Psychology Research and Practice* (psychology, multidisciplinary), *Psychological Services* (psychology, clinical), Psycho-Oncology (psychological aspects of oncology), *Frontiers in Psychology* (psychology, multidisciplinary), and *Journal of Pediatric Psychology* (child psychology).

Figure 4 shows a cluster analysis of co-citations among the most relevant journals in this field of research. This analysis is based on the existence of thematic similarity between two or more documents that are co-cited in a third and subsequent work. Thus, the higher the frequency of co-citation, the greater the affinity between them. Three main clusters were identified. Two of them are directly related to aspects of psychology led *by Professional Psychology Research and Practice* and *Journal of Pediatric Psychology*. The other cluster is more focused on health and medicine, with a central axis in the journal *Social Science & Medicine*, which has close relationships with *Journal of Health Communication* and with *Patient Education and Counseling* among others.

With regard to the articles with the largest number of citations (Table 5), three of the top ten were published in *Information & Management*, a journal mainly focused on the field of information systems and applications which, in this case, are focused on eHealth. The four articles with the most citations have a common central element, the analysis of the technology acceptance model (TAM). The first article, "Why do people play on-line games? An extended TAM with social influences and flow experience" [67] analyzes the reasons why people play online games using the TAM model, connecting social influence, psychology, and telemedicine technology (778 citations). The second article (with 756 citations), "Examining the technology acceptance model using physician acceptance of telemedicine technology" [68], studies the applicability of the TAM model for explaining physicians' decisions for accepting telemedicine technology in the healthcare context, providing some implications for user technology acceptance research and telemedicine management. The third article, with 548 citations, "Information technology acceptance by individual professionals: A model comparison approach" [69] represents a conceptual replication of several model comparison studies, TAM, theory of planned behavior (TPB), and a deconstructed TPB model, by analyzing the responses to a survey on telemedicine technology acceptance. The fourth article, "Investigating healthcare professionals' decisions to accept telemedicine technology: an empirical test of competing theories" [70], has 425 citations and evaluates the extent to which prevailing intention-based models, including TAM, TPB, and an integrated model, could explain physicians' acceptance of telemedicine technology.

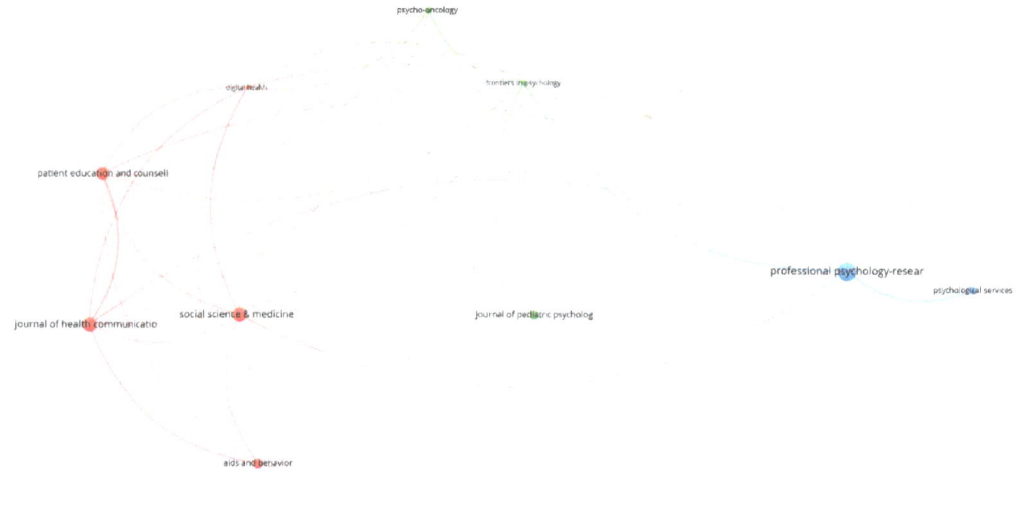

Figure 4. Cluster analysis of co-citations among the most relevant journals.

Table 5. Articles with the largest number of citations on eHealth and social sciences.

R	Article	C	Journal	Reference	C/Y
1	Why do people play on-line games? An extended TAM with social influences and flow experience	778	Information & Management	Hsu, C.L.; Lu, H.P. (2004) [67]	51.87
2	Examining the technology acceptance model using physician acceptance of telemedicine technology	756	Journal of Management Information Systems	Hu, P.J.; Chau, P.Y.K.; Sheng, O.R.L.; Tam, K.Y. (1999) [68]	37.80
3	Information technology acceptance by individual professionals: A model comparison approach	548	Decision Sciences	Chau, P.Y.K.; Hu, P.J.H. (2001) [69]	30.44
4	Investigating healthcare professionals' decisions to accept telemedicine technology: an empirical test of competing theories	425	Information & Management	Chau, P.Y.K.; Hu, P.J.H. (2002) [70]	25.00

Table 5. Cont.

R	Article	C	Journal	Reference	C/Y
5	mHealth for Mental Health: Integrating Smartphone Technology in Behavioral Healthcare	375	Professional Psychology-Research and Practice	Luxton, D.D.; McCann, R.A.; Bush, N.E.; Mishkind, M.C.; Reger, G.M. (2011) [71]	46.88
6	Zooming In and Out: Studying Practices by Switching Theoretical Lenses and Trailing Connections	273	Organization Studies	Nicolini, D. (2009) [73]	27.30
7	A Behavior Change Model for Internet Interventions	266	Annals of Behavioral Medicine	Ritterband, L.M.; Thorndike, F.P.; Cox, D.J.; Kovatchev, B.P.; Gonder-Frederick, L.A. (2009) [74]	26.60
8	Examining a model of information technology acceptance by individual professionals: An exploratory study	259	Journal of Management Information Systems	Chau, P.Y.K.; Hu, P.J. (2002) [75]	15.24
9	Interdisciplinary Chronic Pain Management Past, Present, and Future	215	American Psychologist	Gatchel, R.J.; McGeary, D.D.; McGeary, C.A.; Lippe, B. (2014) [72]	43.00
10	Technology acceptance model for internet banking: an invariance analysis	208	Information & Management	Lai, V.S.; Li, H.L. (2005) [76]	14.86

R: rank; C: total citations; C/Y: citations per year.

Another featured article is "mHealth for Mental Health: Integrating Smartphone Technology in Behavioral Healthcare" [71], which provides an overview of smartphone use in behavioral healthcare and discusses options for integrating mobile technology into clinical practice (375 citations; 4688 citations per year). The article "Interdisciplinary Chronic Pain Management Past, Present, and Future" [72], with 215 citations, is the third document with a large number of citations per year (43). This research discussed the major components of a true interdisciplinary pain management program, providing future directions in this field, including telehealth.

3.4. Relevant Areas of Knowledge

Given that eHealth is an issue that cuts across many disciplines, it is not surprising that research on this issue is of interest to researchers in numerous fields and involves many areas of knowledge within the social sciences. Among these knowledge areas, Psychology is the most relevant, with 778 articles published on this topic and 14,158 citations, having an h-index of 54 (Table 6). This corresponds to the findings on the most relevant journals since, as previously stated, half of those in the top ten have psychology as applied to various fields as their main field of research. Thus, psychology becomes the human dimension of digital health. The future of psychology should be conducted through technology and patient empowerment. Patient social networks are becoming an important instrument for empowering patients and their families in managing their disease. Thus, one of the challenges faced by eHealth with online interventions is for people to change their attitude and/or their behavior. Among the many articles of Psychology on this topic, there are 19 that have more than 100 citations, two of which even exceed 250 citations: "mHealth for Mental Health: Integrating Smartphone Technology in Behavioral Healthcare" [69] and "A Behavior Change Model for Internet Interventions" [74].

Table 6. Relevance of areas of knowledge on eHealth and social sciences.

Area of Knowledge	Articles	Citations	h-Index	Average
Psychology	778	14,158	54	18.20
Education & Educational Research	248	2513	25	10.13
Biomedical Social Sciences	234	3878	34	16.57
Business & Economics	189	5911	32	31.28
Social Sciences—Other Topics	170	2010	25	11.82
Communication	135	2207	26	16.35
Social Work	59	482	13	8.17
Government & Law	57	364	9	6.39
Linguistics	52	888	18	17.08
Family Studies	40	431	13	10.78
Social Issues	31	486	11	15.68
Sociology	25	756	12	30.24
Public Administration	19	195	7	10.26
Women's Studies	16	161	6	10.06
Development Studies	15	68	5	4.53
Criminology & Penology	12	71	5	5.92
Geography	10	110	5	11.00
International Relations	4	16	2	4.00
Urban Studies	4	6	1	1.50
Area Studies	3	6	2	2.00
Ethnic Studies	3	51	2	17.00
Demography	1	3	1	3.00

Other areas which play a prominent role in research on this topic are *Education & Educational Research* (248 articles); *Biomedical Social Sciences* (234); *Business & Economics* (189); *Social Sciences—Other Topics* (170); and *Communication* (135). In relation to *Education & Educational Research*, it is observed that medical care has evolved from more disease-focused care to patient-directed care, including in the field of health education. The works published in this area mainly investigate aspects related to the design, implementation and evaluation of eHealth education. The aim is to empower health professionals and the general public in terms of health education and digital skills, to promote healthy lifestyle habits and achieve a more active and participatory role in relation to individual and community health and well-being. The article with the most citations (168) in this field is entitled "Internet use for health information among college students" [77].

Of import within the field of *Biomedical Social Sciences* is the development of methods of analysis and processing of biomedical signals and images to aid the diagnosis of different pathologies, as well as the generation of predictive models based on bio-signals and symptoms with applications in the field of eHealth. "Quantifying the body: monitoring and measuring health in the age of mHealth technologies" [78] is the paper with the largest number of citations in this area (189).

While the Business & Economics area ranks fourth in terms of the number of articles published, this field has the largest average number of citations per paper (31.28), which shows the interest of academia in this topic. In fact, the paper with the largest number of citations on this topic is precisely from the Business & Economics area, the aforementioned work by Hsu and Lu [67] "Why do people play on-line games? An extended TAM with social influences and flow experience". Another of the great challenges of research in this field is an efficient integration of eHealth within public systems, with special focus on the reduction of costs and, at the same time, of patient waiting times.

Another aspect to consider is the interrelation between the areas of knowledge, that is, papers related to social sciences and medicine that are framed in more than one area at the same time. For this, a Venn diagram was used, considering the six research areas with more than 100 papers published in this field (Figure 5). Once again, it can be seen that Psychology plays the central role as it is linked with the other five areas, highlighting its close relationship with Biomedical Social Sciences, sharing 51 papers, and with Education

& Educational Research (20). Psychology shares other papers with Social Sciences—Other Topics (10), Communication (10), and Business (1).

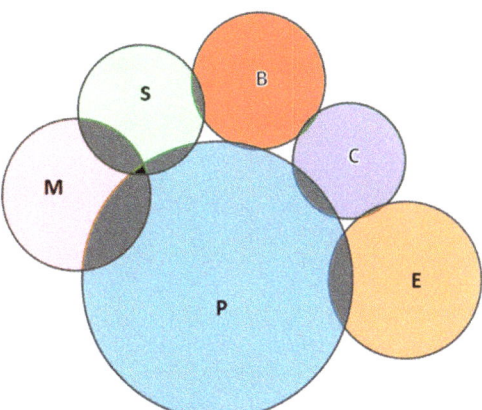

Figure 5. Venn diagram of the interrelations between areas of knowledge. P: Psychology; E: Education & Educational Research; M: Biomedical Social Sciences; B: Business & Economics; S: Social Sciences—Other Topics; C: Communication.

Furthermore, the Social Sciences—Other Topics area, given its transversal nature, shares research with other fields, such as Biomedical Social Sciences (26), and Business & Economics (4). Specifically, there is a paper by Fraser [79] published in International Journal of Transgenderism, which is framed within three different research areas: Psychology, Biomedical Social Sciences, and Social Sciences—Other Topics.

3.5. Keywords and Trends

The analysis found 105 keyword terms that appeared a minimum of 25 times. It seems logical that the most used terms are "care", "technology", "Internet", and "health". It is noteworthy that the fifth most used term is "depression", a finding that seems consistent with the fact that Psychology was the most relevant area of knowledge found in the analysis. On the other hand, despite Education & Educational Research being the second most relevant area, the first term related with this area, "education", was ranked 15th.

The analysis of the terms showed five clearly identified clusters (Figure 6). The cluster in red color is focused on the nuclear terms related to eHealth, with keywords that define the concept, like "information", "communication", "management", "technology", "online", or "digital health". The technology and innovation features of eHealth are also represented by keywords like "implementation", "innovation", "services", "system", or "technology", as these are essential aspects of the very concept of eHealth. Other important keywords found were "challenges", "barriers", or "ethics", which reflect some of the problems that the eHealth can deliver. Finally, one of the most important aspects of eHealth, the users, is featured in this cluster with terms like "patient" or "people", but also with "attitude", "perceptions", "satisfaction", or "user acceptance".

The cluster in green is focused on three aspects related with the social features of the use of eHealth. Keywords like "adolescents", "adults", "behavior", "behavior-change", "engagement", "smartphone", or "self-efficacy" are related with aspects of the users that use eHealth interventions. Keywords like "alcohol", "health", "HIV", "obesity", "physical activity", or "prevention" reflect the medical aspects that concern people. Finally, keywords like "smartphone", "social support", or "text messaging" reflect how eHealth has the potential to allow people to access community support.

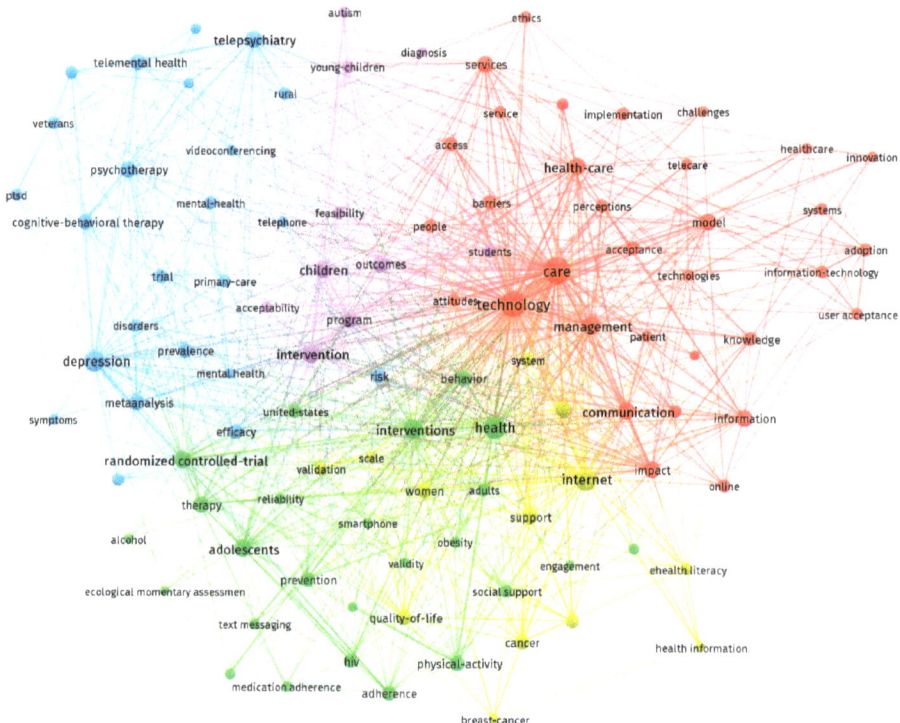

Figure 6. Cluster visualization of co-occurrence of keywords.

The cluster in blue highlights the importance of psychological and mental health aspects in this field, grouping keywords like "anxiety", "depression", "mental health", "psychotherapy", or "telepsychiatry". This seems logical as Psychology is the most relevant area of knowledge found in the analysis, reflecting that this field is an important part of the eHealth literature when analyzed from the point of view of the social sciences.

The cluster in yellow reflects two related aspects, women and health literacy, as women use more eHealth and have more health and eHealth literacy. Finally, the fifth cluster (purple color) is related to children, with keywords like "autism", "children", "students", and "young children".

A trend analysis showed that some of these terms currently being used most frequently are "acceptance", "acceptability", "engagement", "eHealth literacy", or "barriers". As has been found in the literature, this seems to confirm that the main guidelines for future research concern acceptance, increasing eHealth literacy of users, and overcoming barriers.

4. Conclusions

Social sciences play an increasingly important role in eHealth. From the information obtained, the time-based progression of the number of articles published is particularly significant, showing the interest of the scientific community in this topic and a constant increase in research works. The USA is the country with the largest number of published articles and citations. China has the largest mean number of citations per article, although the highest h-index belongs to the USA. Only three of the ten countries (USA, China, and UK) have 11 articles with more than 250 citations. Finally, Australia is the country with most citations considering the population of the country.

With regard to the number of articles and the h-index, Professional Psychology Research and Practice is the most influential journal on eHealth in Social Sciences, followed by Patient Education and Counseling and Journal of Health Communication. However, Social Science & Medicine has the largest number of citations per article. A cluster analysis of co-citations in the most relevant journals identified three main clusters. Two of them are focused on different aspects of Psychology, which is very significant since 50% of the most relevant journals in this field are closely related to this area of knowledge. The other cluster is directly related to Health and Medicine. Most (96.52%) of the articles on these topics have been published in the 21st century. The analysis of the TAM is the central axis of some of the most cited articles. Nevertheless, there are other subjects of great interest, such as the information systems field oriented to eHealth, the use of smartphones in behavioral healthcare, the applications for integrating mobile technology into clinical practice, or an interdisciplinary pain management program in eHealth.

It is notable that the relationship of patients with the health system has changed. The concept of the passive patient has fallen by the wayside in favor of people who are more active and involved in all processes. As a result, eHealth is a very transversal field for the different areas of social sciences. Although there are many areas of knowledge and different fields of Social Sciences related to research on eHealth, Psychology stands out above all others. One of the important research trends in this field will continue to be the empowerment of patients (and people in general) through technology, as well as helping change people's attitudes and behaviors, based on psychological theories and principles. This will offer new opportunities for both theoretical and applied research.

Other relevant areas in this field are Education & Educational Research; Biomedical Social Sciences; Business & Economics; Social Sciences—Other Topics; and Communication. Education & Educational Research is focused on the design, implementation, and evaluation of eHealth education. Based on the findings of this research, it appears that in the future, there will be a growing interest in the acquisition of knowledge at different levels related to both health education and digital skills addressed to different groups, both medical professionals and people in general (particularly, in certain targeted population groups, such as elderly or ethnic groups).

The potential of eHealth as a professional training instrument will improve the quality of care provided to the population, as well as develop new sources of knowledge and research. In Biomedical Social Sciences, there are still good opportunities for research with regard to the methods of processing biomedical signals and the development of predictive models in eHealth. Business & Economics is the area with the largest average number of citations per paper. One of the challenges of research in this field is the analysis of the eHealth TAM (as well as the extended version), including cultural and social factors, to empirically assess the validity of its constructs, mainly its level of helpfulness, usability, and intention to use eHealth services. Other important research lines are the efficient integration of eHealth within public systems, efficient budget management, or the improvement in the quality of service for patients, and improved perception by all stakeholders. In addition, social sciences have tools to measure different types of outcomes.

Furthermore, it is important to highlight the interaction between the different areas of knowledge. Once again, Psychology plays a central role, sharing research with the other most relevant areas, mainly with Biomedical Social Sciences and Education & Educational Research. For future research, it would be necessary to promote even more synergy between different disciplines.

The most used terms were grouped into five main clusters focused on nuclear terms related to eHealth are "care", "technology", "Internet", and "health"; aspects related to social features and the use of eHealth; and psychological and mental health aspects in this field. The main trends found are studying acceptability, increasing eHealth literacy of users, and overcoming barriers.

This work is not exempt from some limitations, some of which could be the basis for future research. Thus, in addition to the use of WoS, other quantitative and/or qualitative tools could also be utilized. Finally, other terms related to eHealth, including broader concepts, could be analyzed.

Author Contributions: Conceptualization, J.L.R.-R. and J.U.-T.; methodology, J.U.-T.; validation, J.L.R.-R. and J.U.-T.; formal analysis, J.L.R.-R., J.U.-T. and B.J.N.-S.; writing—original draft preparation, J.L.R.-R., J.U.-T. and B.J.N.-S.; writing—review and editing, J.L.R.-R., J.U.-T. and B.J.N.-S.; supervision, J.L.R.-R. All authors have read and agreed to the published version of the manuscript.

Funding: This research received no external funding.

Institutional Review Board Statement: Not applicable.

Informed Consent Statement: Not applicable.

Data Availability Statement: The data presented in this study are available on request from the corresponding author.

Conflicts of Interest: The authors declare no conflict of interest.

References

1. Bujnowska-Fedak, M.M. Trends in the use of the Internet for health purposes in Poland. *BMC Public Health* **2015**, *15*, 194. [CrossRef]
2. Von Rosen, A.J.; Von Rosen, F.T.; Tinnemann, P.; Müller-Riemenschneider, F. Sexual Health and the Internet: Cross-Sectional Study of Online Preferences Among Adolescents. *J. Med. Internet Res.* **2017**, *19*, e379. [CrossRef] [PubMed]
3. Bates, D.W.; Wright, A. Evaluating eHealth: Undertaking robust international cross-cultural eHealth research. *PLoS Med.* **2009**, *6*, e1000105. [CrossRef] [PubMed]
4. Li, F.; Li, M.; Guan, P.; Ma, S.; Cui, L. Mapping publication trends and identifying hot spots of research on Internet health information seeking behavior: A quantitative and co-word biclustering analysis. *J. Med. Internet Res.* **2015**, *17*, e81. [CrossRef] [PubMed]
5. Diviani, N.; van den Putte, B.; Giani, S.; van Weert, J.C. Low health literacy and evaluation of online health information: A systematic review of the literature. *J. Med. Internet Res.* **2015**, *17*, e112. [CrossRef] [PubMed]
6. Zhang, H.; Wang, X.; Yang, Z.; Zhao, Y. Analysis of Requirements for Developing an mHealth-Based Health Management Platform. *JMIR mHealth uHealth* **2017**, *5*, e117. [CrossRef]
7. Sebelefsky, C.; Voitl, J.; Karner, D.; Klein, F.; Voitl, P.; Böck, A. Internet use of parents before attending a general pediatric outpatient clinic: Does it change their information level and assessment of acute diseases? *BMC Pediatr.* **2016**, *16*, 129. [CrossRef]
8. Stellefson, M.; Hanik, B.; Chaney, B.; Chaney, D.; Tennant, B.; Chavarria, E.A. eHealth literacy among college students: A systematic review with implications for eHealth education. *J. Med. Internet Res.* **2011**, *13*, e102. [CrossRef]
9. Eysenbach, G. What is e-health? *J. Med. Internet Res.* **2001**, *3*, e20. [CrossRef]
10. Boogerd, E.A.; Arts, T.; Engelen, L.J.; Van De Belt, T.H. "What is eHealth": Time for an update? *JMIR Res. Protoc.* **2015**, *4*, e29. [CrossRef]
11. Pagliari, C.; Sloan, D.; Gregor, P.; Sullivan, F.; Detmer, D.; Kahan, J.P.; Oortwijn, W.; MacGillivray, S.A. What is eHealth (4): A scoping exercise to map the field. *J. Med. Internet Res.* **2005**, *7*, e9. [CrossRef] [PubMed]
12. Catwell, L.; Sheikh, A. Evaluating eHealth interventions: The need for continuous systemic evaluation. *PLoS Med.* **2009**, *6*, e1000126. [CrossRef] [PubMed]
13. Estrada, Y.; Rojas, L.M.; Murray, A.; Drumhiller, K.; Tapia, M.; Sardinas, K.M.; Rosen, A.; Pantin, H.; Perrino, T.; Sutton, M.; et al. eHealth Familias Unidas: Pilot Study of an Internet Adaptation of an Evidence-Based Family Intervention to Reduce Drug Use and Sexual Risk Behaviors Among Hispanic Adolescents. *Int. J. Environ. Res. Public Health* **2017**, *14*, 264. [CrossRef] [PubMed]
14. Van Der Gugten, A.C.; De Leeuw, R.J.; Verheij, T.J.; Van Der Ent, C.K.; Kars, M.C. E-health and health care behaviour of parents of young children: A qualitative study. *Scand. J. Prim. Health Care* **2016**, *34*, 135–142. [CrossRef]
15. Vogel, T.K.; Kleib, M.; Davidson, S.J.; Scott, S.D. Parental Evaluation of a Nurse Practitioner-Developed Pediatric Neurosurgery Website. *JMIR Res. Protoc.* **2016**, *5*, e55. [CrossRef]
16. Walsh, A.M.; Hamilton, K.; White, K.M.; Hyde, M.K. Use of online health information to manage children's health care: A prospective study investigating parental decisions. *BMC Health Serv. Res.* **2015**, *15*, 131. [CrossRef]
17. Iacono, T.; Stagg, K.; Pearce, N.; Hulme Chambers, A. A scoping review of Australian allied health research in ehealth. *BMC Health Serv. Res.* **2016**, *16*, 543. [CrossRef]
18. Ingersoll, B.; Berger, N.I. Parent Engagement with a Telehealth-Based Parent-Mediated Intervention Program for Children with Autism Spectrum Disorders: Predictors of Program Use and Parent Outcomes. *J. Med. Internet Res.* **2015**, *17*, e227. [CrossRef]
19. Mackert, M.; Kahlor, L.; Tyler, D.; Gustafson, J. Designing e-health interventions for low-health-literate culturally diverse parents: Addressing the obesity epidemic. *Telemed. J. E Health* **2009**, *15*, 672–677. [CrossRef]
20. Fortier, M.A.; Bunzli, E.; Walthall, J.; Olshansky, E.; Saadat, H.; Santistevan, R.; Mayes, L.; Kain, Z.N. Web-based tailored intervention for preparation of parents and children for outpatient surgery (WebTIPS): Formative evaluation and randomized controlled trial. *Anesth. Analg.* **2015**, *120*, 915–922. [CrossRef]

21. Gómez Quiñonez, S.; Walthouwer, M.J.; Schulz, D.N.; De Vries, H. mHealth or eHealth? Efficacy, Use, and Appreciation of a Web-Based Computer-Tailored Physical Activity Intervention for Dutch Adults: A Randomized Controlled Trial. *J. Med. Internet Res.* **2016**, *18*, e278. [CrossRef] [PubMed]
22. Powell, J.; Inglis, N.; Ronnie, J.; Large, S. The characteristics and motivations of online health information seekers: Cross-sectional survey and qualitative interview study. *J. Med. Internet Res.* **2011**, *13*, e20. [CrossRef]
23. Van der Gugten, A.C.; Uiterwaal, C.S.; Verheij, T.J.; van der Ent, C.K. E-health and consultation rates for respiratory illnesses in infants: A randomised clinical trial in primary care. *Br. J. Gen. Pract.* **2015**, *65*, e61–e68. [CrossRef] [PubMed]
24. Kasparian, N.A.; Lieu, N.; Winlaw, D.S.; Cole, A.; Kirk, E.; Sholler, G.F. eHealth literacy and preferences for eHealth resources in parents of children with complex CHD. *Cardiol. Young* **2017**, *27*, 722–730. [CrossRef] [PubMed]
25. Park, E.; Kim, H.; Steinhoff, A. Health-Related Internet Use by Informal Caregivers of Children and Adolescents: An Integrative Literature Review. *J. Med. Internet Res.* **2016**, *18*, e57.
26. Beck, F.; Richard, J.B.; Nguyen-Thanh, V.; Montagni, I.; Parizot, I.; Renahy, E. Use of the internet as a health information resource among French young adults: Results from a nationally representative survey. *J. Med. Internet Res.* **2014**, *16*, e128. [CrossRef]
27. Osei Asibey, B.; Agyemang, S.; Boakye Dankwah, A. The Internet Use for Health Information Seeking among Ghanaian University Students: A Cross-Sectional Study. *Int. J. Telemed. Appl.* **2017**, *2017*, 1–9. [CrossRef]
28. Shroff, P.L.; Hayes, R.W.; Padmanabhan, P.; Stevenson, M.D. Internet Usage by Parents Prior to Seeking Care at a Pediatric Emergency Department: Observational Study. *Interact. J. Med. Res.* **2017**, *6*, e17. [CrossRef]
29. Chen, J.; Jagannatha, A.N.; Fodeh, S.J.; Yu, H. Ranking Medical Terms to Support Expansion of Lay Language Resources for Patient Comprehension of Electronic Health Record Notes: Adapted Distant Supervision Approach. *JMIR Med. Inform.* **2017**, *5*, e42. [CrossRef]
30. Burke, B.L.; Hall, R.W. Telemedicine: Pediatric Applications. *Pediatrics* **2015**, *136*, e293–e308. [CrossRef]
31. Latulippe, K.; Hamel, C.; Giroux, D. Social Health Inequalities and eHealth: A Literature Review with Qualitative Synthesis of Theoretical and Empirical Studies. *J. Med. Internet Res.* **2017**, *19*, e136. [CrossRef]
32. Hall, C.M.; Bierman, K.L. Technology-assisted Interventions for Parents of Young Children: Emerging Practices, Current Research, and Future Directions. *Early Child. Res. Q.* **2015**, *33*, 21–32. [CrossRef]
33. Glasgow, R.E. eHealth evaluation and dissemination research. *Am. J. Prev. Med.* **2007**, *32*, S119–S126. [CrossRef] [PubMed]
34. Car, J.; Tan, W.S.; Huang, Z.; Sloot, P.; Franklin, B.D. eHealth in the future of medications management: Personalisation, monitoring and adherence. *BMC Med.* **2017**, *15*, 73. [CrossRef] [PubMed]
35. Swallow, V.; Hall, A.; Carolan, I.; Santacroce, S.J.; Webb, N.J.A.; Smith, T.; Hanif, N. Designing a web-application to support home-based care of childhood CKD stages 3-5: Qualitative study of family and professional preferences. *BMC Nephrol.* **2014**, *15*, 34. [CrossRef] [PubMed]
36. Wu, Y.P.; Steele, R.G.; Connelly, M.A.; Palermo, T.M.; Ritterband, L.M. Commentary: Pediatric eHealth interventions. Common challenges during development, implementation, and dissemination. *J. Pediatr. Psychol.* **2014**, *39*, 612–623. [CrossRef]
37. Neill, S.J.; Jones, C.H.; Lakhanpaul, M.; Roland, D.T.; Thompson, M.J. Parent's information seeking in acute childhood illness: What helps and what hinders decision making? *Health Expect.* **2015**, *18*, 3044–3056. [CrossRef]
38. Risling, T.; Martinez, J.; Young, J.; Thorp-Froslie, N. Evaluating Patient Empowerment in Association With eHealth Technology: Scoping Review. *J. Med. Internet Res.* **2017**, *19*, e329. [CrossRef]
39. Andreassen, H.K.; Bujnowska-Fedak, M.M.; Chronaki, C.E.; Dumitru, R.C.; Pudule, I.; Pekurinen, M.; Voss, H.; Wynn, R. European citizens' use of E-health services: A study of seven countries. *BMC Public Health* **2007**, *7*, 53. [CrossRef]
40. Eisenberg, L.; Kleinman, A. *The Relevance of Social Science for Medicine*; D. Reidel Publishing Company: Dordrecht, The Netherlands, 1981.
41. Jiang, C.; Wang, Z.Z.; Peng, T.Q.; Zhu, J.H. The divided communities of shared concerns: Mapping the intellectual structure of e-Health research in social science journals. *Int. J. Med. Inform.* **2014**, *84*, 24–35. [CrossRef]
42. Mechanic, D. Emerging Trends in the Application of the Social Sciences to Health and Medicine. *Soc. Sci. Med.* **1995**, *40*, 1491–1496. [CrossRef]
43. Meier, C.A.; Fitzgerald, M.C.; Smith, J.M. eHealth: Extending, enhancing, and evolving health care. *Ann. Rev. Biomed. Eng.* **2013**, *15*, 359–382. [CrossRef] [PubMed]
44. De Rouck, S.; Jacobs, A.; Leys, M. A methodology for shifting the focus of e-health support design onto user needs: A case in the homecare field. *Int. J. Med. Inf.* **2008**, *77*, 589–601. [CrossRef] [PubMed]
45. Pagliari, C. Design and evaluation in eHealth: Challenges and implications for an interdisciplinary field. *J. Med. Internet Res.* **2007**, *9*, e15. [CrossRef]
46. Peek, S.T.M.; Wouters, E.J.M.; van Hoof, J.; Luijkx, K.G.; Boeije, H.R.; Vrijhoef, H.J.M. Factors influencing acceptance of technology for aging in place: A systematic review. *Int. J. Med. Inform.* **2014**, *83*, 235–248. [CrossRef] [PubMed]
47. Atienza, A.A.; Hesse, B.W.; Baker, T.B.; Abrams, D.B.; Rimer, B.K.; Croyle, R.T.; Volckmann, L.N. Critical issues in eHealth research. *Am. J. Prev. Med.* **2007**, *32*, S71–S74. [CrossRef]
48. Brørs, G.; Norman, C.D.; Norekvål, T.M. Accelerated importance of eHealth literacy in the COVID-19 outbreak and beyond. *Eur. J. Cardiovasc. Nurs.* **2020**, *19*, 458–461. [CrossRef]
49. Raghupathi, W.; Nerur, S. Research Themes and Trends in Health Information Systems. *Methods Inf. Med.* **2008**, *47*, 435–442. [CrossRef]

50. Peng, T.Q.; Zhang, L.; Zhong, Z.J.; Zhu, J.H. Mapping the landscape of Internet Studies: Text mining of social science journal articles 2000–2009. *New Media Soc.* **2013**, *15*, 644–664. [CrossRef]
51. Kokol, P.; Saranto, K.; Vosner, H.B. eHealth and health informatics competences: A systemic analysis of literature production based on bibliometrics. *Kybernetes* **2018**, *47*, 1018–1030. [CrossRef]
52. Müller, A.M.; Maher, C.; Vandelanotte, C.; Hingle, M.; Middelweerd, A.; Lopez, M.L.; Desmet, A.; Short, C.E.; Nathan, N.; Hutchesson, M.J.; et al. Physical Activity, Sedentary Behavior, and Diet-Related eHealth and mHealth Research: Bibliometric Analysis. *J. Med. Internet Res.* **2018**, *20*, e122. [CrossRef] [PubMed]
53. Shen, L.N.; Xiong, B.; Li, W.; Lan, F.Q.; Evans, R.; Zhang, W. Visualizing Collaboration Characteristics and Topic Burst on International Mobile Health Research: Bibliometric Analysis. *JMIR mHealth uHealth* **2018**, *6*, e135. [CrossRef] [PubMed]
54. Kan, W.C.; Chou, W.; Chien, T.W.; Yeh, Y.T.; Chou, P.H. The Most-Cited Authors Who Published Papers in JMIR mHealth and uHealth Using the Authorship-Weighted Scheme: Bibliometric Analysis. *JMIR mHealth uHealth*. **2020**, *8*, e11567. [CrossRef]
55. Son, Y.J.; Jeong, S.; Kang, B.G.; Kim, S.H.; Lee, S.K. Visualization of e-Health Research Topics and Current Trends Using Social Network Analysis. *Telemed. E-Health* **2015**, *21*, 436–442. [CrossRef]
56. Garfield, E. Citation Index for Science. A New Dimension in Documentation through Association of Ideas. *Science* **1955**, *122*, 108–111. [CrossRef]
57. Pritchard, A. Statistical bibliography or bibliometrics. *J. Doc.* **1969**, *25*, 348–349.
58. Hirsch, J.E. An index to quantify an individual's scientific research output. *Proc. Natl. Acad. Sci. USA* **2005**, *102*, 16569–16572. [CrossRef]
59. Moed, H.F. *Citation Analysis in Research Evaluation*; Springer: Dordrecht, The Netherlands, 2005.
60. Brereton, P.; Kitchenham, B.A.; Budgen, D.; Turner, M.; Khalil, M. Lessons from applying the systematic literature review process within the software engineering domain. *J. Syst. Softw.* **2007**, *80*, 571–583. [CrossRef]
61. Perianes-Rodriguez, A.; Waltman, L.; Van Eck, N.J. Constructing bibliometric networks: A comparison between full and fractional counting. *J. Informetr.* **2016**, *10*, 1178–1195. [CrossRef]
62. Van Eck, N.J.; Waltman, L. Text. mining and visualization using VOSviewer. *ISSI Newsl.* **2011**, *7*, 50–54.
63. Van Eck, N.J.; Waltman, L. Visualizing bibliometric networks. In *Measuring Scholarly Impact: Methods and Practice*; Ding, Y., Rousseau, R., Wolfram, D., Eds.; Springer: Cham, Switzerland, 2014; pp. 285–320. [CrossRef]
64. Leydesdorff, L.; Park, H.W. Full and fractional counting in bibliometric networks. *J. Infometrics* **2016**, *11*, 117–120. [CrossRef]
65. Park, B.; Bashshur, R. Some Implications of Telemedicine. *J. Commun.* **1975**, *25*, 161–166. [CrossRef] [PubMed]
66. United Nations Department of Economic and Social Affairs. Available online: https://population.un.org/wpp (accessed on 10 January 2021).
67. Hsu, C.L.; Lu, H.P. Why do people play on-line games? An extended TAM with social influences and flow experience. *Inf. Manag.* **2004**, *41*, 853–868. [CrossRef]
68. Hu, P.J.; Chau, P.Y.K.; Liu Sheng, O.R.; Tam, K.Y. Examining the Technology Acceptance Model Using Physician Acceptance of Telemedicine Technology. *J. Manag. Inf. Syst.* **1999**, *16*, 91–112. [CrossRef]
69. Chau, P.Y.K.; Hu, P.J. Information technology acceptance by individual professionals: A model comparison approach. *Decis. Sci.* **2001**, *32*, 699–719. [CrossRef]
70. Chau, P.Y.K.; Hu, P.J. Investigating healthcare professionals' decisions to accept telemedicine technology: An empirical test of competing theories. *Inf. Manag.* **2002**, *39*, 297–311. [CrossRef]
71. Luxton, D.D.; McCann, R.A.; Bush, N.E.; Mishkind, M.C.; Reger, G.M. mHealth for Mental Health: Integrating Smartphone Technology in Behavioral Healthcare. *Prof. Psychol. Res. Pract.* **2011**, *42*, 505–512. [CrossRef]
72. Gatchel, R.; Mcgeary, D.; Mcgeary, C.; Lippe, B. Interdisciplinary Chronic Pain Management Past, Present, and Future. *Am. Psychol.* **2014**, *69*, 119–130. [CrossRef]
73. Nicolini, D. Zooming in and out: Studying practices by switching theoretical lenses and trailing connections. *Org. Stud.* **2009**, *30*, 1391–1418. [CrossRef]
74. Ritterband, L.M.; Thorndike, F.P.; Cox, D.J.; Kovatchev, B.P.; Gonder-Frederick, L.A. A behavior change model for internet interventions. *Ann. Behav. Med.* **2009**, *38*, 18–27. [CrossRef]
75. Chau, P.Y.K.; Hu, P.J. Examining a model of information technology acceptance by individual professionals: An exploratory study. *J. Manag. Inform. Syst.* **2002**, *18*, 191–229. [CrossRef]
76. Lai, V.S.; Li, H. Technology acceptance model for internet banking: An invariance analysis. *Inform. Manag.* **2005**, *42*, 373–386. [CrossRef]
77. Escoffery, C.; Miner, K.M.; Adame, D.D.; Butler, S.; Mccormick, L.; Mendell, E. Internet Use for Health Information Among College Students. *J. Am. Coll. Health* **2005**, *53*, 183–188. [CrossRef] [PubMed]
78. Lupton, D. Quantifying the Body: Monitoring and Measuring Health in the Age of mHealth Technologies. *Crit. Public Health* **2013**, *23*, 393–403. [CrossRef]
79. Fraser, L. Etherapy: Ethical and Clinical Considerations for Version 7 of the World Professional Association for Transgender Health's Standards of Care. *Int. J. Transgend.* **2009**, *11*, 247–263. [CrossRef]

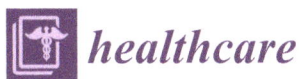

Article

Comparison of Intaglio Surface Trueness of Interim Dental Crowns Fabricated with SLA 3D Printing, DLP 3D Printing, and Milling Technologies

Keunbada Son [1,2], Jung-Ho Lee [3] and Kyu-Bok Lee [2,4,*]

1. Department of Dental Science, Graduate School, Kyungpook National University, Daegu 41940, Korea; sonkeunbada@gmail.com
2. Advanced Dental Device Development Institute, Kyungpook National University, Daegu 41940, Korea
3. SAESHIN, 52, Secheon-ro 1-gil, Dasa-eup, Dalseong-gun, Daegu 42941, Korea; president@saeshin.com
4. Department of Prosthodontics, School of Dentistry, Kyungpook National University, Daegu 41940, Korea
* Correspondence: kblee@knu.ac.kr; Tel.: +82-053-600-7674

Abstract: This study aimed to evaluate the intaglio surface trueness of interim dental crowns fabricated with three 3-dimensional (3D) printing and milling technologies. Dental crown was designated and assigned as a computer-aided design (CAD) reference model (CRM). Interim dental crowns were fabricated based on CRM using two types of 3D printer technologies (stereolithography apparatus and digital light processing) and one type of milling machine ($n = 15$ per technology). The fabricated interim dental crowns were obtained via 3D modeling of the intaglio surface using a laboratory scanner and designated as CAD test models (CTMs). The alignment and 3D comparison of CRM and CTM were performed based on the intaglio surface using a 3D inspection software program (Geomagic Control X). Statistical analysis was validated using one-way analysis of variance and Tukey HSD test ($\alpha = 0.05$). There were significant differences in intaglio surface trueness between the three different fabrication technologies, and high trueness values were observed in the milling group ($p < 0.05$). In the milling group, there was a significant difference in trueness according to the location of the intaglio surface ($p < 0.001$). In the manufacturing process of interim dental crowns, 3D printing technologies showed superior and uniform manufacturing accuracy than milling technology.

Keywords: trueness; 3D printing; milling; interim dental crown; digital dentistry; dental device

1. Introduction

The introduction of dental computer-aided design and computer-aided manufacturing (CAD/CAM) systems in dental clinics is rapidly increasing [1–3]. Errors in operator experience and materials have been reduced due to the dental CAD/CAM system compared with the conventional methods [4,5]. Moreover, the CAD/CAM method is superior to the conventional method in terms of production time efficiency [6]. The CAD/CAM process manufactures dental prostheses in the order of scanning, CAD, and CAM processes [7,8]. The steps of CAD/CAM workflow are as follows: acquire a virtual work model using a 3-dimensional (3D) scanner and produce a working cast using a 3D printer, milling machine, or design a prosthesis in CAD software without a model and then use 3D printing and milling technologies to fabricate dental prostheses [9,10].

The manufacturing industry verifies that manufactured products are accurately manufactured [11–13]. Compared with visual inspection, this can save time, and the use of a 3D scanner makes accurate and quantitative analysis possible [14]. Because of the spread of dental CAD/CAM technology, several studies have evaluated the 3D data [15–18]. The accuracy was evaluated by measuring the distance from any reference point or shape [19,20]. Furthermore, in many previous studies, 3D analysis was performed by an overlapping CAD reference model (CRM), which is the basis of evaluation, and CAD test model (CTM),

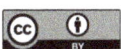

which is the subject of evaluation, and calculating the distances of the corresponding 3D modeling points [21–23]. The alignment process, overlapping with CRM on software, is an important point in the 3D analysis, and the overlapping process is generally studied via best fit alignment [24].

In the dental CAD/CAM system, CAM can be largely divided into milling and additive technologies, and 3D printing, an additive technology, is widely used for manufacture of dental interim prosthesis [25–28]. Srinivasan et al. [29] and Kalberer et al. [30] evaluated the 3D trueness to verify the volume change of the intaglio surface of the fabricated dental prosthesis. Jang et al. [31] has reported that the intaglio surface trueness of dental prostheses can affect marginal and internal fit [31]. Additionally, previous studies reported that, considering the cement space of dental prostheses, intaglio surface trueness of <100 μm was considered as a clinically applicable range [32,33]. Therefore, evaluation of the intaglio surface trueness according to various CAM technologies is still necessary for application to dental clinical practice.

Various 3D printer technologies are being applied for the fabrication of dental prostheses [25–28]. In the fabrication of dental prostheses using 3D printing with photosensitive resin, stereolithography apparatus (SLA), and digital light processing (DLP) technologies are popularly used [25–28]. The DLP 3D printer is a technology that uses a light projector to project an image to polymerize photosensitive resin [28]. The SLA 3D printer is a technology that performs layer-by-layer polymerization using ultraviolet laser to polymerize photosensitive resin [27]. Previous studies evaluated the trueness of dental prostheses using SLA and DLP techniques [25–28], but studies evaluating both SLA and DLP technologies are still lacking. Also, studies evaluating trueness according to specific areas of intaglio surface of interim crowns are still lacking, except for the present study.

Thus, this study aimed to evaluate the intaglio surface trueness of interim dental crowns manufactured with two types of 3D printer technologies (SLA and DLP) and one type of milling machine. The null hypothesis of this study was that there is no difference in the intaglio surface trueness of interim dental crowns manufactured with three types of CAM technologies.

2. Materials and Methods

A maxillary typodont model (D85DP-500B.1; Nissin dental, Kyoto, Japan) was used for the fabrication of resin abutment. The abutment of maxillary right first molar was prepared with an occlusal reduction of 1.5 mm, an axial reduction of 1.2 mm, a finish line design of the chamfer, and a convergence angle of 6°. The abutment was prepared using diamond bur (852.FG.014; Jota AG, Rüthi, SG, Switzerland) with a diameter of 1.4 mm round end taper shape, and medium roughness. A dental CAD software program (3Shape Dental System, version 17.3.0, 3Shape, Copenhagen, Denmark) was used to design a virtual crown with cement space of 80 μm based on the abutment scanned using a desktop scanner (E1, 3Shape, Copenhagen, Denmark) and acquired virtual model was designated as CRM (Figure 1).

Based on CRM, interim crowns were fabricated through the three manufacturing technologies (n = 15 per technology). For 3D printing technology, SLA (ZENITH U, Dentis, Daegu, Korea) with photopolymer resin for interim crown (ZMD-1000B; Dentis, Daegu, Korea) and DLP (RAYDENT Studio, Ray, Seoul, Korea) with photopolymer resin for interim crown (RAYDENT C&B; Ray, Seoul, Korea) were used (Figure 1). The 3D printing conditions were the same for both SLA and DLP, and CRM was printed under the condition of a 180° building angle with the occlusal surface facing the platform and a layer thickness of 25 μm. The manufacturer did not provide any information about the value or compensation for shrinkage that occurs during polymerization of the photopolymer resin. The interim crowns were fabricated with milling technology using a milling machine (CORITEC 250i, imes-icore GmbH, Eiterfeld, Germany). The milling rotary instruments were set to the smallest size of 0.6 mm, and wet processing was performed with prefabricated resin block (PMMA DISK; Yamahachi dental mpg, Aichi Pref, Japan). The tool path was automatically set using standard CAM software programs (iCAM V4.6; imes-icore GmbH, Eiterfeld, Germany), and the milling process was performed under the following conditions (machine configuration: five axis; milling strategy: one spindle using different instruments in z-level; diameters rotary instruments (mm): 2.5, 1.0, 0.6). The fabricated interim crowns were washed to remove all residual resin following the manufacturer's recommendations. After interim crowns were fabricated, each interim crown was rinsed with 95% isopropyl alcohol for 5 min using an ultrasonic cleaner, followed by post-polymerization using a curing unit (CUREDEN; Kwang Myung DAICOM, Seoul, Korea) for 15 min [28]. A desktop scanner (E1, 3Shape, Copenhagen, Denmark) was used to scan the fabricated interim crowns under high-precision scan mode by designating the intaglio surface using, and the scanned virtual crowns were designated as CTMs (Figure 1). The desktop scanner used in this study was calibrated before the scanning process, and according to the manufacturer, it has a scanning accuracy of less than 10 μm. The acquisition of CTMs was completed within 2 h after the second curing in consideration of the volume change according to the passage of time.

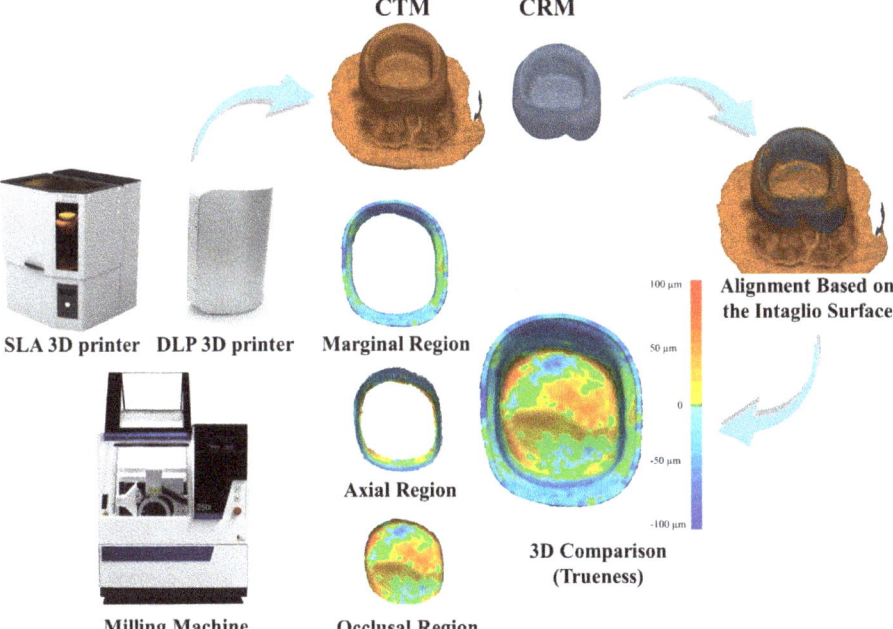

Figure 1. Procedure for intaglio surface trueness of interim crowns fabricated with SLA 3D printing, DLP 3D printing, and milling technologies.

The 3D trueness analysis was performed using 3D inspection software (Geomagic Control X v2018.0.0, 3D Systems Inc., Rock Hill, SC, USA). The CRM was loaded in the 3D inspection software, and three regions were segmented to compare the 3D trueness according to the location of the intaglio surface (Figure 1). The marginal region was the region from the crown margin to 1 mm, the axial region was the region from the end of the margin region through the axial to the point where the flat surface of the occlusal region began, and the occlusal region was the region remaining from the end of the axial region (Figure 1).

After preparing CRM, CTMs were imported and initial alignment was performed. Based on the segmented intaglio surface, best fit alignment was performed, and the sampling rate was set to all point clouds (100%) of the intaglio surface (Figure 1). Analysis of 3D trueness was performed by calculating all point cloud points of the segmented intaglio surface of CRM. At this time, each corresponding data point in CRM and CTM was calculated as the root mean square (RMS) value as shown in Formula (1):

$$RMS = \frac{1}{\sqrt{n}} \cdot \sqrt{\sum_{i=1}^{n}(X_{1,i} - X_{2,i})^2} \qquad (1)$$

For all data points, $X_{1,i}$ is the CRM, $X_{2,i}$ is the coordinate at i time in the CTM, and n is the number of all data points measured in each analysis. The RMS value shows how the shapes of different virtual models are different in 3D, and a low RMS value means a high degree of matching of the superimposed virtual models. The 3D comparison was shown as a color difference map, and a range of ±100 µm (20 color segments) and a tolerance range of ±10 µm (green) were specified (Figure 1).

To determine the sample size, an appropriate sample size was calculated as 15 using power analysis (G*Power v3.1.9.4, Heinrich-Heine-Universität, Dusseldorf, Germany) based on the results of five pilot experiments (SLA group: 24.7 ± 6.0 µm; DLP group: 30.8 ± 2.8 µm; milling group: 49.0 ± 2.1 µm; effect size [f] = 0.86; actual power = 99.94%; power = 99.9%; α = 0.05). All data analyses were performed using statistical software (IBM SPSS Statistics v23.0, IBM Corp, Armonk, NY, USA). First, the normal distribution of the data was investigated using the Shapiro–Wilk test, and the normal distribution of the obtained data was confirmed. Therefore, the differences between groups were confirmed using one-way analysis of variance (ANOVA) and analyzed using the Tukey HSD test as a post hoc test (α = 0.05). The interaction effect between the evaluated region and the manufacturing technology was verified using two-way ANOVA (α = 0.05).

3. Results

There were significant differences in intaglio surface trueness in all regions among SLA, DLP, and milling groups (Table 1; $p < 0.001$). Except for the occlusal region, there was no significant difference between SLA and DLP in the whole, marginal, and axial regions (Table 1; $p > 0.05$), but there was a significant difference between the milling and 3D printing group (Table 1; $p < 0.05$). SLA (23.6 ± 5.3 µm), DLP (29.0 ± 3.6 µm), and milling groups (36.9 ± 4.4 µm) showed significantly higher intaglio surface trueness in the order in the occlusal region (Table 1; $p < 0.05$). According to the results of two-way ANOVA, there was a significant interaction effect between the evaluated region and the manufacturing technology (F = 3.699; $p = 0.002$).

Table 1. Comparison of intaglio surface trueness (µm) of interim crowns fabricated with SLA 3D printing, DLP 3D printing, and milling technologies.

Evaluated Region	Manufacturing	Mean	SD	95% Confidence Interval (CI)		Minimum	Maximum	F	p
				Lower	Upper				
Whole region	SLA	25.7 A	5.1	22.8	28.6	18	34.2	66.684	<0.001 *
	DLP	29.5 A	3.3	27.6	31.3	24.4	36.8		
	Milling	44.8 B	5.5	41.7	47.9	33	53.2		
Marginal region	SLA	26.7 A	4.4	24.2	29.2	20.2	34	45.267	<0.001 *
	DLP	27.0 A	4.7	24.3	29.6	20.4	37.3		
	Milling	45.2 B	8.2	40.6	49.8	35.8	59.4		
Axial region	SLA	27.6 A	6.5	24	31.3	17.6	40.9	47.674	<0.001 *
	DLP	30.9 A	5.6	27.8	34	23.6	40.6		
	Milling	50.5 B	8.3	45.9	55.2	34	63.1		

Table 1. Cont.

Evaluated Region	Manufacturing	Mean	SD	95% Confidence Interval (CI)		Minimum	Maximum	F	p
				Lower	Upper				
Occlusal region	SLA	23.6 A	5.3	20.6	26.5	17	33.4	32.288	<0.001 *
	DLP	29.0 B	3.6	26.9	31	24.3	35.5		
	Milling	36.9 C	4.4	34.4	39.3	29.1	45.5		

* Significant difference by one-way ANOVA; $p < 0.05$. Different letters indicate significant differences among the three methods by the Tukey HSD test ($p < 0.05$).

There was no significant difference between SLA ($p = 0.219$) and DLP groups according to the locations of the intaglio surface ($p = 0.122$) (Table 2). However, the milling group showed a significant difference according to the locations of the intaglio surface and showed lower intaglio surface trueness in the occlusal region than that in the marginal and axial regions (Table 2; $p < 0.001$).

Table 2. Comparison of intaglio surface trueness (μm) of interim crowns according to the evaluated regions.

Evaluated Region	SLA	DLP	Milling
Whole region	25.7 ± 5.1	29.5 ± 3.3	44.8 ± 5.5 A
Marginal region	26.7 ± 4.4	27.0 ± 4.4	45.2 ± 8.2 A
Axial region	27.6 ± 6.5	30.9 ± 5.6	50.5 ± 8.3 A
Occlusal region	23.6 ± 5.3	29.0 ± 3.6	36.9 ± 4.4 B
F	1.52	2.016	10.025
p	0.219	0.122	<0.001 *

* Significant difference by one-way ANOVA; $p < 0.05$. Different letters (A and B) indicate significant differences among the evaluated regions by the Tukey HSD test ($p < 0.05$).

In the color difference map, SLA and DLP did not have a specific color distribution in any region, but in the milling group, there was a high amount of trueness (red color) in the axial and angular regions of the intaglio surface (Figure 2).

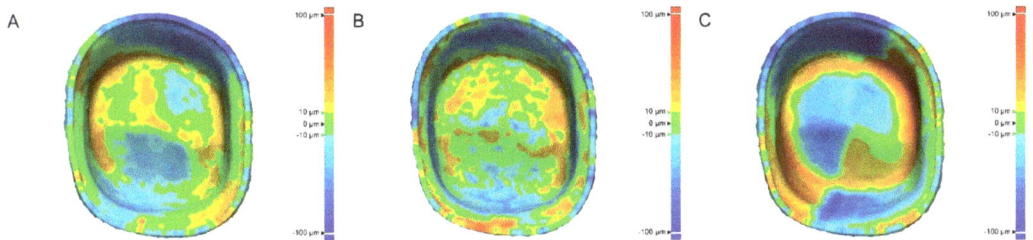

Figure 2. Schematic of color difference map of intaglio surface trueness of interim crowns. (**A**) SLA. (**B**) DLP. (**C**) Milling.

4. Discussion

In this study, three types of fabrication technologies were used to fabricate interim dental crowns and the intaglio surface trueness was evaluated. The null hypothesis of this study was rejected because there was a significant difference in the intaglio surface trueness of interim dental crowns manufactured with the three types of CAM technologies ($p < 0.05$). Previous studies have evaluated the intaglio surface trueness of dental crowns [29,30]. In a previous study, the 3D trueness of zirconia crowns fabricated using 3D printing was evaluated to investigate the potential application of 3D printing technology in a study on dental ceramic restorations [34]. In another study, the 3D printing group (38 ± 12 μm) showed significantly better intaglio surface trueness than the milling group (43 ± 12 µm) ($p < 0.001$), and the 3D printing group showed the same results as those reported in this study that showed superior results in the 3D printing group (Table 1) [25]. Another previous study evaluated the trueness of zirconia crowns fabricated by printing with 3D gel deposition technology [26]. The results of this study (Table 1) and the study by Wang et al. [25] showed that the 3D printing group showed significantly better intaglio surface trueness than the milling group. In light of the results of previous studies and this study, 3D printing technology is considered to have sufficient manufacturing accuracy for clinical application.

The intaglio surface trueness of dental prostheses fabricated with various materials and methods have been reported in many previous studies [25–30,34]. A previous study has reported the intaglio surface trueness (28.5 ± 6.0 µm) of interim crowns fabricated by printing with SLA technology [27]. These results showed similar trueness to that of this study (SLA: 25.7 ± 5.1 µm) (Table 1). Another previous study has reported the intaglio surface trueness (24.91 ± 3.62 µm) of interim crowns fabricated by printing with DLP technology [28]. These results showed trueness similar to that observed in this study (DLP: 29.5 ± 3.3 µm) (Table 1). Furthermore, another previous study has reported the intaglio surface trueness (42.9 ± 4.4 µm) of crowns fabricated with milling technology [7]. These results showed trueness similar to that observed in this study (milling: 44.8 ± 5.5 µm) (Table 1). Therefore, despite the differences in in vitro experimental conditions, the results of previous studies and this study showed similar trends. Additionally, previous clinical studies evaluated the intaglio surface trueness (43.8 ± 11.7 µm) of ceramic crowns fabricated with milling technology [8] and showed trueness similar to that observed in this study (milling: 44.8 ± 5.5 µm). In previous studies, the intaglio surface trueness of <100 µm was recommended based on the cement space of the fixed dental prosthesis as an error may occur in the manufacturing process [32,33]. Therefore, in terms of intaglio surface trueness, interim crowns evaluated in this study can be considered appropriate for clinical use, and 3D printing can be considered to have superior intaglio surface trueness than milling technology.

The trueness evaluation of interim crowns performed in previous studies compared the results of milling technology and 3D printing technology [27,28]. The present study compared the results of SLA and DLP of 3D printing technology, including the comparison of milling technology and 3D printing technology, and reported the similar trueness of interim crowns between SLA and DLP (Table 1). The results of this study showed that the interim crowns fabricated with 3D printing technology showed the same results regardless of the evaluated region, but the milling technology showed different results of trueness according to the locations of the intaglio surface (Table 2). Furthermore, a previous study reported that milling technology could have different trueness according to the region of the intaglio surface of the crown [7]. In this study, Figure 2C shows an error in the angle region between the axial and occlusal regions, and these results are similar to those reported in previous studies [6,7]. During the milling process, this machining error was reported as a machining limitation due to the size of the diameter of the burr used and may appear when machining angle region of the intaglio surface [6,7]. Milling technology reported that the number of burrs affects the accuracy, and trueness is better when using many burs [6]. Using a smaller diameter bur increases manufacturing time due to increased tool path, but may yield better trueness results because a wider range of bur diameters is created [6]. For this reason, using a smaller diameter burr allows for more accurate milling of the angle region of the intaglio surface [7]. Therefore, the error in the angle region between the axial and occlusal regions in crowns must be considered during milling. Additional studies through trueness evaluation using burs of various diameters are needed.

SLA and DLP technologies are one of the most used additive manufacturing processes in dentistry, offering the highest accuracy and resolution of any printing technology, superior detail and smooth surface finish [35]. It is then built through the deposition of successive layers of a photosensitive material that polymerizes easily [35]. SLA is the first rapid prototyping technology with a reliable printing process [27]. So far, SLA is the only photocurable 3D printing technology that can print large-format models, but SLA has a low printing rate due to the curing rate caused by the movement of the laser beam, so the larger the model, the slower the printing speed [36]. However, DLP 3D printing uses a digital projector screen to flash an image in layers across the entire platform, curing all points at the same time, so it has the advantages of high precision and fast manufacturing times [37]. However, only small sized objects can be printed because the projection size is limited to ensure high precision. Volume shrinkage is also reported as a disadvantage of photocurable 3D printing [28]. Milling technology, a subtractive manufacturing process, reproduces shapes by cutting using milling equipment and burs [30]. Therefore, the material loss is relatively large, and the reproducibility is limited by the diameter of the burr [30].

This study has some limitations. First, the effect of intaglio surface trueness on the actual clinical environment should be investigated via additional clinical studies. Second, 3D printers and milling equipment from more diverse manufacturers should be used to confirm additional results. Third, the trueness of external surfaces including intaglio surfaces should be evaluated via additional studies.

5. Conclusions

Based on the findings of this in vitro study, the following conclusions were drawn. The 3D printing and milling technologies used in this study showed clinically acceptable intaglio surface trueness (<100 μm) of interim crowns. The milling technology showed inferior trueness in the reproduction of angle region than occlusal region. However, interim crowns fabricated with 3D printing technologies (SLA and DLP) can reproduce more uniform and superior intaglio surface trueness than milling technology.

Author Contributions: Conceptualization, K.S.; methodology, K.S.; validation, K.-B.L.; formal analysis, K.S.; investigation, K.S.; data curation, K.-B.L.; writing—original draft, K.S.; writing—review and editing, J.-H.L. and K.S.; statistical analysis, J.-H.L.; visualization, K.S.; supervision, K.-B.L.; project administration, K.-B.L. All authors have read and agreed to the published version of the manuscript.

Funding: This work was supported by the Industrial Strategic Technology Development Program (10062635, New hybrid milling machine with a resolution of less than 10 μm development, using open CAD/CAM S/W integrated platforms for one-day prosthetic treatment of 3D smart medical care system) funded by the Ministry of Trade, Industry and Energy (MOTIE, Korea). This work was also supported by Industrial Infrastructure Program of Laser Industry Support (Grant N0000598) funded by the Ministry of Trade, Industry and Energy (MOTIE, Korea).

Institutional Review Board Statement: Not applicable.

Informed Consent Statement: Not applicable.

Data Availability Statement: Data are included within the article.

Acknowledgments: The authors thank the researchers of the Advanced Dental Device Development Institute, Kyungpook National University, for their time and contributions to the study.

Conflicts of Interest: The authors declare no conflict of interest. The funders had no role in the design of the study; in the collection, analyses, or interpretation of the data; in the writing of the manuscript; or in the decision to publish the results.

References

1. Kale, E.; Cilli, M.; Özçelik, T.B.; Yilmaz, B. Marginal fit of CAD-CAM monolithic zirconia crowns fabricated by using cone beam computed tomography scans. *J. Prosthet. Dent.* **2020**, *123*, 731–737. [CrossRef] [PubMed]
2. Son, K.; Lee, K.B. Effect of finish line locations of tooth preparation on the accuracy of intraoral scanners. *Int. J. Comput. Dent.* **2021**, *24*, 29–40.
3. Angwarawong, T.; Reeponmaha, T.; Angwaravong, O. Influence of thermomechanical aging on marginal gap of CAD-CAM and conventional interim restorations. *J. Prosthet. Dent.* **2020**, *124*, 566.e1–566.e6. [CrossRef] [PubMed]
4. Ahn, J.J.; Bae, E.B.; Lee, J.J.; Choi, J.W.; Jeon, Y.C.; Jeong, C.M.; Huh, J.B. Clinical evaluation of the fit of lithium disilicate crowns fabricated with three different CAD-CAM systems. *J. Prosthet. Dent.* **2020**, in press. [CrossRef] [PubMed]

5. Baba, N.Z.; Goodacre, B.J.; Goodacre, C.J.; Müller, F.; Wagner, S. CAD/CAM complete denture systems and physical properties: A review of the literature. *J. Prosthodont.* **2021**, *30*, 113–124. [CrossRef] [PubMed]
6. Kirsch, C.; Ender, A.; Attin, T.; Mehl, A. Trueness of four different milling procedures used in dental CAD/CAM systems. *Clin. Oral Investig.* **2017**, *21*, 551–558. [CrossRef]
7. Son, K.; Yu, B.Y.; Yoon, T.H.; Lee, K.B. Comparative study of the trueness of the inner surface of crowns fabricated from three types of lithium disilicate blocks. *Appl. Sci.* **2019**, *9*, 1798. [CrossRef]
8. Lee, J.J.; Son, K.; Bae, E.B.; Choi, J.W.; Lee, K.B.; Huh, J.B. Comparison of the trueness of lithium disilicate crowns fabricated from all-in-one and combination CAD/CAM systems. *Int. J. Prosthodont.* **2019**, *32*, 352–354. [CrossRef]
9. Taha, D.; Nour, M.; Zohdy, M.; El-Etreby, A.; Hamdy, A.; Salah, T. The effect of different wax pattern fabrication techniques on the marginal fit of customized lithium disilicate implant abutments. *J. Prosthodont.* **2019**, *28*, 1018–1023. [CrossRef]
10. Kim, M.K.; Son, K.; Yu, B.Y.; Lee, K.B. Effect of the volumetric dimensions of a complete arch on the accuracy of scanners. *J. Adv. Prosthodont.* **2020**, *12*, 361–368. [CrossRef] [PubMed]
11. Martínez, S.; Cuesta, E.; Barreiro, J.; Álvarez, B. Analysis of laser scanning and strategies for dimensional and geometrical control. *J. Adv. Manuf. Technol.* **2010**, *46*, 621–629. [CrossRef]
12. Choi, Y.K.; Banerjee, A. Tool path generation and tolerance analysis for free-form surfaces. *Int. J. Mach. Tools Manuf.* **2007**, *47*, 689–696. [CrossRef]
13. Xiao, Z.; Yang, Y.; Xiao, R.; Bai, Y.; Song, C.; Wang, D. Evaluation of topology-optimized lattice structures manufactured via selective laser melting. *Mater. Des.* **2018**, *143*, 27–37. [CrossRef]
14. Bosch, G.; Ender, A.; Mehl, A. A 3-dimensional accuracy analysis of chairside CAD/CAM milling processes. *J. Prosthet. Dent.* **2014**, *112*, 1425–1431. [CrossRef] [PubMed]
15. Jeong, Y.G.; Lee, W.S.; Lee, K.B. Accuracy evaluation of dental models manufactured by CAD/CAM milling method and 3D printing method. *J. Adv. Prosthodont.* **2018**, *10*, 245–251. [CrossRef]
16. Park, H.N.; Lim, Y.J.; Yi, W.J.; Han, J.S.; Lee, S.P. A comparison of the accuracy of intraoral scanners using an intraoral environment simulator. *J. Adv. Prosthodont.* **2018**, *10*, 58–64. [CrossRef]
17. Tan, F.B.; Wang, C.; Dai, H.W.; Fan, Y.B.; Song, J.L. Accuracy and reproducibility of 3D digital tooth preparations made by gypsum materials of various colors. *J. Adv. Prosthodont.* **2018**, *10*, 8–17. [CrossRef] [PubMed]
18. Wong, K.Y.; Esguerra, R.J.; Chia, V.A.P.; Tan, Y.H.; Tan, K.B.C. Three-dimensional accuracy of digital static interocclusal registration by three intraoral scanner systems. *J. Prosthodont.* **2018**, *27*, 120–128. [CrossRef]
19. Motel, C.; Kirchner, E.; Adler, W.; Wichmann, M.; Matta, R.E. Impact of different scan bodies and scan strategies on the accuracy of digital implant impressions assessed with an intraoral scanner: An in vitro study. *J. Prosthodont.* **2020**, *29*, 309–314. [CrossRef]
20. Fluegge, T.; Att, W.; Metzger, M.; Nelson, K. A novel method to evaluate precision of optical implant impressions with commercial scan bodies—An experimental approach. *J. Prosthodont.* **2017**, *26*, 34–41. [CrossRef]
21. Zarone, F.; Ruggiero, G.; Ferrari, M.; Mangano, F.; Joda, T.; Sorrentino, R. Accuracy of a chairside intraoral scanner compared with a laboratory scanner for the completely edentulous maxilla: An in vitro 3-dimensional comparative analysis. *J. Prosthet. Dent.* **2020**, *124*, 761.e1–761.e7. [CrossRef] [PubMed]
22. Mejía, J.B.C.; Wakabayashi, K.; Nakamura, T.; Yatani, H. Influence of abutment tooth geometry on the accuracy of conventional and digital methods of obtaining dental impressions. *J. Prosthet. Dent.* **2017**, *118*, 392–399. [CrossRef]
23. Jeong, I.D.; Kim, W.C.; Park, J.; Kim, C.M.; Kim, J.H. Ceramic molar crown reproducibility by digital workflow manufacturing: An in vitro study. *J. Adv. Prosthodont.* **2017**, *9*, 252–256. [CrossRef] [PubMed]
24. Revilla-León, M.; Subramanian, S.G.; Özcan, M.; Krishnamurthy, V.R. Clinical study of the influence of ambient light scanning conditions on the accuracy (trueness and precision) of an intraoral scanner. *J. Prosthodont.* **2020**, *29*, 107–113. [CrossRef]
25. Wang, W.; Yu, H.; Liu, Y.; Jiang, X.; Gao, B. Trueness analysis of zirconia crowns fabricated with 3-dimensional printing. *J. Prosthet. Dent.* **2019**, *121*, 285–291. [CrossRef]
26. Li, R.; Chen, H.; Wang, Y.; Zhou, Y.; Shen, Z.; Sun, Y. Three-dimensional trueness and margin quality of monolithic zirconia restorations fabricated by additive 3D gel deposition. *J. Prosthodont. Res.* **2020**, *64*, 478–484. [CrossRef]
27. Yu, B.Y.; Son, K.; Lee, K.B. Evaluation of intaglio surface trueness and margin quality of interim crowns in accordance with the build angle of stereolithography apparatus 3-dimensional printing. *J. Prosthet. Dent.* **2020**, in press. [CrossRef]
28. Lee, B.I.; You, S.G.; You, S.M.; Kang, S.Y.; Kim, J.H. Effect of rinsing time on the accuracy of interim crowns fabricated by digital light processing: An in vitro study. *J. Adv. Prosthodont.* **2021**, *13*, 24–35. [CrossRef]
29. Srinivasan, M.; Cantin, Y.; Mehl, A.; Gjengedal, H.; Müller, F.; Schimmel, M. CAD/CAM milled removable complete dentures: An in vitro evaluation of trueness. *Clin. Oral Investig.* **2017**, *21*, 2007–2019. [CrossRef] [PubMed]
30. Kalberer, N.; Mehl, A.; Schimmel, M.; Müller, F.; Srinivasan, M. CAD-CAM milled versus rapidly prototyped (3D-printed) complete dentures: An in vitro evaluation of trueness. *J. Prosthet. Dent.* **2019**, *121*, 637–643. [CrossRef]
31. Jang, D.; Son, K.; Lee, K.B. A Comparative study of the fitness and trueness of a three-unit fixed dental prosthesis fabricated using two digital workflows. *Appl. Sci.* **2019**, *9*, 2778. [CrossRef]
32. Ender, A.; Attin, T.; Mehl, A. In vivo precision of conventional and digital methods of obtaining complete-arch dental impressions. *J. Prosthet. Dent.* **2016**, *115*, 313–320. [CrossRef]
33. Fukazawa, S.; Odaira, C.; Kondo, H. Investigation of accuracy and reproducibility of abutment position by intraoral scanners. *J. Prosthodont. Res.* **2017**, *61*, 450–459. [CrossRef] [PubMed]

34. Methani, M.M.; Revilla-León, M.; Zandinejad, A. The potential of additive manufacturing technologies and their processing parameters for the fabrication of all-ceramic crowns: A review. *J. Esthet. Dent.* **2020**, *32*, 182–192. [CrossRef]
35. Quan, H.; Zhang, T.; Xu, H.; Luo, S.; Nie, J.; Zhu, X. Photo-curing 3D printing technique and its challenges. *Bioact. Mater.* **2020**, *5*, 110–115. [CrossRef] [PubMed]
36. Wang, J.; Goyanes, A.; Gaisford, S.; Basit, A.W. Stereolithographic (SLA) 3D printing of oral modified-release dosage forms. *Int. J. Pharm.* **2016**, *503*, 207–212. [CrossRef] [PubMed]
37. Wu, L.; Zhao, L.; Jian, M.; Mao, Y.; Yu, M.; Guo, X. EHMP-DLP: Multi-projector DLP with energy homogenization for large-size 3D printing. *Rapid Prototyp. J.* **2018**, *24*, 1500–1510. [CrossRef]

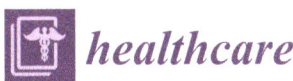

Article

Development of a System for Storing and Executing Bio-Signal Analysis Algorithms Developed in Different Languages

Moon-Il Joo [1], Satyabrata Aich [2] and Hee-Cheol Kim [1,2,*]

[1] Institute of Digital Anti-Aging Healthcare, Inje University, Gimhae-si 50834, Korea; joomi@inje.ac.kr
[2] Department of Computer Engineering, Inje University, Gimhae-si 50834, Korea; satybrataaich@gmail.com
* Correspondence: heeki@inje.ac.kr; Tel.: +82-55-320-3720

Abstract: With the development of mobile and wearable devices with biosensors, various healthcare services in our life have been recently introduced. A significant issue that arises supports the smart interface among bio-signals developed by different vendors and different languages. Despite its importance for convenient and effective development, however, it has been nearly unexplored. This paper focuses on the smart interface format among bio-signal data processing and mining algorithms implemented by different languages. We designed and implemented an advanced software structure where analysis algorithms implemented by different languages and tools would seem to work in one common environment, overcoming different developing language barriers. By presenting our design in this paper, we hope there will be much more chances for higher service-oriented developments utilizing bio-signals in the future.

Keywords: data mining; bio-signal analysis; bio-signal repository; execution engine; bio-signal monitoring

1. Introduction

With the incoming of the fourth industrial revolution, the technological development of the Internet of Things (IoT) and smart infrastructure makes us pay more attention to the technology in order to collect and analyze a huge amount of information [1,2]. Particularly in medical and healthcare fields, there has been a paradigm shift from cure-oriented to prevention-oriented medical practices, partly due to the emergence of wearable devices that can measure and acquire vital signs wherever and whenever the users are [3–6]. Wearables are now part of every individual since these devices provide more concrete analytics decisions about the individuals using the individual data, which could help in better decision making connection with the bio-signals [7]. Naturally, it enables better and high-quality medical and healthcare services utilizing the vital signs acquired.

Recently, such data have been accumulated exponentially with the help of the devices [8]. It is not that difficult to imagine the potential knowledge and information inferred by the analysis of the big data for disease prevention, health management, diagnosis, therapies, etc. [9–12]. Artificial intelligence has created a lot of positive impacts in clinical decision making, diagnosis, predictive medicine, etc., which is a good sign for developing personalized systems [13].

Personalized and customized healthcare services are expected to be common sooner or later. Since smartphones and wearable healthcare devices are already employed, the technology for collection and analysis of health information gathering is easier and advanced enough [14,15]. This situation promotes more research on various healthcare services utilizing and analyzing vital signs [16,17]. Global IT giants including Apple, Google, and Samsung are carrying out huge projects where healthcare platforms and services as well as wearable devices with biosensors are designed and developed [18,19].

The development of a bio-signal analysis algorithm is of prime importance to provide a seamless healthcare service. All bio-signal data have no meaning on their own. For

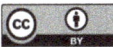

example, electrocardiogram (ECG) signals and pulse wave data are time-series data, and health status cannot be analyzed using data alone. In this case, to analyze the health status, it is necessary to extract feature values by applying an analysis algorithm suitable for the data, since these services can be provided to the healthcare system using these characteristic values. Moreover, due to the fact that the development of bio-signal analysis algorithms is performed in multiple languages such as MATLAB and R, the source code conversion technology is a requirement to make the system development independent of the programming language. However, source code conversion techniques are primarily a very complex and redundant process and also depend heavily on the development tool which is used for deployment. Furthermore, due to the complexity, the management of the source codes of algorithms and the reusability of the source codes becomes very difficult. Therefore, to overcome the complex manual conversion process, this work implemented an algorithm specification for developing bio-signal analysis algorithms in different languages and a common execution engine that will be able to execute the algorithms written in different languages. The proposed architecture provides software architecture, by which one can reuse the bio-signal analysis algorithms developed by other developers in different languages such as MATLAB and R, without building a transformation process between multiple development environments.

The primary objective of the study is to develop a smart interface to run bio-signal analysis algorithms developed in different languages. An execution engine is developed to apply the smart interface. The execution engine can easily apply the bio-signal analysis technology developed in various algorithm development languages to the system using the source code conversion technology. This technology is expected to increase the reusability of analysis algorithms and the efficiency of system development.

When such a smart interface is provided, healthcare system developers can have more room to go further to higher service-oriented development using bio-signals. In addition, it is judged that the execution engine proposed in this paper can be used in various fields that require signal processing other than the healthcare field.

The remainder of this paper is organized as follows. First, we present the related works and backgrounds. Second, we describe the design of bio-signal storage where bio-signals with big sizes are stored and managed. Third, we discuss an architecture to support a smart interface among heterogeneous mining algorithms implemented in different languages. Fourth, the results and discussion of this paper are presented. Finally, we conclude with a description of the results.

2. Related Works

The conversion technique of the analysis of the vital sign algorithm source code is the task of changing the algorithm source code to match the system that provides healthcare services. Typically, the algorithms developed by MATLAB and Python are converted to C/C++ and applied to the system [20,21]. However, applying the source code converted to C/C++ to the system requires additional work by the developer to accommodate the system environment. We developed a system that can execute the source code of algorithms from multiple programming languages in the Java environment. The interface developed in the work is a Java-based interface, that can execute various bio-signal analysis algorithms from a single service definition. The work proposed in the paper allows the execution of bio-signal analysis source codes developed in the MATLAB and R programming using Java-based libraries running on Java Runtime Environment.

R programming was conducted to secure the interoperability between Java and R programming using rJava [22]. An interoperability study using rJava uses Java's graphical user interface (GUI) to overcome the delicate graphic task, which is a disadvantage of R programming. This is a graphical representation of the data analyzed using JavaFX by R programming [23]. The study also analyzes the disease data of patients using R programming and shows the analyzed data using the GUI in Java [24].

The MATLAB control library can connect to the MATLAB engine in Java and execute the MATLAB source code [25]. A typical remote connection to a server installed with MATLAB was made to execute the MATLAB command using Java and MATLAB control [26].

The technology of executing the algorithm source code itself has been studied to perform more sophisticated graphical tasks or to use development tools remotely. As such, most studies have been conducted by choosing the development tool for the system environment being developed. So far, research into applying development tools developed in different languages is insufficient. Therefore, research needs to be done by applying the source code developed with various development tools to the system and executing the desired algorithms. This study will be the basic research to apply various algorithm managements to the system.

This paper proposes an architecture for executing the source code itself, which is developed by MATLAB and R programming in the system, as shown in Figure 1. The proposed architecture is divided into an execution engine that executes the vital signs algorithm and a repository that stores the bio-signals.

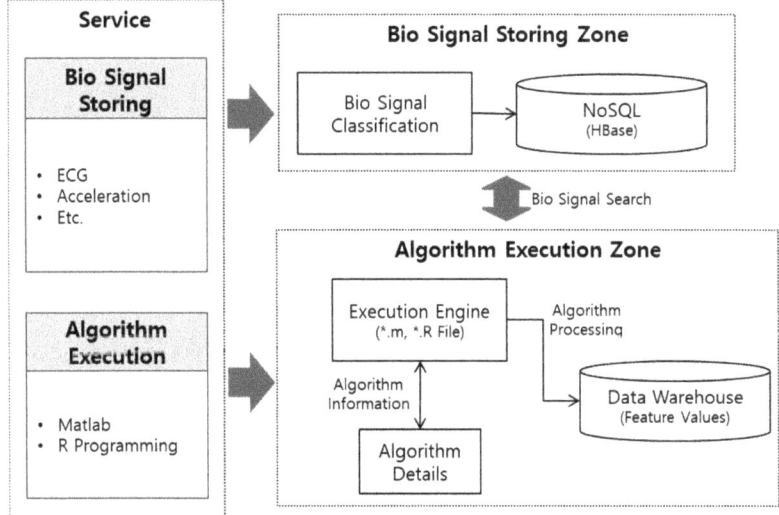

Figure 1. Architecture for analyzing bio-signal data by MATLAB and R programming.

3. Materials and Methods

The bio-signal analysis system proposed in this paper has two services, as shown in Figure 1. First, the bio-signal storage service collects bio-signals and stores the collected bio-signals in big bata-based NoSQL. Second, the algorithm execution service develops an execution engine for executing the bio-signal analysis algorithms developed in various development languages.

3.1. Bio-Signal Storage Design

The data accumulated by wearable health devices typically form big data. For instance, when the ECG sampling rate is 500 Hz, the system collects 500 pieces of data per second from an individual. Suppose it can gather them for a day. Then, the amount is 43,200,000 pieces of data. If it gathers them from more than 1000 people for a year or so, the amount of ECG data increases exponentially. The database storing such big data must secure scalability. As we know it, however, the relational database management system (RDBMS) has difficult aspects of processing such explosive vital sign data. Since RDBMS stores structured data, it uses data consistency and normalization and provides high performance. However, we face a huge problem to process unstructured data and big data beyond zettabytes [27]. There is a need for a new way of storing and processing big unstructured or semi-structured data, which we call NoSQL. NoSQL is a non-relational database where its table schema is not fixed, join operation is not supported, and its horizontal expansion is easy. Therefore, NoSQL is more suitable for processing a vast number of data [28].

NoSQL can be divided into three ways of storing: Key-value store, document store, and column store. The key-value store database stores, retrieves, and manages data as a key/value pair. A document store NoSQL database retrieves data by more complex conditions than key/value types, and its typical examples are MongoDB and CouchDB. Column store databases have a more powerful scalability in, for example, Cassandra and HBase.

In this paper, according to the bio-signal characteristics of Figure 2, the bio-signal raw data and feature data are stored in a storage. Bio-signal raw data is stored in NoSQL based on big data, and feature data is stored in Datawarehouse for big data analysis. Since recent bio-signals reflect various bio-signals such as electrocardiogram, respiration, respiration, SpO2, etc. to analyze disease or health conditions. To facilitate the search and analysis of bio-signals, raw data and feature data should be stored separately. In addition, this bio-signal classification method is easy to further expand feature data according to various bio-signal analysis techniques.

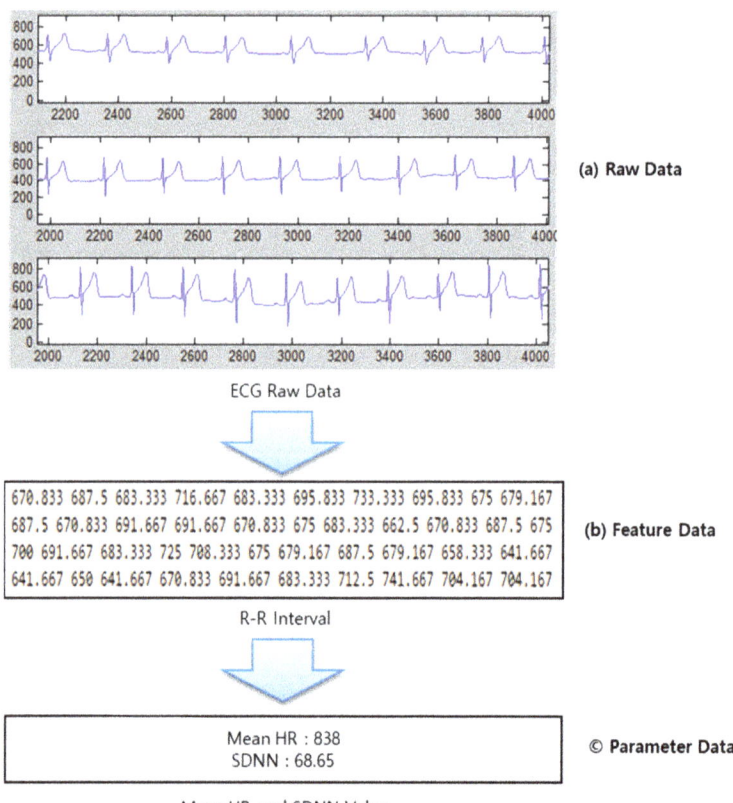

Figure 2. Characteristics of data according to the ECG signal analysis.

3.1.1. Design of Bio-Signal Raw Data Storage

In this paper, we designed a wide column database based on big data to store raw bio-signal data. This is due to the fact that the wide column database has excellent compression, distributed processing, aggregation processing (sum, count, avg, etc.), and query operation speed and scalability of large amounts of data. In addition, it is important to analyze bio-signals in units of year/month/week/day. Therefore, the column-oriented wide column database is easy to retrieve only the information of raw bio-signal data. In addition, this paper designed a bio-signal raw data storage using HBase, which is mainly used in the wide column database.

Raw data on their own have no meaning. They must have more meaningful attributes together such as the time when raw data are measured, whose data are, sampling rates, types of bio-signals, etc., as well as the raw bio-signals such as ECG, respiration, and acceleration data. Table 1 shows an example of the data table that we have designed, using HBase. HBase stores data in a key-value format. Therefore, 'Row-Key' specifies the measurement date and ID. The 'Data' column is the bio-signal information. The 'User' column is the user information that measured the bio-signals. We need information about the types of bio-signals such as electrocardiogram, acceleration, respiration, etc., and the hertz (Hz) which is the sampling frequency of the signal to analyze bio-signals. Moreover, 'User' information includes age and gender, since the analysis techniques of bio-signal analysis algorithms vary according to age and gender.

Table 1. HBase table structure.

Row-Key (Measurement Time ID)	Data				User	
	Raw Data	Hz	Type	Overall Time (s)	Age	Gender
2021.03.06.17.420.07_JOO	100 110 112	200	ECG	125	38	Man
2021.03.06.19.01.07_JOO	120 131 110	200	ECG	100	38	Man
2021.03.06.21.28.07_JOO	121 111 120	200	ECG	111	38	Man

3.1.2. Design of Data Warehouse for Feature Data

Our approach uses HBase to store the vast amount of bio-signal data, depending on the column family. The extracted data (e.g., heart rate variability (HRV)) from raw data (e.g., ECG) are sometimes large as well, and they are stored in the data warehouse. Moreover, we use SQL-On-Hadoop [29] to search and analyze the mined data, which processes the data in a familiar way of interfacing SQL, working with data warehouse-based Hive. Hive uses a similar interface to SQL called HiveQL, and it can be used for statistical analysis.

Since Hive is Hadoop-based, its processing speed is much slower if it searches and accesses all the data. Therefore, we use the partitioning method to improve the speed. There is also a need to connect three heterogeneous information types to store the mined and analyzed data in Figure 3. First, the information about the given algorithm to analyze bio-signals in the algorithm information table of MySQL. Second, the information about bio-signals used to analyze in HBase. Third, the extracted feature data in Hive.

Table 2 shows the table structure of Hive. The data are expressed by algorithm ID, algorithm name, the mined data value, and date. In addition, since it is partitioned by bio-signal ID, the acquired year, and month, the search time can be shorter.

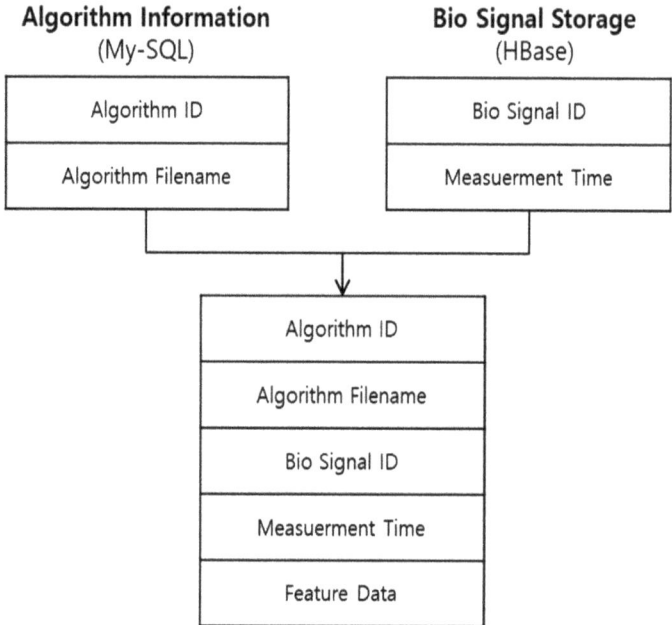

Figure 3. Design of data warehouse structure.

Table 2. The table structure of Hive.

Partition	Column Name	Data Type	Explanation
X	algorithm_id	String	Algorithm ID
X	algorithm_filename	String	Algorithm file name
X	output	array<String>	Output value
X	day	int	Day
X	hour	int	Hour
X	minute	int	Minute
X	second	int	Second
O	id	String	User ID
O	year	int	Year
O	month	int	Month

3.2. Architecture of Bio-Signal Data Mining

Many researchers employ MATLAB to analyze bio-signals, and there is also a recent tendency to use an open-source programming R for big data analysis. Some develop signal processing and mining techniques with MATLAB, others with R programming or with other languages or tools. Data mining techniques are developed in various environments. However, when developers try to use components developed in another language environment than the current development environment, the process of transforming sources in one language to the ones in another is needed, which demands a substantial amount of time for implementing its processor for coding the components working in the development language.

For this reason, it is of great meaning to provide an execution engine enabling to skip the source transforming process, which supports interoperability between different sources. It is particularly important and desirable when one wants to develop systems using vital sign data mining techniques developed in various languages and environments previously. We describe a flow to support interoperability between different (bio-signal) data mining techniques. The execution engine that we designed requires data mining technique specifications where input/output parameters and tool (or language) types are specified to interact with the engine. With such specifications, the execution engine makes the data mining algorithms implemented in different languages work as if they operated in one common environment, resulting in features and other values after executing the sources.

Among the many development languages, we concentrated on two popular languages, MATLAB and R, which are most frequently used to implement data mining algorithms, as well as Java which is our development language. Both MATLAB and R programming have the advantage in that they support many libraries, GUI, and various ways of expressing the analyzed data and enable the bio-signal analysis with the usage of function-based source files, simultaneously. In our approach, the execution engine helps execute *.m files of MATLAB and *.R of R programming and get feature values from the given bio-signals.

The proposed architecture is based on a web service model based on a service oriented architecture (SOA) in Figure 4. SOA can be integrated and used without a redundant development of applications that provide various bio-signal services. Therefore, SOA can minimize development costs, and users can easily receive biometric information monitoring services in an integrated environment. In this paper, an SOA-based bio-signal analysis system was developed. The architecture for interoperating among the components consists of the following four processes:

1. Service request for executing the bio-signal analysis algorithm through the simple object access protocol (SOAP) message.
2. Input value, output value, and algorithm explanation for supporting the mining specification of the bio-signal analysis algorithm.
3. Execution engine to run the bio-signal analysis algorithm.
4. Design a data warehouse that stores and classifies the results from the execution engine.

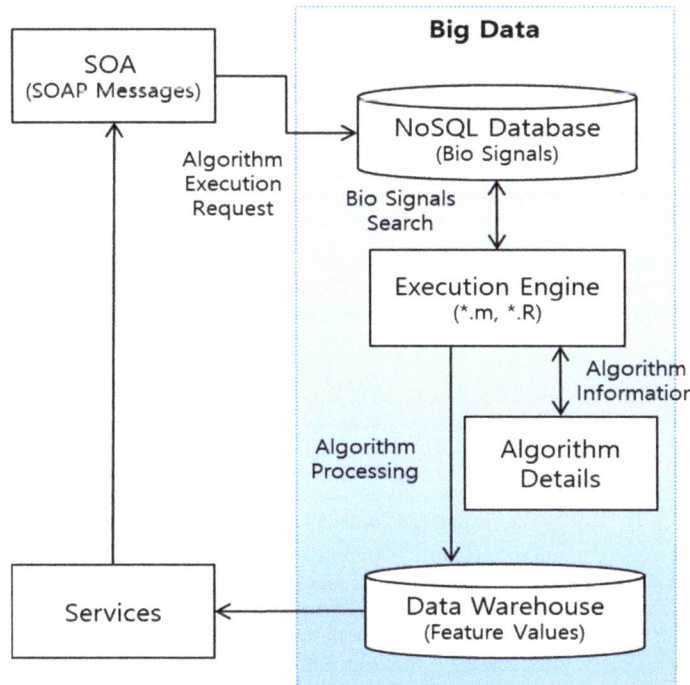

Figure 4. SOA-based bio-signal analysis system architecture.

The web-based simple object access protocol (SOAP) message offers the service for executing the bio-signal analysis algorithm. It includes a request to search for raw bio-signals data, a request that uploads the bio-signal algorithm source file developed by using MATLAB or R programming, and a request that extracts the bio-signal feature value by executing the bio-signal analysis algorithm.

To run the bio-signal analysis algorithm in the system, the parameters and variables of the bio-signal analysis algorithm should be defined. Hence, the algorithm specification describes the information on types of bio-signals to be analyzed (such as ECG, respiration, and acceleration signals), an input value of the bio-signals, result value after the execution of the algorithm, clear explanation of the algorithm, and the developer.

The data warehouse stores the results from the execution engine. The data extracted by applying the bio-signal analysis algorithm may be a great amount in a single column. Therefore, the data is needed to save into the data warehouse for big data analysis.

3.2.1. Data Modeling Specification

To execute data mining modules, an accurate specification of the mining techniques is necessary, since the execution engine works according to the specification in which a type of language (or tool), input/output values, and explanation of the mining algorithms are described. Our study focuses on two well-known languages, MATLAB and R. To understand the execution of source files in these languages, we need to be aware of 'function' in MATLAB and R. They help analyze the bio-signal data by providing the functions where various input values are represented, stored, and visualized.

Figure 5 shows an example of MATLAB source code to extract HRV from ECG raw data. In the source, two input values appear such as data (ECG data) and FS (sampling rate). The output values are maxIdx (R-R interval index), maxVal (value of R-R interval), and endIdx (last R-R interval index). MATLAB has a vector data structure so that it can process different types of both input and output variables. For example, it supports several variables to handle ECG such as int, int array, double, and double array.

In general, software specification is a summary of the requirements and functions demanded in the design phase. The mining technique specifications proposed in our work are needed to define and execute the mining techniques in the system. In addition, the mining technique specifications are used to insert, delete, and update input/output parameters, as well as describe the techniques themselves.

Our approach uses the relational database management system (RDBMS) for specification concerning functions in MATLAB and R programming, so that various input/output values can be defined, inserted, and updated systematically. Figure 6 presents the related database modeling. Table 'algorithm_details' represents basic information about a data mining algorithm including 'id' (who uploads it), file name, explanation, type of bio-signal, type of analysis tool, and registration date. Here, 'vitalsign_type' is a column needed to process various bio-signals, whose values are ECG, respiration, acceleration data, etc. In addition, the tool_type's values are MATLAB or R to express which bio-signal analysis tool is employed. The table 'algorithm_inp_out' is the table where definitions of input/output values are, and one registers what algorithm is applied, the order of parameters (if it is an input value or output value), parameter type, and parameter explanation.

3.2.2. Source File Strategy for the Mining Technique

Hadoop's Hadoop distributed file system (HDFS) plays a role in storing mining algorithm source files developed in MATLAB and R, which is suitable for the safe storage of sources. Figure 7 illustrates how source files are stored in Hadoop. It shows that mining algorithm source files are stored under the Hadoop's folder '/AlgorithmDB/' in Linux to execute algorithm source files ('joo@wellness.com/AlgorithmFile'). Here, it is necessary to copy the source files in HDFS to Linux or Windows OS by downloading the files in a browser used in HDFS or writing a command.

```
function [maxIdx, maxVal, endIdx] = evalQRSDetection(data, FS)
if nargin<2
    FS=100;
end
fs=FS;
fl=60;
fh=5;
maxIdx = [];
maxVal = [];
eIndex = [];
rawData = data;
dcRemData = rawData-mean(rawData);
lpData = lpassfilter(dcRemData, fl, fs);
hpData = hpassfilter(lpData, fh, fs);
diffData = diff(hpData);
sqrData = diffData.*diffData;
window= ones(1,30);
integral= medfilt1(filter(window,1,sqrData),10);
delay = ceil(length(window)/2);
integralData = integral(delay:length(integral));
max_h=max(integralData);
thresh = 0.3;
peak_reg = integralData>(thresh*max_h);
sIndex = find(diff([0 peak_reg'])==1);
eIndex = find(diff([peak_reg' 0])==-1);

for i=1:length(sIndex)
    [maxVal(i) maxIdx(i)] = max( hpData(sIndex(i):eIndex(i)) );
    maxIdx(i) = maxIdx(i)-1+sIndex(i); % offset
end
if ~isempty(eIndex)
    endIdx = eIndex(1);
else
    endIdx=1;
end
if isempty(maxIdx)
    maxIdx = [1];
end
```

Figure 5. Example of MATLAB source to extract HRV from ECG.

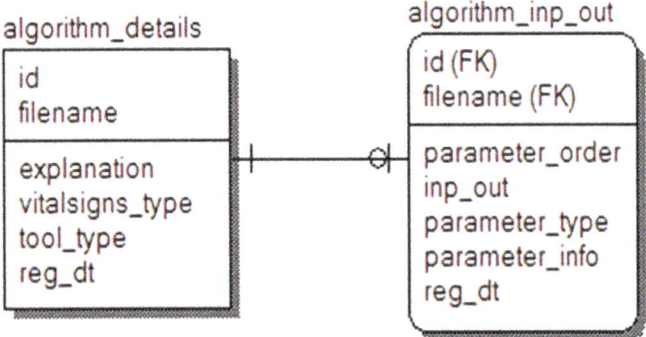

Figure 6. Database modeling for a mining algorithm.

/AlgorithmDB/joo@wellness.com/AlgorithmFile   Go!

Permission	Owner	Group	Size	Last Modified	Replication	Block Size	Name
-rw-r--r--	hadoop	supergroup	136 B	4/10/2017, 1:52:02 PM	3	128 MB	average_pw.m
-rw-r--r--	hadoop	supergroup	382 B	4/10/2017, 3:27:18 PM	3	128 MB	dfilt2.m
-rw-r--r--	hadoop	supergroup	3.01 KB	4/10/2017, 2:13:13 PM	3	128 MB	evalQRSDetection.m
-rw-r--r--	hadoop	supergroup	693 B	4/10/2017, 3:04:45 PM	3	128 MB	filtspec.m
-rw-r--r--	hadoop	supergroup	631 B	4/10/2017, 2:54:50 PM	3	128 MB	hpassfilter.m

Figure 7. Example of the list of algorithm source files.

3.2.3. Bio-Signal Analysis Algorithm Execution Engine

The bio-signal analysis algorithm source execution technology is a technology that executes a bio-signal analysis algorithm developed by a user, utilizing a bio-signal analysis tool developed in different languages in the system. By omitting the source conversion technology according to the system environment, the environment and interface to execute the source file itself in the system are provided.

In this paper, we design an architecture that performs the functions developed in MATLAB and R programming using Java, as shown in Figure 8.

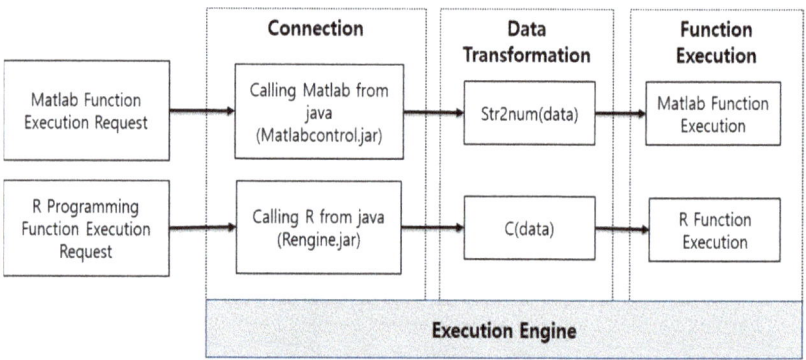

Figure 8. The architecture of functions developed in MATLAB and R programming through Java.

The execution technology of the bio-signal analysis algorithm runs the source code developed by MATLAB and R programming in Java. The bio-signal analysis algorithm developed by MATLAB is executed using the MATLAB control library. In addition, the bio-signal analysis algorithm developed by R programming is executed using the Rengine library. Each library is the application programming interface between Java and the development tools.

To run MATLAB in Java, use the MATLAB control library. The MATLAB control can use MATLAB commands in Java using the eval and f eval methods. The MATLAB control eval and f eval methods can be passed to the MATLAB workspace to execute MATLAB commands. In addition, the result value executed in MATLAB can be returned to Java. The result value returned from MATLAB is returned using the returning eval method of MATLAB controls. This paper accesses MATLAB using Java to execute MATLAB functions. Since the input value to execute the function is inputted through Java, it is inputted in a text format. Therefore, as shown in Figure 9, the input value needs to be converted to a number format through str2 num, a MATLAB method. If the entered value is a text, it can be used as it is. After inputting the input value, execute the MATLAB function, and return the result value to Java for processing.

```
>> text='1 2 3 4 5 6 7';
>> data=str2num(text);
>> rst=standardDeviation(data)
rst =
    2.1602
```

Figure 9. MATLAB function execution command.

To execute R programming, we use a method similar to MATLAB. Java uses the Rengine library to access R programming. Rengine can use R programming commands in Java using eval. The R programming eval method can be passed to the R programming workspace to execute R programming instructions. In addition, the result value executed in R programming can be returned to Java. The result value returned from R programming is returned using the eval method. In this paper, we access R programming using Java to execute the R programming function. The input value for executing the function is converted into an R programming input instruction through Java and inputted immediately. Therefore, as shown in Figure 10, since the input value is converted to the c format, there is no need to use a separate conversion function. After entering the input value, execute the R programming function, and return the result value to Java for processing.

```
> data=c(1,2,3,4,5,6,7)
> source("standardDeviation(data)
> rst=standardDeviation(data)
> rst
[1]  2.160247
```

Figure 10. R function execution command.

Since R programming is an open-source type of development tool, various R packages exist. This is important since developers can freely install and use the R packages they need. Therefore, this paper developed a service that can install the R package. However, the R package installation cannot use the Java JRI, since JRI is a Java and R programming interface that allows you to run R in Java applications with a single thread. Here, JRI operates as a single thread, thus installing the R package is physically impossible. Therefore, in this paper, we created the R function in Figure 11 and installed the R package using the Rscirpt of R programming.

```
args <- commandArgs(TRUE)
Install.packages(args, repos=
      'http://healthstat.snu.ac.kr/CRAN')
```

Figure 11. R packages install function.

4. Results

Table 3 measures the execution time of the algorithm source code. It was measured using an electrocardiogram signal among the biological signals. Using data from 60,000 to 150,000 ECG data, one source code was executed a hundred times to obtain an average. The algorithm source code used a lowpass filter developed by MATLAB and R programming to secure universality. As shown in Table 3, the source code is executed directly in R programming and MATLAB runs faster than the source code executed in conjunction with the development tool in Java. The difference in execution speed is to create an input value and pass it to the development tool to execute it in Java. This is due to the fact that it takes time to generate the input value. In addition, it is judged that there is no time difference felt when the bio-signal analysis system is executed.

Table 3. Comparison of execution time using MATLAB, R programming, and Java interface.

ECG Data Amount	R Running Time (s)	JRI Running Time (s)	MATLAB Running Time (s)	MATLAB Control Running Time (s)
60,000	0.01129	0.07554	0.001117402	0.018959
70,000	0.012122	0.07925	0.002032382	0.020659
80,000	0.015542	0.08802	0.002297501	0.021919
90,000	0.014942	0.09725	0.002646774	0.023969
100,000	0.018541	0.12115	0.002932099	0.026389
110,000	0.020813	0.14253	0.003061065	0.029939
120,000	0.022766	0.14519	0.003414657	0.032159
130,000	0.023421	0.15199	0.003779691	0.034149
140,000	0.023759	0.16123	0.004370618	0.036269
150,000	0.025931	0.17423	0.004643073	0.038039

5. Discussion

We can check the results of the feature values through analysis and visualization using the ECG signal. Currently, bio-signals can be measured using various sensors. For example, there are data such as electrocardiogram, brain wave, pulse wave, and acceleration signal. These data have a process of making feature values from raw data and servicing them using feature values. Therefore, the system proposed in this paper can apply various bio-signal data. However, since the algorithm is analyzed using only electrocardiogram data, it is necessary to analyze various bio-signal data such as brain waves and pulse waves. Bio-signal analysis processing can be used in all the versions using a basic analysis module. However, while doing an analysis the version compatibility such as licenses have to be checked, which is a necessary condition. Our framework can be used for all kinds of bio-signals with little customization and also different kinds of analyses can be performed with little or no modification.

In addition, this paper was developed with an emphasis on analyzing feature values through signal processing. However, recently, artificial intelligence technology using train sets and test sets have been widely used. It is necessary to develop a technology that automatically converts the train set and test set to match the bio-signal development language through further research.

6. Implementation

We have implemented a bio-signal analysis system that can execute SOA-based MATLAB and R programming source codes. The bio-signal analysis system consists of a service that transmits the algorithm developed by MATLAB and R programming to a server and a service that executes the algorithm. In this paper, we have implemented the evalQRSDetection function in Figure 5. Figure 12a is a request SOAP message to execute a function, which includes the function name, input data, and development language. The input values are electrocardiogram data and sampling frequency. The input value can be inputted as the input value of the bio-signal data stored in the bio-signal storage. Moreover, you can input the direct input value. Furthermore, Figure 12b is the response SOAP message. This SOAP message contains the result of executing the function.

```
<soapenv:Envelope xmlns:soapenv="http://schemas.xmlsoap.org/soap/envelope/"
    xmlns:ser="http://service.wellness">
    <soapenv:Header/>
    <soapenv:Body>
        <ser:getApplyAlgorithm>
            <!--Optional:-->
            <ser:id>joo@wellness.com</ser:id>
            <!--Optional:-->
            <ser:filename>evalQRSDetection.m</ser:filename>
            <!--Zero or more repetitions:-->
            <ser:input>1337 1359 1383 1409 1434 1457 1481 1505 1527 1545 1558 1564 1564
            1555 1542 1525 1503 1480 1457 1433 1406 1375 1339 1298 1251 1203 1156 1111
            1068 1025 986 949 916 887 863 843 827 814 803 795 789 783 779 780 783 791 801
            813 824 836 847 857 868 879 891 901 909 917 925 933 944 954 965 977 987 995
            1003 1009 1016 1023 1027 1029 1031 1036 1044 1051 1058 1064 1072 1082 1092
            1099 1104 1110 1114 1115 1115 1116 1114 1114 1115 1117 1118 1121 1124 1129
            1135 1141 1147 1153 1162 1174 1191 1224 1278 1355 1448 1505 1480 1407 1331
            </ser:input>
            <ser:input>250</ser:input>
            <!--Optional:-->
            <ser:toolType>matlab</ser:toolType>
        </ser:getApplyAlgorithm>
    </soapenv:Body>
</soapenv:Envelope>
```

(a) Algorithm Execution SOAP Message

```
<soapenv:Envelope xmlns:soapenv="http://schemas.xmlsoap.org/soap/envelope/">
    <soapenv:Body>
        <ns:getApplyAlgorithmResponse xmlns:ns="http://service.wellness" xmlns:ax27="http://report.wellness/xsd">
            <ns:return>15.0 91.0</ns:return>
            <ns:return>54.85248454132336 32.8066721884158</ns:return>
            <ns:return>22.0</ns:return>
        </ns:getApplyAlgorithmResponse>
    </soapenv:Body>
</soapenv:Envelope>
```

(b) Response SOAP Message

Figure 12. SOAP message of vital sign analysis algorithm execution; (**a**) SOAP message to request the algorithm execution; (**b**) response SOAP message with the algorithm executed.

Figure 13 shows the UI for executing the evalQRSDetection function developed in MATLAB and the result UI. Figure 13a is the request UI for executing the evalQRSDetection function. Figure 13b is the response UI showing the result of executing the evalQRSDetection function. The evalQRSDetection function displays three result values. Therefore, we show three UIs for the result values, which show the result data and chart in data format.

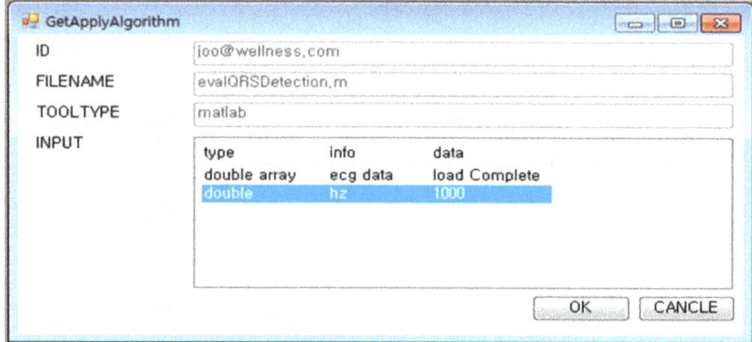

(a) Algorithm Execution Request UI

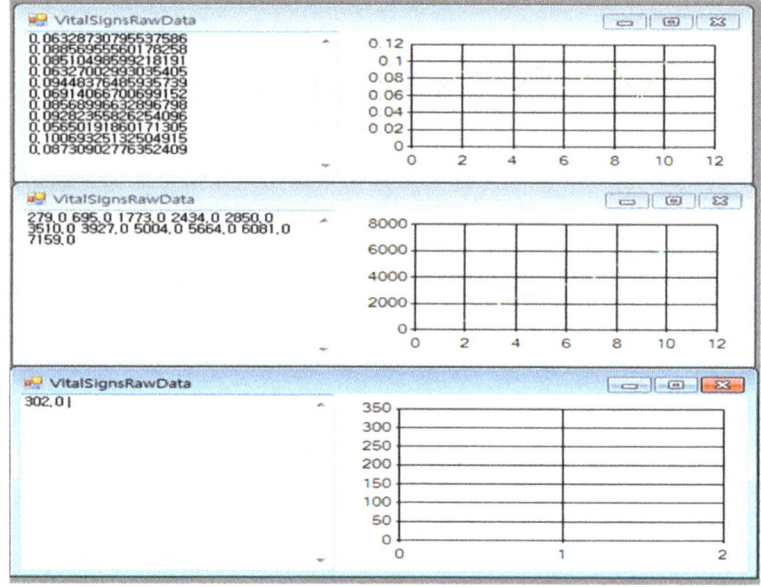

(b) Response UI

Figure 13. Implementation of vital sign system user interfaces; (**a**) UI for requesting the algorithm execution; (**b**) response UI where the algorithm was executed.

7. Conclusions

This paper presented an architecture that manages and executes bio-signal analysis algorithms more effectively, with a special focus on interoperability between data mining algorithms developed in heterogeneous environments. While bio-signal analysis components are implemented in different languages such as MATLAB, R, and Java, the proposed platform helps the design teams develop such components and systems as if they were developed in one common language.

Until now, bio-signal analysts have paid little attention to bio-signals as big data. However, as IoT and wearable technology are rapidly developing, the issue of bio-signals has high potentiality as a research theme for big data processing. Therefore, we need a repository for bio-signals as big data. Secondly, we designed mining algorithm specifications to share algorithms implemented in heterogeneous environments among developers. When design teams implement systems according to such specifications, they are expected to have many benefits, e.g., acquisition of many open algorithms, the overcoming of development restrictions caused by different environments, effective management of bio-signals, and application of the mining algorithms to various and wider environments and languages. In particular, it is expected that healthcare and medical system developers will be able to shorten the system development time using the algorithm execution engine technology. In addition, the real-time execution of various algorithms on the system will be very helpful for system maintenance and management. Thirdly, we developed the execution engine, naturally leading to an advantage that one can execute so many heterogeneous mining techniques with one common system. It also brings about a reduction of the development time and would make people and bio-signal analysts developing in different languages work together. We also hope that communication and competition between algorithms developers are enhanced, and thus higher quality mining technology will be eventually promoted. However, the system presented in this paper has limitations in applying artificial intelligence based on supervised learning. Supervised learning-based artificial intelligence needs to collect and transform a large amount of train set data. The difficulty of transferring large amounts of image files and the study on the application of the conversion technology to train set data are still insufficient. It is judged that such data transmission and conversion technology will be able to find a solution through future research.

Finally, we hope that this research will be fundamental, in which we can go one more step to high-quality, service-oriented research beyond simple signal processing for biodata, by utilizing and developing mining algorithms easily regardless of whatever environments are available.

Author Contributions: Conceptualization, M.-I.J. and H.-C.K.; methodology, M.-I.J.; software, M.-I.J.; validation, M.-I.J., S.A., and H.-C.K.; formal analysis, S.A.; investigation, M.-I.J.; resources, S.A.; data curation, S.A.; writing—original draft preparation, M.-I.J.; writing—review and editing, S.A. and H.-C.K.; visualization, M.-I.J.; supervision, H.-C.K.; project administration, H.-C.K.; funding acquisition, M.-I.J. All authors have read and agreed to the published version of the manuscript.

Funding: This research was supported by the Basic Science Research Program through the National Research Foundation of Korea (NRF) funded by the Ministry of Education (NRF2021R1I1A1A01050306) and by the Ministry of Science, ICT, and Future Planning (NRF2017R1D1A3B04032905).

Institutional Review Board Statement: Not applicable.

Informed Consent Statement: Not applicable.

Data Availability Statement: The data are available on request.

Conflicts of Interest: The authors declare no conflict of interest.

References

1. Lee, J.; Kao, H.A.; Yang, S. Service innovation and smart analytics for industry 4.0 and big data environment. *Procedia Cirp.* **2014**, *16*, 3–8. [CrossRef]
2. Morrar, R.; Arman, H.; Mousa, S. The fourth industrial revolution (Industry 4.0): A social innovation perspective. *Technol. Innov. Manag. Rev.* **2017**, *7*, 12–20. [CrossRef]
3. Trossen, D.; Pavel, D.; Platt, G.; Wall, J.; Valencia, P.; Graves, C.A.; Zamarripa, M.S.; Gonzalez, V.M.; Favela, J.; Lovquist, E.; et al. Sensor networks, wearable computing, and healthcare applications. *IEEE Pervasive Comput.* **2007**, *6*, 58–61. [CrossRef]
4. Bonato, P. Wearable sensors and systems. *IEEE Eng. Med. Biol. Mag.* **2010**, *29*, 25–36. [CrossRef] [PubMed]
5. Buenaflor, C.; Kim, H.C. Wearable computers in human perspective: The decision process of innovation acceptance with user issues and concerns. *Int. J. Emerg. Technol. Adv. Eng.* **2012**, *2*, 573–580.
6. Gimhae, G.N. Six human factors to acceptability of wearable computers. *Int. J. Multimed. Ubiquitous Eng.* **2013**, *8*, 103–114.
7. Yetisen, A.K.; Martinez-Hurtado, J.L.; Ünal, B.; Khademhosseini, A.; Butt, H. Wearables in medicine. *Adv. Mater.* **2018**, *30*, 1706910. [CrossRef] [PubMed]
8. Khan, Y.; Ostfeld, A.E.; Lochner, C.M.; Pierre, A.; Arias, A.C. Monitoring of vital signs with flexible and wearable medical devices. *Adv. Mater.* **2016**, *28*, 4373–4395. [CrossRef] [PubMed]
9. Pantelopoulos, A.; Bourbakis, N.G. A survey on wearable sensor-based systems for health monitoring and prognosis. *IEEE Trans. Syst. Man Cybern. Part C Appl. Rev.* **2009**, *40*, 1–12. [CrossRef]

10. Kim, T.W.; Park, K.H.; Yi, S.H.; Kim, H.C. A big data framework for u-healthcare systems utilizing vital signs. In Proceedings of the 2014 International Symposium on Computer, Consumer and Control, Taichung, Taiwan, 10–12 June 2014.
11. Raghupathi, W.; Raghupathi, V. Big data analytics in healthcare: Promise and potential. *Health Inf. Sci. Syst.* **2014**, *2*, 1–10. [CrossRef] [PubMed]
12. Joo, M.I.; Ko, D.H.; Kim, H.C. Development of smart healthcare wear system for acquiring vital signs and monitoring personal health. *J. Korea Multimed. Soc.* **2016**, *19*, 808–817. [CrossRef]
13. Secinaro, S.; Calandra, D.; Secinaro, A.; Muthurangu, V.; Biancone, P. The role of artificial intelligence in healthcare: A structured literature review. *BMC Med. Inform. Decis. Mak.* **2021**, *21*, 1–23. [CrossRef] [PubMed]
14. Boulos, M.N.K.; Wheeler, S.; Tavares, C.; Jones, R. How smartphones are changing the face of mobile and participatory healthcare: An overview, with example from ecAALYX. *Biomed. Eng. Online* **2011**, *10*, 1–14. [CrossRef] [PubMed]
15. Kim, H.; Kim, T.; Joo, M.; Yi, S.; Yoo, C.; Lee, K.; Kim, J.; Chung, G. Design of a calorie tracker utilizing heart rate variability obtained by a nanofiber technique-based wellness wear system. *Appl. Math. Inf. Sci.* **2011**, *5*, 171S–177S.
16. Luxton, D.D.; McCann, R.A.; Bush, N.E.; Mishkind, M.C.; Reger, G.M. mHealth for mental health: Integrating smartphone technology in behavioral healthcare. *Prof. Psychol. Res. Pract.* **2011**, *42*, 505. [CrossRef]
17. Ozdalga, E.; Ozdalga, A.; Ahuja, N. The smartphone in medicine: A review of current and potential use among physicians and students. *J. Med. Internet Res.* **2012**, *14*, e128. [CrossRef] [PubMed]
18. Farshchian, B.A.; Vilarinho, T. Which mobile health toolkit should a service provider choose? A comparative evaluation of Apple HealthKit, Google Fit, and Samsung Digital Health Platform. In Proceedings of the 13th European Conference on Ambient Intelligence, Malaga, Spain, 26–28 April 2017. [CrossRef]
19. Park, S.J.; Park, B.S.; Kang, S.A.; Kang, S.Y. The Application of Digital Health Content Using Mobile Device. In Proceedings of the Information Science and Applications (ICISA) 2016, Ho Chi Minh, Vietnam, 16 February 2016. [CrossRef]
20. Vikström, A. A Study of Automatic Translation of MATLAB Code to C Code Using Software from MathWorks. Master's Thesis, Lulea University, Luleå, Sweden, 2009.
21. Aycock, J. Converting Python virtual machine code to C. In Proceedings of the 7th International Python, Houston, TX, USA, 10–13 November 1998.
22. Satman, M.H. RCaller: A software library for calling R from Java. *J. Adv. Math. Comput. Sci.* **2014**, 2188–2196. [CrossRef]
23. Ignatchenko, V.; Ignatchenko, A.; Sinha, A.; Boutros, P.C.; Kislinger, T. VennDIS: A JavaFX-based Venn and Euler diagram software to generate publication quality figures. *Proteomics* **2015**, *15*, 1239–1244. [CrossRef] [PubMed]
24. Furtună, T.F.; Vinte, C. Integrating R and Java for Enhancing Interactivity of Algorithmic Data Analysis Software Solutions. *Rom. Stat. Rev.* **2016**, *64*, 29–41.
25. Wu, C.H. A patient-centered self-care support system for diabetics. In Proceedings of the 2014 IEEE 11th International Conference on e-Business Engineering, Guangzhou, China, 5–7 November 2014. [CrossRef]
26. Bisták, P. Remote laboratory server based on Java Matlab interface. In Proceedings of the 2011 14th International Conference on Interactive Collaborative Learning, Piestany, Slovakia, 21–23 September 2011. [CrossRef]
27. Cattell, R. Scalable SQL and NoSQL data stores. *Acm Sigmod Rec.* **2011**, *39*, 12–27. [CrossRef]
28. Han, J.; Haihong, E.; Le, G.; Du, J. Survey on NoSQL database. In Proceedings of the 2011 6th International Conference on Pervasive Computing and Applications, Port Elizabeth, South Africa, 26–28 October 2011. [CrossRef]
29. Chen, Y.; Qin, X.; Bian, H.; Chen, J.; Dong, Z.; Du, X.; Gao, X.; Liu, D.; Lu, J.; Zhang, H. A study of SQL-on-Hadoop systems. In Proceedings of the Workshop on Big Data Benchmarks, Performance Optimization, and Emerging Hardware, Salt Lake City, UT, USA, 1 March 2014. [CrossRef]

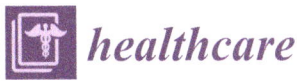

Article

The Use of Modern Technologies by Dentists in Poland: Questionnaire among Polish Dentists

Mateusz Świtała [1,*], Wojciech Zakrzewski [1], Zbigniew Rybak [1], Maria Szymonowicz [1] and Maciej Dobrzyński [2,*]

1. Pre-Clinical Research Centre, Wroclaw Medical University, Bujwida 44, 50-345 Wrocław, Poland; wojciech.zakrzewski@student.umw.edu.pl (W.Z.); zbigniew.rybak@umw.edu.pl (Z.R.); maria.szymonowicz@umw.edu.pl (M.S.)
2. Department of Pediatric Dentistry and Preclinical Dentistry, Wroclaw Medical University, Krakowska 26, 50-425 Wrocław, Poland
* Correspondence: m.switala97@gmail.com (M.Ś.); maciej.dobrzynski@umw.edu.pl (M.D.); Tel.: +48-511-42-59-00 (M.Ś.); +48-71-7840-378 (M.D.)

Abstract: Background: From one year to another, dentists have access to more procedures using modern techniques. Many of them can improve the effectiveness of dental procedures and frequently facilitate and accelerate them. Objectives: Technically advanced devices are an important part of modern dentistry. Over the years, there were developed technologies like ultrasounds, lasers, air abrasion, ozonotherapy, caries diagnostic methods, chemomechanical caries removal (CMCR), pulp vitality tests, computer-controlled local anesthetic delivery (CCLAD). The aim of this study was to investigate the requirement of Polish dentists for such technologies. Methods: An anonymous questionnaire was posted on a social media group of dentists from Poland. 187 responses were obtained. Results: It turned out that almost every respondent uses ultrasounds, but other technologies are not as popular. 43% use CCLAD, 33% use diagnostic methods, 28% use air abrasion, 25% use dental lasers, 21% use CMCR, 18% use pulp vitality tests and 6% use ozonotherapy. The most common reason for not using the aforementioned technologies were their high cost and the sufficient effectiveness of traditional methods. There was a correlation between use of a dental laser and CCLAD and size of office, CMCR use and dentists' work time and air abrasion use and gender. Many dentists claim that they will try one of the modern technologies in the future. Conclusions: It can be concluded that Polish dentists tend to use ultrasounds and CCLAD more than any other technology. In the future this may change, so more studies in this topic are needed.

Keywords: dentistry; computer-controlled local anesthetic delivery; ultrasounds; chemomechanical caries removal; modern technologies; laser; ozone

Citation: Świtała, M.; Zakrzewski, W.; Rybak, Z.; Szymonowicz, M.; Dobrzyński, M. The Use of Modern Technologies by Dentists in Poland: Questionnaire among Polish Dentists. *Healthcare* **2022**, *10*, 225. https://doi.org/10.3390/healthcare10020225

Academic Editor: Marco P. Soares dos Santos

Received: 16 December 2021
Accepted: 23 January 2022
Published: 25 January 2022

Publisher's Note: MDPI stays neutral with regard to jurisdictional claims in published maps and institutional affiliations.

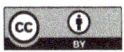

Copyright: © 2022 by the authors. Licensee MDPI, Basel, Switzerland. This article is an open access article distributed under the terms and conditions of the Creative Commons Attribution (CC BY) license (https://creativecommons.org/licenses/by/4.0/).

1. Introduction

Dentistry is a branch of medicine which dynamically develops new technologies. From one year to another, dentists have access to more procedures using modern techniques. Many of them can improve and the effectiveness of dental procedures. And accelerate the related procedures. Some of the technologies were introduced to dentistry years ago. For example, ozone in the form of ozonated water was used in dentistry for the first time by Dr. E.A. Fisch and in surgery by Dr Erwin Payr. They reported their results in 1935 [1]. Another technology that was also developed years ago is lasers, which were introduced in the 1960s by Miaman [2].

On the other hand, some technologies are quite new. Lussi et al., in 1999, validated the use of the DIAGNOdent system (KaVo, Biberach, Germany) for the detection and quantification of caries on occlusal surfaces [3]. The pulse oximetry was invented by Takuo Aoyagi in the early 1970s and in 2007 V. Gopikrishna et al. constructed a pulse oximeter dental probe for assessment of pulp vitality [4]. A computer-controlled local anesthetic delivery system (CCLAD) was introduced in 1997 by Milestone Scientific Inc. as the Wand [5].

This shows that dentists need to constantly keep up on their knowledge about new technologies. In times where the Internet is a great source of knowledge, practitioners have a great opportunity to learn about newly developed technologies and adapt them to their work. The aim of this study was to investigate modern technique use by Polish dentists by posting an online survey in a social-media group for Polish dentists. Another purpose of study is to give information, which can be utilized to streamline the usage of technologies in Polish dental practices. The authors tried to identify factors which correlate with new technology use patterns (like sex, years in practice, size of office). The authors assume that there will not be statistically important difference in terms of sex and expect a difference in terms of years in practice and size of office. We also identified reasons which might lead dentistry practitioners to stop using new technologies.

2. Materials and Methods

An anonymous questionnaire was posted in a social media group of Polish dentists in January 2019. Before publication, the aspects of privacy and data security were addressed. The survey was planned to be anonymous. The survey only concerned opinions and the expression of thoughts of respondents and not clinical trials on humans. Due to this, it was considered unnecessary to proceed with the formal approval procedures. The generation of the questionnaire and collection of responses were done through Google Forms (Google LLC, Mountain View, CA, USA). Members were given four weeks to respond.

The survey had 10 sections. The first section included questions about the biometric data of the respondents. In this section, the authors asked about gender, years in practice, type of employment and size of their offices. Respondents with more than one year in practice were considered in this study. Sections 2 to 9 had five questions each, investigating the use of each technology, including laser, ultrasounds, air abrasion, ozone, diagnostic methods, chemo-mechanical caries removal, pulp vitality tests, and computer-controlled local anesthetic delivery. The tenth section included general questions about reasons for not using the mentioned technologies, patients attitudes about new technologies, and sources of knowledge about new technologies (Table 1). The online form is visible in [6].

Collected data were tabulated using Microsoft Excel (Microsoft, Redmond, WA, USA). Only the authors had access to data collected from the survey.

All analyses were performed with the help of Statistica for Windows (version 13.3, TIBCO Software, Palo Alto, CA, USA). A chi-squared test was used to assess the statistical significance. Probabilities less than 0.05 were accepted as statistically significant.

Table 1. Questions included in the survey.

Questions in Survey	Responds
Biometric questions	
1. Gender (choice question)	Male/Female
2. Years in practice (graded question)	<5/5–10/10–20/>20
3. specialization (multiple choice question)	- restorative dentistry - dental surgery - periodontology - orthodontics - pedodontics - prosthetics - no specialization
4. Form of employment (choice question)	- own office - hired in office
5. Size of office (graded question)	one unit/two to five units/>five units

Table 1. Cont.

Questions in Survey	Responds
Questions in each technology section	
1. Have you access to this technology in your practice? (graded question)	Yes/No
2. How often do you use this technology? (graded question)	- don't use - less often than conventional method - as often as conventional method - more often than conventional method - use only modern method
3. How do you rate efficiency of this technology? (graded question)	- More efficient - as efficient as conventional method - less efficient - don't know
4. How do you rate difficulty of this technology? (graded question)	- More difficult - as difficult as conventional method - less difficult - don't know
5. Will you use this technology in the future? (choice question)	Yes/No/Maybe
General questions	
1. About how many methods you didn't know? (graded question)	1–5/6–10/>10
2. Why don't you use mentioned technologies? (multiple choice question)	- high cost - more complicated method - less efficient method - sufficient effectiveness of conventional method - lack of knowledge
3. What is the attitude of patients to innovative technologies? (choice question)	- They are interested - They are inert - They refuse treatment with these technologies
4. Which sources of knowledge do you use to acquire competency about mentioned technologies? (multiple choice question)	- journals/research - courses - college/ specialization courses - internet - books - other (open question)

3. Results

187 responses were acquired over January and February 2019. The biometrics of the respondents are shown in Figure 1. A significant portion of the respondents were women (82.9%), which reflects gender proportion of dentists in Poland. There were roughly equal responses in terms of years in practice groups, with fewer dentists in the >20 years in practice group. Most of the respondents worked in an office with two to five units. A major portion of the respondents (79.5%) had their own office. 82.9% of respondents did not have any specialization. There were 10 dentists with prosthetic specialization, 10 dentists with restorative specialization, seven with surgery, three with orthodontics, two with pedodontics, and two with periodontics.

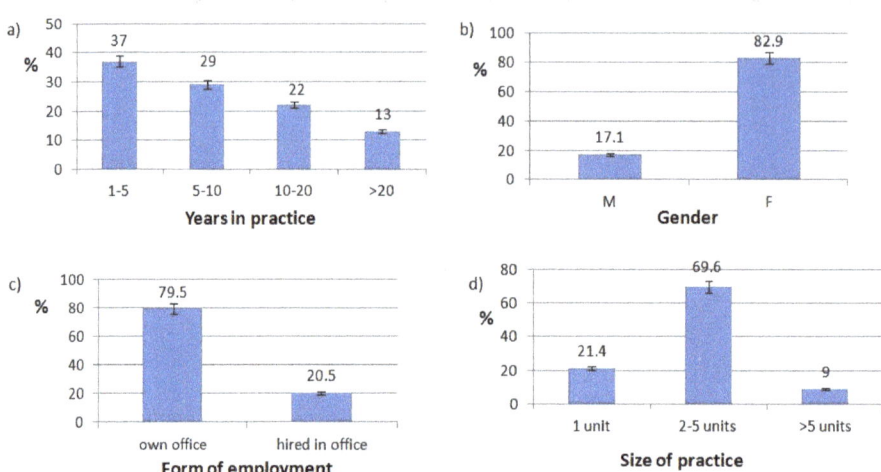

Figure 1. Respondents biometrics. (**a**) Years In practice distribution, (**b**) gender of responding dentists, (**c**) dentist's form of employment, (**d**) size of practice.

The percentage use of each investigated technology is shown in Table 2.

Table 2. Percentage of respondents who declare use of each technology.

Technology	Percentage of Use
Laser	25
Ultrasounds	97
Air abrasion	28
Ozone	6
CDM	33
CMCR	21
PVT	18
CCLAD	43

The ratings of effectiveness and difficulty of each technology are shown in Figures 2–9. Most dentists rate ultrasounds as less difficult (59%) and more effective (76%) in comparison with manual methods. Air abrasion was rated by the most dentists as comparatively difficult in comparison with the traditional method. In case of other methods, the most respondents didn't know how difficult and effective they are.

Procedures in which dentists use ultrasounds are shown in Figure 3b. The most popular ultrasonic procedure is scaling (96%). Endodontic treatment (canals irrigation) (85%) and prosthetic procedures (teeth preparation for crowns, inlays etc., post-and-cores removal) (80%) are popular fields to use ultrasounds. This technology is used by fewer respondents in surgery (piezosurgery) (24%) and in caries removal (32%).

The most respondents use lasers in surgery (18%) and teeth whitening. The least popular laser procedure is caries removal (4%) (Figure 2b).

Respondents use ozone for the following procedures: surgery (wounds disinfection, dry socket, abscesses)–5.36%, periodontology (gingivitis, periodontitis)–3.57%, endodontic treatment (canals disinfection)–3.57%, prosthetic (disinfection of prepared teeth)–1.79% (Figure 5b).

The most popular caries diagnostic method (CDM) is FOTI/Di-FOTI (27%) (Figure 6a).

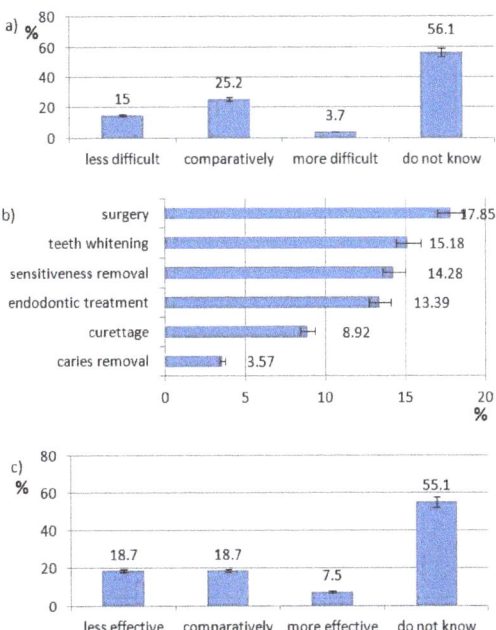

Figure 2. Laser use pattern of responding dentists. (**a**) difficulty of laser procedures, (**b**) type of laser procedures, (**c**) effectiveness of laser procedures.

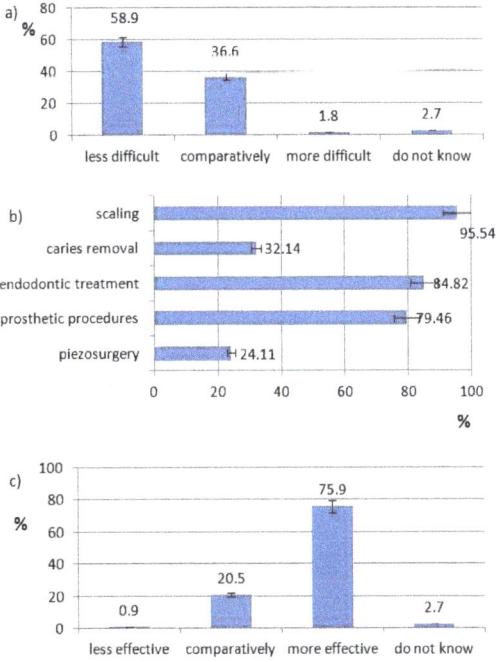

Figure 3. Ultrasounds use pattern of responding dentists; (**a**) difficulty of ultrasonic procedures, (**b**) type of ultrasonic procedures, (**c**) effectiveness of ultrasonic procedures.

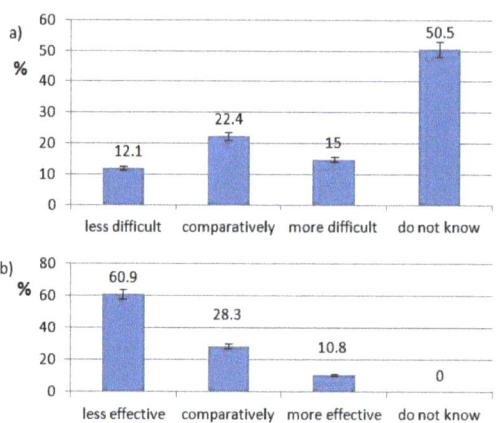

Figure 4. Air abrasion use pattern of responding dentists; (**a**) difficulty of air abrasion procedures, (**b**) effectiveness of air abrasion procedures.

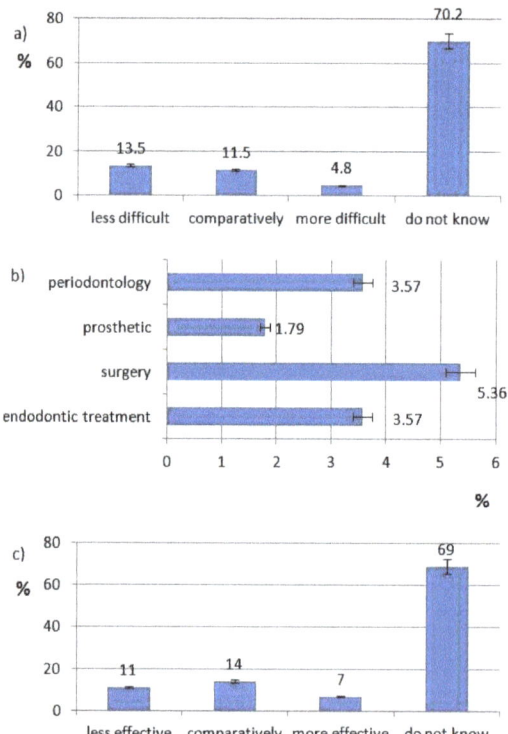

Figure 5. Ozone use pattern of responding dentists; (**a**) effectiveness of ozone procedures, (**b**) type of ozone procedures, (**c**) difficulty of ozone procedures.

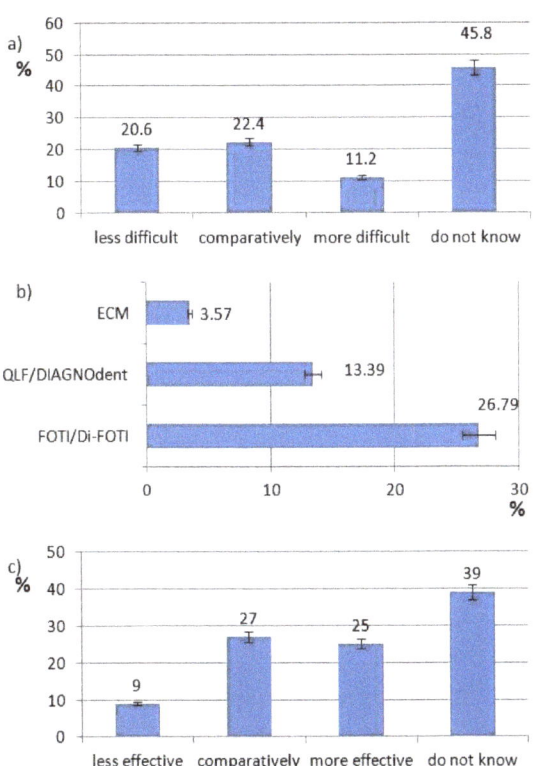

Figure 6. Caries diagnostics methods use pattern of responding dentists; (**a**) use of each method, (**b**) difficulty of caries diagnostics methods, (**c**) effectiveness of caries diagnostics methods.

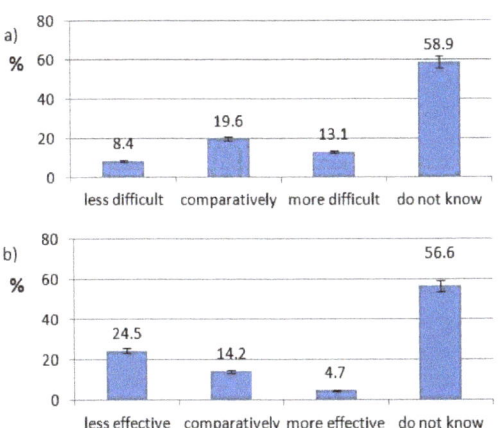

Figure 7. Chemo-mechanical caries removal use pattern of responding dentists; (**a**) effectiveness of CMCR, (**b**) difficulty of CMCR.

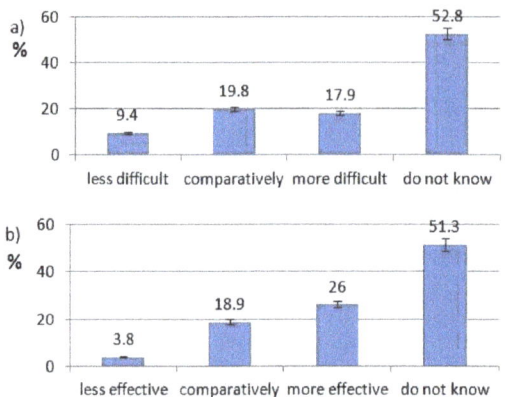

Figure 8. Pulp vitality tests use pattern of responding dentists; (**a**) effectiveness of pulp vitality tests, (**b**) difficulty of pulp vitality tests.

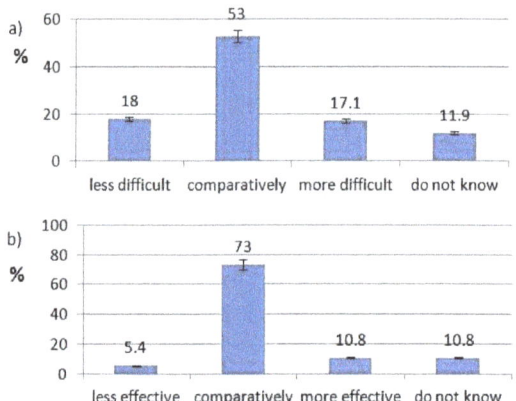

Figure 9. Computer controlled local anesthetic delivery use pattern of responding dentists; (**a**) effectiveness of CCLAD, (**b**) difficulty of CCLAD.

In our survey, we also asked dentists if they would use each technology in the future. Almost every respondent claimed that they may use ultrasounds (99%). Also, many dentists show interest in using other technologies in the future: CDM (91%), laser (86%), pulp vitality tests (PVT) (86%), air abrasion (85%), CCLAD (82%), ozone (80%), chemo-mechanical caries removal (CMCR) (64%).

A dental laser was present in the offices of only 30% of respondents. All dentists had an ultrasonic device in their offices.

An air abrasion unit was present in 35% of offices. Only 7% of dentists has access to a device for ozonotherapy.

85.7% of respondents didn't know about one to five of the methods mentioned in the questionnaire, 9% didn't know about six to ten of the techniques, and six percent didn't know about more than ten of them. There wasn't a statically relevant difference between groups of dentists with different work schedules.

In our study we also investigated the reasons for not using modern technologies in dental practices. The most dentists (51%) don't use a dental laser because of the high cost. High cost was also reason for not using ozone (41%), caries diagnostic methods (30%), pulp vitality tests (30%) and computer-controlled local anesthetic delivery (29%). Lack of knowledge was a reason for not using a dental laser for 9% of respondents, ozonoterapy for 12%, caries diagnostic methods for 10%, and chemo-mechanical caries removal for 14%.

The sufficient effectiveness of traditional methods was a reason to not use air abrasion (22%), caries diagnostic methods (CDM) (21%), CMCR (28%), PVT (29%) and CCLAD (24%).

Because of higher complexity in use in comparison with traditional methods, respondents do not use CDM (20%), PVT (16%), CMCR (14%), air abrasion (11%) and ozonoterapy (8%).

For respondents, the most popular source of knowledge were: courses (89%), the Internet (75%), science magazines and research (69%), knowledge earned during college, specialized courses (42%), and books (41%).

A majority of respondents (57%) say that their patients show interest in innovative methods of dental treatment. 39% claim that method of treatment is inert for their patients and only 4.5% respondents claim that their patients refuse treatment with these methods.

A chi-squared test showed statistical differences in the use of CMCR in different years in practice groups. Dentists that have worked for more than 20 years seems to not use CMCR. Differences in laser use in groups of office sizes was also statistically important. In smaller offices with only one dental unit, lasers were less popular than in bigger offices. The same situation was observed with regard to CCLAD use patterns. A statistical assessment showed that female dentists use air abrasion more often than male dentists–Table 3.

Table 3. The number of respondents (percentage) who use each technology.

CCLAD	PVT	CMCR	CDM	Ozone	Air Abrasion	Ultrasounds	Laser	Technology	
33 (43)	11 (16)	20 (29)	18 (26)	2 (3)	20 (29)	65 (94)	13 (19)	<5 (n = 69)	
23 (43)	7 (13)	8 (15)	18 (33)	6 (11)	15 (28)	54 (100)	17 (31)	5–10 (n = 54)	Years in practice
11 (27)	8 (20)	12 (29)	15 (37)	2 (5)	13 (32)	41 (100)	12 (29)	10–20 (n = 41)	
13 (57)	7 (30)	0 (0)	11 (48)	2 (9)	5 (22)	22 (96)	12 (29)	>20 (n = 23)	
0.08	0.03	0.009 *	0.261	0.288	0.862	0.142	0.373	P	
8 (20)	7 (18)	7 (18)	15 (38)	2 (5)	8 (20)	37 (93)	2 (5)	1 unit (n = 40)	
64 (49)	23 (18)	28 (22)	42 (32)	8 (6)	41 (32)	128 (98)	41 (32)	2–5 u. (n = 130)	Size of office
8 (47)	3 (18)	5 (29)	5 (29)	2 (12)	3 (18)	17 (100)	4 (24)	>5 u. (n = 17)	
0.004 *	0.999	0.603	0.782	0.619	0.224	0.096	0.003 *	P	
67 (43)	28 (18)	33 (21)	55 (35)	12 (8)	50 (32)	152 (97)	37 (24)	F (n = 157)	
13 (43)	5 (17)	7 (23)	7 (23)	0 (0)	3 (10)	30 (100)	10 (33)	M (n = 30)	Gender
0.947	0.878	0.777	0.212	0.118	0.015 *	0.322	0.259	P	

CDM–caries diagnostic methods, CMCR–chemo-mechanical caries removal, PVT–pulp vitality tests, CCLAD–computer-controlled local anesthetic delivery. P–based on chi squared test, * $p < 0.05$.

4. Discussion

In 2012, Verma, S. et al. predicted that specific laser procedures would become essential components of contemporary dental practice over the next decade [7]. In 2019, the dental laser was present in only 30% of Polish offices and 75% dentists did not use the laser in their practice. Mentioned authors in research review showed that laser can be used in many dental procedures, for example: cavity preparation, caries and restorative removal, treatment of dentinal hypersensitivity, and surgical procedures. Cozean et al. concluded that using the Er:YAG laser is both safe and effective for caries removal and cavity preparation [8]. Valenti et al. evaluated the ability of the Er:YAG laser in reducing the microbial population in carious lesions. The authors showed that the use of lasers resulted in greater reduction of bacterial CFU than traditional preparations [9]. These conclusions don't affect the use of lasers by Polish dentists for the mentioned procedures, as only 3.75% of respondents use it.

Verma, S. et al. mentioned surgical procedures which can be performed with the use of a laser, which include aesthetic gingival re-contouring, crown lengthening, exposure of unerupted teeth, removal of inflamed, hypertrophic tissue, and frenectomies [7]. Laser dental surgery was used by 17.85% dentists.

The authors claim that these procedures, with the help of a laser, can be performed without bleeding, sutures and with no need for special postoperative care. This correlates with the opinion of Polish dentists: 40.2% of them think that laser procedures are less or as difficult as classical ones and 37.4% dentists claim that this procedure has better or equal effectiveness.

Schwarz et al. investigated the ability of lasers to treat dentinal hypersensitivity. He proved that the Er:YAG laser is effective in this procedure, and that the results lasted longer than when the traditional procedure was used [10]. For this procedure, 14.28% of respondents use a laser. In conclusion, the research reveals that a laser can be a valuable method in modern dentistry and can enhance the effectiveness of many procedures, but it is not a popular method among Polish dentists.

In a review of the literature, Walmsley et al. pointed out that research showed that both methods, manual and ultrasonic, are effective in calculus removal on a clinical level, but scanning microscopy studies have suggested that ultrasonic methods are more effective. Ultrasonic scalers are also more effective in the more inaccessible areas of the oral cavity such as the posterior molars [11]. Polish dentists agree with that opinion, as 95.54% of them use ultrasounds for scaling and 75.9% rate it as more effective.

In the opinion of Plotino et al., in endodontic treatment, ultrasounds can be used for access refinement, finding calcified canals, removal of intracanal obstructions, activation of irrigating solutions, and root canal preparation. The authors mention many benefits of ultrasonic procedures, such as improved visualization combined with a more conservative approach when selectively removing tooth structure, specific angulation or tip design [12]. In 2020, Abu Hasna A et al. showed that passive ultrasonic irrigation decreased levels of *Enterococcus faecalis, Esherichia coli* and endotoxins in combination with NaOCl [13]. Verma et al. provided a randomized controlled trail of endodontic treatment with the help of ultrasonic and laser-activated irrigation. They observed a 100% success rate of periapical periodontitis healing after endodontic treatment with the addition of additional activation [14]. Thanks to their effectiveness, ultrasonic procedures are very popular in Polish dentistry. 84.82% of respondents use it for endodontic treatment.

Another field of dentistry where ultrasounds can be used is surgery. Thomas M. et al. mention oral and maxillofacial surgery procedures, which can be done with the help of piezosurgery. These are: sinus lift, bone graft harvesting, periodontal surgery, cyst removal, ridge expansion, osteogenic distraction, unilateral condylar hyperplasia, dental extraction and impacted tooth removal [15]. Agarwal et al. show advantages of piezosurgery as being precise and selective bone cutting, faster healing, less invasive, reduced post-operative pain, and better tactile sensitivity [16]. As the largest disadvantage, the authors consider increased operating time [15,16]. These observations were also confirmed by Otake Y et al. In an experimental study, the authors determined a difference in the time of osteotomy done with piezosurgery and rotary instruments. Piezosurgery required three times longer to cut the bone, but did not cut soft tissues [17]. In Poland, piezosurgery is not as widely used. Only 24.11% of respondents use it.

Hegde VS and Khatavkar RA mention indications for air abrasion: removal of superficial enamel defects, detection of pit and fissure caries suspect, preparation of cavities restricted only to small section of the tooth, surface preparation of abfractions and abrasions, the removal of existing restorations, and the avoidance of local anesthesia [18]. Air abrasion is used by only 28% of questioned Polish dentists. In our study, 60.9% of dentists rate air abrasion as effective as traditional techniques. Similar conclusions were drawn by Bhushan and Goswami. In their study, air abrasion pretreatment did not result in a statistically significant difference in sealant retention in both primary and permanent molars after three and six months follow-up [19].

Ozonotherapy was an area of research for William C. Domb. He gathered indications for using ozone in dentistry. These were: treating caries, periodontal disease, endodontics treatment, perioral viral and fungal infections, sinusitis and even temporomandibular joint dysfunctions. He also takes ozone as proper treatment in osteonecrotic lesions after bisphosphonate medications [20]. Gupta and Mansi had reviewed many cases where ozone was successfully used in periodontal disease. They confirm the disinfecting ability of ozone and suggest using it in daily dental practice [21]. In Polish dentistry, ozone seems not to be popular, as only 6.25% of respondents use it, (3.57% in periodontology). This may change, as 80% claim that they will or may use ozone in the future.

Gomez J. discusses the current available methods to detect early caries lesions. She mention methods like quantitative light-inducted fluorescence (QLF), DIAGNOdent, fibre-optic transillumination (FOTI) and its digital version–Di-FOTI, and electrical conductance measurement (ECM). In the opinion of the authors, these methods should be used as an adjunct to well-established and evidence-based methods such as visual assessment and radiographs [22]. In our study, 32.14% respondents use one of the caries diagnostic methods. Cho KH et al. showed that quantitative light-induced fluorescence (QLF) has the ability to detect caries of occlusal surfaces in primary teeth [23]. In the opinion of 52% of our respondents, new caries diagnostic methods are more or comparatively effective in comparison with visual or radiographic methods.

Chemomechanical caries removal (CMCR) seems to be the optimal method in treating caries, especially in children who are anxious about dental procedures. In Venkataraghavan and Karthik et al.'s study, the use of CMCR resulted in decreasing pain complaints and the reduced need for anesthesia. The only disadvantage of CMCR was an increase in cleaning duration [24]. Similar conclusions was drawn by Sontakke, Priyanka et al. in 2019. The authors report an overall absence of bad smell/taste in CMCR [25]. A CMCR was compared to Er:YAG and carbid burs in terms of the ability to remove microorgams from cavities. CMCR showed the lowest ability and the Er:YAG laser was the most capable of decreasing the size of the cavital biome [26]. In a systemic review, Cardoso et al. compared efficacy and patient acceptance of caries removal with alternative methods. Traditional preparation showed faster caries removal and resulted in larger cavities, which can lead to the unnecessary removal of healthy tissues. Rotary instrumentation often was related with a need for anesthesia. Patients were experiencing less negative emotions (pain, fear) when alternative methods were used [27]. 78.6% of our respondents do not use chemomechanical methods in their dental practice. Efficiency of CMCR was rated as "less effective" by 24.5% of questioned dentists and 56.6% of them did not know how effective this method is. The low popularity of CMCR may be a result of the lack of knowledge or experience about it among respondents.

Pulp vitality testing is an important step in endodontic treatment. It determinates the best option for treatment. In 2017, Salgar, AR et al. rated electrical tests in comparison with thermal tests. He has shown that thermal tests are a better option in pulp vitality diagnosis than electrical tests [28]. Mainkar A. et al., compared five dental pulp tests: cold pulp testing (CPT), heat pulp testing (HPT), electric pulp testing (EPT), laser Doppler flowmetry (LDF), and pulse oximetry (PO). In their study, LDF and PO were the most accurate diagnostic methods and should be used by clinicians if possible. HPT was the least accurate diagnostic method [29]. In Poland, most of our respondents use traditional cold or heat tests. Only 17.86% use one of the newer tests (EPT, LDF or PO). From these,

EPT is used predominately. 26% of surveyed dentists say that these tests are more reliable than the traditional cold test.

Aggarwal, K et al. compared anxiety and pain levels during local anesthesia using traditional syringe and computer-controlled local anesthetic delivery (CCLAD). In their study, patients reported lower anxiety levels during CCLAD anesthesia. 64.4% of patients preferred CCLAD [30]. Mittal M. et al. have shown, in their study, that intraligamentary anesthesia can be more effective and less painful for children with the help of CCLADS devices [31]. Flisfisch S et al. evaluated patients opinions after local anesthesia with CCLAD and a conventional syringe. Most of the patients rated CCLAD as more acceptable [32]. Pozos-Guillén et al. delivered a meta-analysis about children's pain and fear levels during dental local anesthesia with the use of a standard syringe and CCLAD. The analysis shows that lower levels of negative emotions occurred when CCLAD was used [33]. In our study, 42.86% of respondents use CCLAD, but only 10.8% of them think that it is more effective than local anesthesia with the conventional syringe. Most of Polish dentists (73%) say CCLADS systems are as effective as the syringe.

One of the limitations to the study is that almost 65% of respondents fell into the category of having <5 or 5–10 years of practice, so they could have founding limitations. This can be the reason why more costly technologies are not used as frequently. Practitioners with more years in practice do not use social media as often as their younger colleagues, which could explain the low number of respondents in the category of >20 years of practice. The low numbers of obtained responses is a major limitation in this study. Further studies need to include other options of survey dissemination.

Publications Which Compare Use of Other Modern Technologies by Dentists in Europe

Nassar HM et al. conducted a survey about novel caries diagnostic technologies among restorative dentists. In their study, most dentists chose optical translumination (FOTI/DIFOTI) as the preferred method, saying that it has the widest clinical usage (i.e., for detecting enamel cracks) and is easy to use. The main reason for rejecting other methods was their high cost [34]. These findings greatly complement the results of our survey.

D. Tran et al. formed 1031 online surveys that were sent to a sample of UK dentists. 385 practitioners responded. Most users did not use any CAD/CAM technology and the main barriers to use this technology were, according to them, the lack of perceived benefit and initial costs as disadvantages. CAD/CAM technology was mainly used by dentists delivering private work. Most users of CAD/CAM technology were trained either by themselves or by companies, but on the other hand, a significant number of CAD/CAM users felt that their training was insufficient. 89% of respondents think that CAD/CAM has an important role in the future of dentistry [35].

Van der Zande et al. investigated the degree of digital technology use among general dental practitioners. A questionnaire was created that has reached 1000 practitioners in the Netherlands. The response rate was 31.3%. Dentists have adopted an average number of 6.3 ± 2.3 technologies. 22.5% were low technology users (0–4 technologies), 46.2% were intermediate technology users (5–7 technologies) and 31.3 were high technology users (8–12 technologies). What was interesting was that high technology users were younger on average ($p = 0.024$), had invested more hours per year in professional activities ($p = 0.026$), were more likely to have a specialization ($p < 0.001$), and also worked for more hours per week ($p = 0.003$) than low technology users. Among technologies that were asked about in a questionnaire were digital intraoral radiography, digital orthopantomogram, digital 3D radiography CBCT, intraoral camera and scanner, CAD/CAM systems, and others. According to the questionnaire, out of the nonclinical technologies, digital registration of patient information is the most frequently used technology (93.2%).

When it comes to clinical and diagnostic technologies, digital intraoral radiography (90%) and digital orthopantomograms (57.2%) are used most often.

The authors of the questionnaire confirm the importance of such a study, saying "Understanding where dentistry is going in terms of digital developments begins with knowing where dentistry stands now, and how digital technologies are incorporated at present." [36].

5. Conclusions

In Poland, dentists tend to use ultrasounds the most. Other technologies are not as popular. This may change in the future, as many dentists say that they will try some of the new technologies. In most cases, the usage of each technology did not depended on the size of office, work experience or sex. The most common reason for not using modern technologies was their high cost. This study showed that even if reports say some technologies are a better option, dentists prefer using conventional ones.

From the above data, it follows that the use of new technologies reduces dental procedure duration and makes treatment more effective. They allow for the detection of diseases in earlier stages, which directly relate to the reduction of therapy costs for patients and for the health care system (insurance system).

The authors are convinced that this research is an important addition in understanding the current state of technologies in dentistry.

Author Contributions: Conceptualization, M.Ś., M.D., M.S. and Z.R.; methodology, M.Ś. and W.Z.; formal analysis, M.Ś.; writing—original draft preparation, M.Ś. and W.Z.; writing—review and editing, M.D., M.S. and Z.R.; supervision, M.D., M.S. and Z.R. All authors have read and agreed to the published version of the manuscript.

Funding: This work was financed by a subsidy from Wroclaw Medical University, number SUBZ. B180.22.091.

Institutional Review Board Statement: Not applicable.

Informed Consent Statement: Not applicable.

Data Availability Statement: Not applicable.

Conflicts of Interest: The authors declare no conflict of interest.

References

1. Azarpazhooh, A.; Limeback, H. The application of ozone in dentistry: A systematic review of literature. *J. Dent.* **2008**, *36*, 104–116. [CrossRef] [PubMed]
2. Maiman, T.H. Stimulated Optical Radiation in Ruby. *Nature* **1960**, *187*, 493–494. [CrossRef]
3. Lussi, A.; Imwinkelried, S.; Pitts, N.B.; Longbottom, C.; Reich, E. Performance and Reproducibility of a Laser Fluorescence System for Detection of Occlusal Caries in vitro. *Caries Res.* **1999**, *33*, 261–266. [CrossRef] [PubMed]
4. Gopikrishna, V.; Tinagupta, K.; Kandaswamy, D. Evaluation of Efficacy of a New Custom-Made Pulse Oximeter Dental Probe in Comparison With the Electrical and Thermal Tests for Assessing Pulp Vitality. *J. Endod.* **2007**, *33*, 411–414. [CrossRef]
5. Friedman, M.J.; Hochman, M.N. A 21st century computerized injection system for local pain control. *Compend. Contin. Educ. Dent.* **1997**, *18*, 995–1003.
6. Available online: https://forms.gle/SKwkp97q1j54N3wF7 (accessed on 22 February 2019).
7. Verma, S.K.; Chaudhari, P.K.; Maheshwari, S.; Singh, R.K. Laser in dentistry: An innovative tool in modern dental practice. *Natl. J. Maxillofac. Surg.* **2012**, *3*, 124–132. [CrossRef]
8. Cozean, C.; Arcoria, C.J.; Pelagalli, J.; Powell, G.L. Dentistry for the 21st century? Erbium:Yag laser for teeth. *J. Am. Dent. Assoc.* **1997**, *128*, 1080–1087. [CrossRef]
9. Valenti, C.; Pagano, S.; Bozza, S.; Ciurnella, E.; Lomurno, G.; Capobianco, B.; Coniglio, M.; Cianetti, S.; Marinucci, L. Use of the Er:YAG Laser in Conservative Dentistry: Evaluation of the Microbial Population in Carious Lesions. *Materials* **2021**, *14*, 2387. [CrossRef]
10. Schwarz, F.; Arweiler, N.; Georg, T.; Reich, E. Desensitizing effects of an Er:YAG laser on hypersensitive dentine. *J. Clin. Periodontol.* **2002**, *29*, 211–215. [CrossRef]
11. Walmsley, D.; Laird, W.; Lumley, P. Ultrasound in dentistry. Part 2—periodontology and endodontics. *J. Dent.* **1992**, *20*, 11–17. [CrossRef]
12. Plotino, G.; Pameijer, C.H.; Grande, N.M.; Somma, F. Ultrasonics in Endodontics: A Review of the Literature. *J. Endod.* **2007**, *33*, 81–95. [CrossRef] [PubMed]
13. Abu Hasna, A.; Da Silva, L.P.; Pelegrini, F.C.; Ferreira, C.L.R.; De Oliveira, L.D.; Carvalho, C.A.T. Effect of sodium hypochlorite solution and gel with/without passive ultrasonic irrigation on Enterococcus faecalis, Escherichia coli and their endotoxins. *F1000Research* **2020**, *9*, 642. [CrossRef] [PubMed]

14. Verma, A.; Yadav, R.-K.; Tikku, A.-P.; Chandra, A.; Verma, P.; Bharti, R.; Shakya, V.-K. A randomized controlled trial of endodontic treatment using ultrasonic irrigation and laser activated irrigation to evaluate healing in chronic apical periodontitis. *J. Clin. Exp. Dent.* **2020**, *12*, e821–e829. [CrossRef] [PubMed]
15. Ealla, K.K.R.; Thomas, M.; Akula, U.; Gajjada, N. Piezosurgery: A boon for modern periodontics. *J. Int. Soc. Prev. Community Dent.* **2017**, *7*, 1–7. [CrossRef] [PubMed]
16. Agarwal, E. Escalating Role of Piezosurgery in Dental Therapeutics. *J. Clin. Diagn. Res.* **2014**, *8*, ZE08–11. [CrossRef] [PubMed]
17. Otake, Y.; Nakamura, M.; Henmi, A.; Takahashi, T.; Sasano, Y. Experimental Comparison of the Performance of Cutting Bone and Soft Tissue between Piezosurgery and Conventional Rotary Instruments. *Sci. Rep.* **2018**, *8*, 17154. [CrossRef] [PubMed]
18. Hegde, V.S.; Khatavkar, A.R. A new dimension to conservative dentistry: Air abrasion. *J. Conserv. Dent.* **2010**, *13*, 4–8. [CrossRef]
19. Bhushan, U.; Goswami, M. Evaluation of retention of pit and fissure sealants placed with and without air abrasion pretreatment in 6-8 year old children—An in vivo study. *J. Clin. Exp. Dent.* **2017**, *9*, e211–e217. [CrossRef]
20. Domb, W.C. Ozone Therapy in Dentistry. *Interv. Neuroradiol.* **2014**, *20*, 632–636. [CrossRef]
21. Gupta, G.; Mansi, B. Ozone therapy in periodontics. *J. Med. Life* **2012**, *5*, 59–67.
22. Gomez, J.L. Detection and diagnosis of the early caries lesion. *BMC Oral Health* **2015**, *15*, S3. [CrossRef]
23. Cho, K.H.; Kang, C.-M.; Jung, H.-I.; Lee, H.-S.; Lee, K.; Lee, T.Y.; Song, J.S. The diagnostic efficacy of quantitative light-induced fluorescence in detection of dental caries of primary teeth. *J. Dent.* **2021**, *115*, 103845. [CrossRef]
24. Venkataraghavan, K.; Kush, A.; Lakshminarayana, C.; Diwakar, L.; Ravikumar, P.; Patil, S.; Karthik, S. Chemomechanical Caries Removal: A Review & Study of an Indigen-ously Developed Agent (Carie Care (TM) Gel) In Children. *J. Int. Oral Health* **2013**, *5*, 84–90.
25. Sontakke, P.; Jain, P.; Patil, A.D.; Biswas, G.; Yadav, P.; Makkar, D.K.; Jeph, V.; Sakina, B.P. A comparative study of the clinical efficiency of chemo-mechanical caries removal using Carie-Care gel for permanent teeth of children of age group of 12-15 years with that of conventional drilling method: A randomized controlled trial. *Dent. Res. J.* **2019**, *16*, 42–46. [CrossRef]
26. Yavagal, C.; Prabhakar, A.; Lokeshwari, M.; Naik, S.V. Efficacy of Caries Removal by Carie-Care and Erbiumdoped Yttrium Aluminum Garnet Laser in Primary Molars: A Scanning Electron Microscope Study. *Int. J. Clin. Pediatr. Dent.* **2018**, *11*, 323–329. [CrossRef]
27. Cardoso, M.; Coelho, A.; Lima, R.; Amaro, I.; Paula, A.; Marto, C.M.; Sousa, J.; Spagnuolo, G.; Ferreira, M.M.; Carrilho, E. Efficacy and Patient's Acceptance of Alternative Methods for Caries Removal—a Systematic Review. *J. Clin. Med.* **2020**, *9*, 3407. [CrossRef]
28. Salgar, A.R.; Singh, S.H.; Podar, R.S.; Kulkarni, G.P.; Babel, S.N. Determining predictability and accuracy of thermal and electrical dental pulp tests: An in vivo study. *J. Conserv. Dent.* **2017**, *20*, 46–49. [CrossRef]
29. Mainkar, A.; Kim, S.G. Diagnostic Accuracy of 5 Dental Pulp Tests: A Systematic Review and Meta-analysis. *J. Endod.* **2018**, *44*, 694–702. [CrossRef]
30. Aggarwal, K.; Lamba, A.K.; Faraz, F.; Tandon, S.; Makker, K. Comparison of anxiety and pain perceived with conventional and computerized local anesthesia delivery systems for different stages of anesthesia delivery in maxillary and mandibular nerve blocks. *J. Dent. Anesthesia Pain Med.* **2018**, *18*, 367–373. [CrossRef]
31. Mittal, M.; Chopra, R.; Kumar, A.; Srivastava, D. Comparison of Pain Perception Using Conventional Versus Computer-Controlled Intraligamentary Local Anesthetic Injection for Extraction of Primary Molars. *Anesth. Prog.* **2019**, *66*, 69–76. [CrossRef]
32. Flisfisch, S.; Woelber, J.P.; Walther, W. Patient evaluations after local anesthesia with a computer-assisted method and a conventional syringe before and after reflection time: A prospective randomized controlled trial. *Heliyon* **2021**, *7*, e06012. [CrossRef] [PubMed]
33. Pozos-Guillén, A.; Loredo-Cruz, E.; Esparza-Villalpando, V.; Martínez-Rider, R.; Noyola-Frías, M.; Garrocho-Rangel, A. Pain and Anxiety Levels Using Conventional versus Computer-Controlled Local Anesthetic Systems in Pediatric Patients: A Meta-Analysis. *J. Clin. Pediatr. Dent.* **2020**, *44*, 371–399. [CrossRef] [PubMed]
34. Nassar, H.M.; Yeslam, H.E. Current Novel Caries Diagnostic Technologies: Restorative Dentists' Attitude and Use Preferences. *Healthcare* **2021**, *9*, 1387. [CrossRef] [PubMed]
35. Tran, D.; Nesbit, M.; Petridis, H. Survey of UK dentists regarding the use of CAD/CAM technology. *Br. Dent. J.* **2016**, *221*, 639–644. [CrossRef]
36. Van Der Zande, M.M.; Gorter, R.C.; Aartman, I.H.A.; Wismeijer, D. Adoption and Use of Digital Technologies among General Dental Practitioners in the Netherlands. *PLoS ONE* **2015**, *10*, e0120725. [CrossRef]

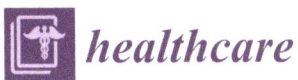

Article

A Design Approach to Optimise Secure Remote Three-Dimensional (3D) Printing: A Proof-of-Concept Study towards Advancement in Telemedicine

Xiao Wen Kok [1], Anisha Singh [2] and Bahijja Tolulope Raimi-Abraham [1,*]

[1] Institute of Pharmaceutical Science, King's College London, School of Cancer and Pharmaceutical Sciences, London SE1 9NH, UK; xwkok0630@gmail.com
[2] Institute for Security Science and Technology (ISST), Imperial Business School, Imperial College London, London W12 7TA, UK; anisha@wippit.net
* Correspondence: bahijja.raimi-abraham@kcl.ac.uk

Citation: Kok, X.W.; Singh, A.; Raimi-Abraham, B.T. A Design Approach to Optimise Secure Remote Three-Dimensional (3D) Printing: A Proof-of-Concept Study towards Advancement in Telemedicine. *Healthcare* 2022, 10, 1114. https://doi.org/10.3390/healthcare10061114

Academic Editor: Marco P. Soares dos Santos

Received: 15 December 2021
Accepted: 4 June 2022
Published: 15 June 2022

Publisher's Note: MDPI stays neutral with regard to jurisdictional claims in published maps and institutional affiliations.

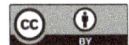

Copyright: © 2022 by the authors. Licensee MDPI, Basel, Switzerland. This article is an open access article distributed under the terms and conditions of the Creative Commons Attribution (CC BY) license (https://creativecommons.org/licenses/by/4.0/).

Abstract: Telemedicine is defined as the delivery of healthcare services at a distance using electronic means. The incorporation of 3D printing in the telemedicine cycle could result in pharmacists designing and manufacturing personalised medicines based on the electronic prescription received. Even with the advantages of telemedicine, numerous barriers to the uptake hinder the wider uptake. Of particular concern is the cyber risk associated with the remote digital transfer of the computer-aided design (CAD) file (acting as the electronic prescription) to the 3D printer and the reproducibility of the resultant printed medicinal products. This proof-of-concept study aimed to explore the application of secure remote 3D printing of model solid dosage forms using the patented technology, DEFEND3D, which is designed to enhance cybersecurity and intellectual property (IP) protection. The size, shape, and colour of the remote 3D-printed model medicinal products were also evaluated to ensure the end-product quality was user-focused. Thermoplastic polyurethane (TPU) and poly(lactic) acid (PLA) were chosen as model polymers due to their flexibility in preventing breakage printing and ease of printing with fused deposition modelling (FDM). Our work confirmed the potential of secure remote 3D (FDM) printing of prototype solid dosage forms resulting in products with good reproducibility, resolution, and quality towards advancements in telemedicine and digital pharmacies. The limitation of the work presented here was the use of model polymers and not pharmaceutically relevant polymers. Further work could be conducted using the same designs chosen in this study with pharmaceutically relevant polymers used in hot-melt extrusion (HME) with shown suitability for FDM 3D printing. However, it should be noted that any challenges that may occur with pharmaceutically relevant polymers are likely to be related to the polymer's printability and printer choice as opposed to the ability of the CAD file to be transferred to the printer remotely.

Keywords: 3D printing; additive manufacturing; telemedicine; patient-centric dosage form

1. Introduction

Telemedicine is defined as the delivery of healthcare services at a distance using electronic means [1]. As a result, telemedicine makes it easier for patients to receive healthcare services remotely, expanding the potential delivery of healthcare to patients across the world [2]. The telemedicine care cycle starts with healthcare providers conducting virtual medical consultations and remote diagnoses with patients using electronic means; electronic prescriptions are then produced and sent remotely to the pharmacies. It is thought that the introduction of three-dimensional (3D) printing (i.e., additive manufacturing method, where the object to be printed is developed through a computer-aided design (CAD)) in the telemedicine care cycle will transform compounding pharmacies into digital pharmacies [2,3] Moreover, 3D printing in pharmaceutical sciences allows for greater flexibility of fabrication capability in manufacturing patient-centric personalised medicines [1,4]. The incorporation of 3D printing in telemedicine could result in pharmacists designing and manufacturing personalised medicines based on the electronic prescriptions received [2]. The customised medicine would then be 3D-printed on-demand in a pharmacy setting [4]. Of concern in this area is the risk to the intellectual property (IP) during the storage, transmission, and execution of 3D printing through digital networks and systems [5,6]. Currently, in 3D printing, the entire digital file is transferred to the manufacturing device, making the digital IP vulnerable to cyberattacks, manipulation, and even theft [7]. Various solutions have been proposed to try and solve the issue of IP exposure, including blockchain, encryption, and licensing business models [8]. However, these solutions still require the complete transfer of the digital file.

The COVID-19 pandemic globally has overwhelmed health systems [9] and telemedicine has been thrust into the spotlight in the fight against COVID-19. The telemedicine approach has been employed in many different ways to better tackle the healthcare challenges that have arisen [10]. Telemedicine will likely have a more permanent place in traditional healthcare delivery long after the COVID-19 pandemic as users and providers recognise its advantages in improving global access to healthcare [9–11]. Even with the advantages of telemedicine, numerous barriers to uptake, such as education, cost, internet access, and patient digital literature, hinder its wider uptake [10]. Of particular concern is the cyber risk associated with the remote digital transfer of the CAD acting as the electronic prescription to the 3D printer and the reproducibility of the resultant printed medicinal products [7]. Additionally, as the shift toward telemedicine increases over time, new issues and risks as they relate to information security and privacy will need to be addressed and sufficiently managed [7].

The work presented in this proof-of-concept study aimed to explore the application of secure remote 3D printing of model solid dosage forms using the patented technology, DEFEND3D. The DEFEND3D platform is a patented secure streaming transfer protocol (SSTP), virtual inventory communications interface (VICI) designed to enhance cybersecurity and intellectual property (IP) protection. The VICI removes the need for file transfer and allows for secure digital resupply of reproduction parts remotely. An additional advantage of this technology means manufacturing and printing on demand can occur without the need for a specialist at the manufacturing or printing site [12]. The resultant remotely 3D-printed products are guaranteed to come out as designed [13].

Here, we focused on the secure remote printability of simple and complex pharmaceutically relevant designs, with a focus on evaluating their properties as they related to the patient experience when taking and accepting medication [14], i.e., visual and physical perception and optimisation of the CAD file and printing parameters (namely layer height and infill density). The size, shape, and colour of the remotely-3D-printed model medicinal products were also evaluated to ensure the end-product quality was user-focused [15]. Thermoplastic polyurethane (TPU) and poly(lactic) acid (PLA) were chosen as model polymers due to their flexibility in preventing breakage printing [16–18] and ease of printing with fused deposition modelling (FDM) [17,19] This proof-of-concept study seeks to explore the considerations in secure remote 3D printing towards optimisation for pharmaceutical use in the advancement of telemedicine and digital pharmacies.

2. Materials and Methods

2.1. Materials

Pink-, blue-, yellow-, and white-coloured 1.75 mm diameter thermoplastic polyurethane (TPU) filaments were purchased from Prima Creator (Malmo, Sweden) and neon pink, blue, and white 1.75 mm diameter poly(lactic) acid (PLA) filaments were purchased from Prima Creator.

2.2. Methods

2.2.1. Computer-Aided Design(s) (CAD)

The geometry of the 3D models to be remotely printed was designed using CAD drawing software, Blender v. 2.80 (Blender Foundation, Amsterdam, The Netherlands). The designs were developed by inserting default shapes and modifying them as required. The four designs (shown in Figure 1) were selected based on work by Goyanes et al. [20] where they investigated patient acceptability of 3D-printed medicines. Their findings showed that disc (design 1), torus (design 2), ring (design 3), and gummy-bear shapes (design 4) were among the most acceptable dosage forms by patients. In our work, designs 2 and 3 represented fixed-dose combination(s) (FDC), defined as two or more drugs combined in a fixed ratio into a single dosage form [21,22]. Innovative geometries [23,24] (i.e., design 4) were also included due to their potential to improve patient compliance. Designs were also chosen for their increasing design and printing complexities to challenge the capacity of the DEFEND3d platform in ensuring the integrity of the CAD design, file, and resultant remote printability.

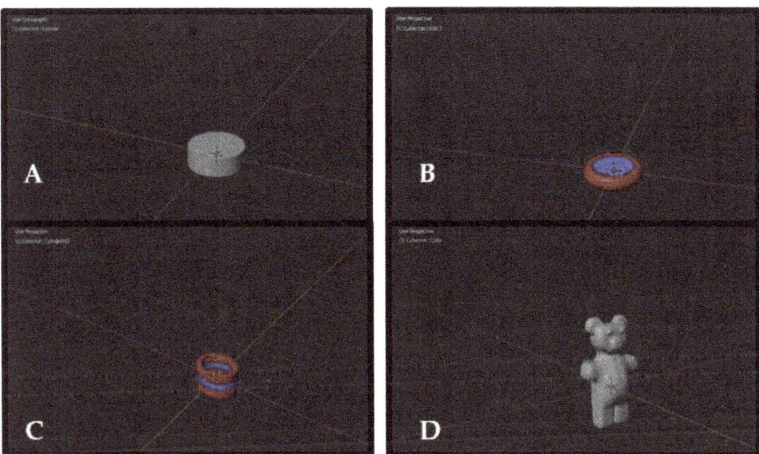

Figure 1. CAD of (**A**) design 1—disc shape ($12 \times 5 \times 4$ mm) (**B**) design 2—torus shape ($12 \times 6 \times 3$ mm) (**C**) design 3—ring shape ($9 \times 5 \times 5$ mm) (**D**) design 4—gummy-bear shape ($11 \times 20 \times 3$ mm), all rendered in Blender v. 2.8.

2.2.2. Remote-Fused Deposition Modelling (FDM) 3D Printing

All designs were remotely 3D-printed using the DEFEND3D platform. Due to the secure nature of the software, the in-depth workings of the algorithm are not able to be published. However, an overview of the workings of the platform can be provided. In brief, the DEFEND3D cybersecurity and transmission protocol allows for a safe remote method for controlled reproduction of an item that is represented by a digital asset stored in a trusted computing environment using a reproduction device (i.e., a 3D printer) in an untrusted computing environment. In practical terms, this is achieved by a continuous secure stream of production instructions to the machine with the use of Microsoft Azure Cloud services. The reproduction instructions are secured by six levels of security with encryption being only one of them. Variables, such as machine type, settings, and the material used, can be preset to enforce high manufacturing standards in the production process. The DEFEND3D platform allows for CAD files to be sliced using pre-defined gcode file pre-printing [14] and, therefore, eliminating the need for complex slicing software for the final CAD file and poor quality of the resultant printed product [25,26].

This study used FDM 3D printing. FDM 3D printing is an extrusion and thermo-based 3D printing technique where thermoplastic polymers are melted at a high temperature and solidified immediately onto the previous layer on the build plate [1,3,22]. Five different printing phases were required, which showed optimisation (namely printing quality and reproducibility to original CAD design) of the model dosage forms. Model solid dosage forms were remoted and printed using a Flashforge Creator Pro Dual Extruder via the DEFEND3D platform. The polymers used, the printer extruder type and the printing parameters are provided in Table 1.

Table 1. Summary of printing phases, polymers used, printer type (i.e., single or dual extruder), and printing parameters.

	Polymer	Printer Type i.e., Single/Dual Extruder	Printing Parameters			
			Nozzle Extrusion Temperature °C	Base Speed mm/s	Layer Height mm	Infill Density %
Phase 1			220	40	0.2	60
Phase 2	TPU	Single extruder		35	60	30
Phase 3			210	20		0, 15, 50, 100
Phase 4	PLA	Dual extruder		50	0.1	15
Phase 5						

2.2.3. Determination of Physical Properties

Visual observation, the physical properties, namely weight, diameter (d), length (l), and thickness (t) surface area (two dimensional (2D) and theoretical), and volume of the model solid dosage forms were recorded. A computerised surface analysis using ImageJ software (Bethesda, Maryland, USA) to calculate the two-dimensional (2D) surface area of printed products was carried out. The scale was calibrated to 300 distance in pixels of a known distance of 1, where the scale was set as 300 pixels/mm. The theoretical surface area (SA) and volume (Vol) were calculated using the equations listed in Table 2.

Table 2. Equations used to calculate the theoretical surface area (SA) and volume (Vol).

Equation	Equation Number
SA of design 1 $= 2\pi r^2 + 2\pi rt$	(1)
SA of design 2 $= 2\pi r^2 + 2\pi rt$	(2)
SA of design 3 $= [2\pi r_1^2 + 2\pi r_1 t] - [2\pi r_2^2 + 2\pi r_2 t]$	(3)
SA of design 4 $= 2dt + 2dl + 2tl$	(4)
Vol of design 1 $= \pi r^2 t$	(5)
Vol of design 2 $= \pi r^2 t$	(6)
Vol of design 3 $= [\pi r_1^2 t] - [\pi r_2^2 t]$	(7)
Vol of design 4 $= d \times l \times t$	(8)

3. Results

The design 1 to 5 prototypes were successfully remotely 3D-printed via the DEFEND3D platform using TPU and PLA printing filaments. Evaluations of the resultant remotely-printed products (general printability, visual appearance, and physical properties) are shown per design (Figures 2–4 and Tables 3–5).

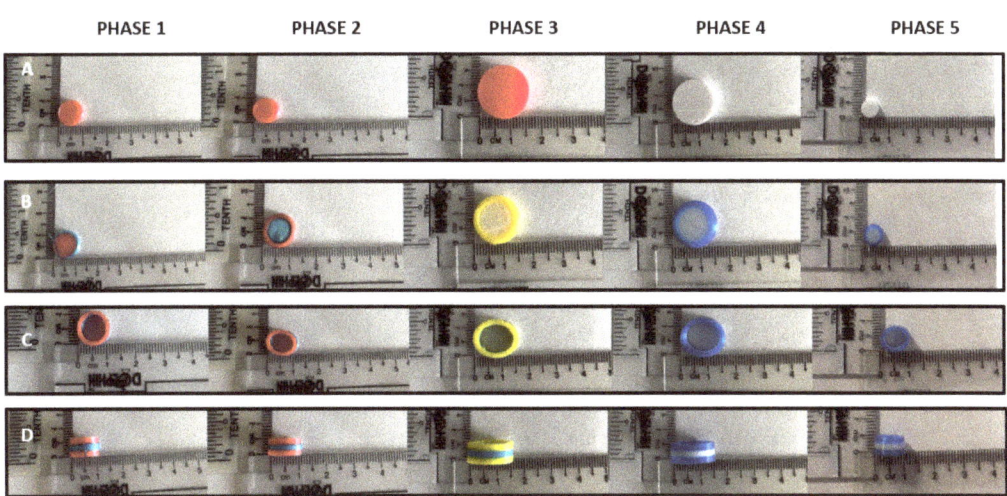

Figure 2. The 2D images of remotely-3D-printed model designs (**A**) 1, (**B**) 2, (**C**) 3—top view and (**D**) 3—side view phases 1 to 5.

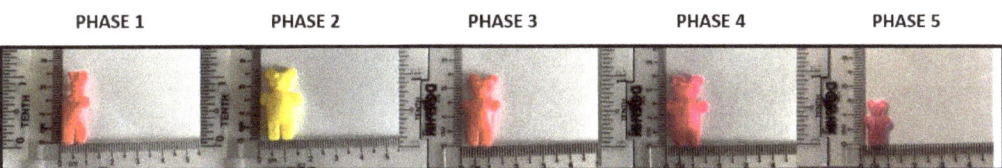

Figure 3. The 2D images of remotely 3D-printed design 4, phases 1 to 5.

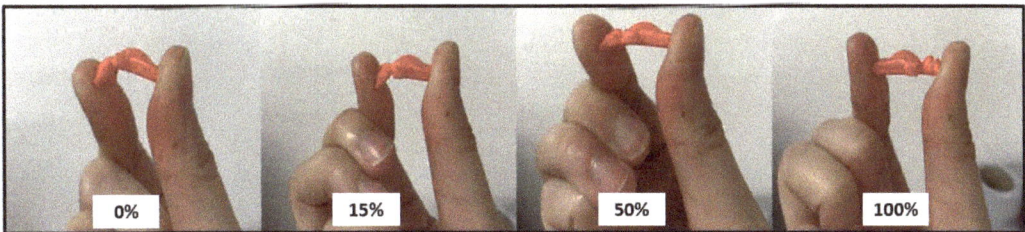

Figure 4. Design 4 (i.e., gummy bear shape) remotely 3D-printed at 0%, 15%, 50%, and 100% infill densities, showing different degrees that the prototypes could be bent manually (as an indication of flexibility).

Table 3. Physical properties of remotely-3D-printed model designs 1 to 3. Data for diameter, length, and thickness represent the mean ± standard deviation.

	Diameter ± SD (mm)	Length ± SD (mm)	Thickness ± SD (mm)	Weight (g)	2D Surface Area (mm^2)	Theoretical Surface Area (mm^2)	Theoretical Volume (mm^3)
Design 1							
Phase 1	10.00 ± 0.71	10.00 ± 0.71	4.50 ± 0.00	0.28	1.38	298.45	353.43
Phase 2	10.00 ± 0.00	10.00 ± 0.00	4.50 ± 0.07	0.26	1.35	298.45	353.43

Table 3. Cont.

	Diameter ± SD (mm)	Length ± SD (mm)	Thickness ± SD (mm)	Weight (g)	2D Surface Area (mm^2)	Theoretical Surface Area (mm^2)	Theoretical Volume (mm^3)
Phase 3	16.00 ± 0.00	16.00 ± 0.71	6.00 ± 0.71	0.67	5.53	703.72	1206.37
Phase 4	15.00 ± 0.00	15.00 ± 0.00	6.00 ± 0.00	0.85	4.11	636.17	1060.29
Phase 5	6.00 ± 0.00	6.00 ± 0.00	3.00 ± 0.00	0.09	0.68	113.10	84.82
Design 2							
Phase 1	12.00 ± 0.71	12.00 ± 0.71	3.00 ± 1.41	0.37	1.33	339.29	339.29
Phase 2	12.00 ± 0.71	12.00 ± 0.71	3.00 ± 1.41	0.43	2.27	339.39	339.39
Phase 3	15.00 ± 0.71	15.00 ± 0.71	6.00 ± 1.41	0.89	4.37	636.17	1060.29
Phase 4	14.00 ± 0.00	14.00 ± 0.00	5.00 ± 0.71	0.81	4.49	527.79	769.69
Phase 5	8.00 ± 2.12	8.00 ± 2.12	3.00 ± 0.71	0.11	0.77	175.93	150.80
Design 3							
Phase 1	11.00 ± 0.00	11.00 ± 0.00	6.00 ± 0.71	0.26	2.21	1.40	146.08
Phase 2	11.00 ± 0.00	11.00 ± 0.00	5.00 ± 0.00	0.33	1.62	1.37	175.93
Phase 3	13.00 ± 1.41	16.00 ± 0.71	6.00 ± 0.71	0.49	3.31	2.56	164.93
Phase 4	13.00 ± 0.71	16.00 ± 0.00	5.00 ± 0.71	0.43	3.52	2.19	155.50
Phase 5	8.00 ± 0.00	10.00 ± 0.00	5.00 ± 0.71	0.14	1.61	1.41	75.40

Table 4. Physical properties of 3D-printed gummy bear shape tablet (design 4). Data for diameter, length, and thickness represent the mean ± standard deviation (SD), where $n = 2$.

DESIGN 4	Diameter (mm)	Length (mm)	Thickness (mm)	Weight (g)	2D Surface Area (mm^2)	Theoretical Surface Area (mm^2)	Theoretical Volume (mm^3)
Phase 1	15.00 ± 0.00	25.00 ± 0.71	2.00 ± 0.71	0.67	3.16	910.00	750.00
Phase 2	15.00 ± 0.00	26.00 ± 0.00	4.00 ± 0.00	0.60	4.27	1168.00	1664.00
Phase 3	14.00 ± 0.71	24.00 ± 0.00	3.00 ± 0.35	0.58	3.92	900.00	1008.00
Phase 4	15.00 ± 0.71	24.00 ± 0.00	3.00 ± 0.35	0.97	4.25	954.00	1080.00
Phase 5	10.00 ± 0.35	15.00 ± 0.00	3.00 ± 0.71	0.21	1.84	450.00	450.00

Table 5. Different infill densities of 3D-printed gummy bear shape tablets (design 4). Data for diameter, length, and thickness represent the mean ± standard deviation (SD), where $n = 2$.

Infill Densities	Diameter (mm)	Length (mm)	Thickness (mm)	Weight (g)	2D Surface Area (mm^2)	Theoretical Surface Area (mm^2)	Theoretical Volume (mm^3)
0%	14.00 ± 0.71	24.00 ± 0.00	3.00 ± 0.35	0.58	3.92	900.00	1008.00
15%	14.00 ± 0.71	24.00 ± 0.71	3.00 ± 0.00	0.62	2.69	900.00	1008.00
50%	13.00 ± 0.00	24.00 ± 0.00	3.00 ± 0.00	0.67	3.20	846.00	936.00
100%	14.00 ± 0.00	25.00 ± 0.71	3.00 ± 0.35	1.16	3.65	934.00	1050.00

3.1. Remote Printability

All designs were remotely printable with varied resolutions, which were optimised with changes in the printing parameters (namely base speed, layer height, infill density, and extrusion temperature) and are shown in Figure 2A–D. Prototypes remotely printed in printing phases 1 to 3 were modified to optimise geometry. The phase 1 model solid dosage form prototypes were of clinical relevance; they were designed to be within the range of size 2 (18 × 6.35 mm) and size 3 capsules (15.9 × 5.82 mm) [14,15,20,27]. Printing phases 4 and 5 involved modifications to optimise the resolution and quality of the remotely-printed model solid dosage forms.

3.2. Visual Observations and Physical Properties of Remotely-Printed Products for Designs 1 to 3

The remotely-3D-printed design 1 (disc shape), shown in Figure 2A, was the simplest design to be printed in this study. Overall, phase 5 models of this design, which involved modifications to optimise the resolution and quality, were found to have the best quality, with the smoothest surfaces, good filament colour distributions, and improved resolutions compared to phases 1–4. Phase 1 remotely-3D-printed model dosage forms had the roughest surfaces to touch compared to phases 2–5 remotely-3D-printed model dosage forms. The remotely-3D-printed model design 2 (phases 1–5), which had an outer torus shape with a flat disc shape inserted into the hollow area achieved by dual extruder FDM printing, is shown in Figure 2B. The phase 1 remotely-printed design 2 model tablets did not have optimal resolutions and well-separated colour distributions. Phases 1 and 2 remotely-printed prototypes had the roughest surfaces upon touching, whereas phase 5 had the smoothest surface among all. Phase 3 to 5 remotely-printed models showed a uniform colour distribution and overall visual appearance.

In general, design 1, 2, and 3 remotely-printed prototypes showed great reproducibility; the mean diameter, length, and thickness had small variations (with a standard deviation of less than 0.8 mm) with the exceptions of design 2–phase 5 and design 3–phase 3 remotely-printed solid dosage form prototypes, which saw larger standard deviation variations at 2.12 and 1.41 mm, respectively. As expected, the overall weight and theoretical volume (mm^3) increased with an increase in prototype dimensions. Images from Figure 2A–D were used to measure the 2D surface areas of the remotely-printed solid dosage form prototypes. The 2D surface area was expected to have a much smaller surface area compared to the theoretical surface area. Results shown in Table 3 support this statement; for example, the design 1–phase 1 remotely-printed tablet 2D surface area (using Figure 2A) was 1.38 mm^2, and 298.45 mm^2 when calculated theoretically.

3.3. Design 4—Gummy Bear Shape

Images of remotely-printed prototypes for design 4 (i.e., 3D-printed gummy bear shape prototype solid dosage forms) phases 1 to 5, and the physical properties, are shown in Figure 3 and Table 4, respectively. The "belly" of the remotely printed design (in phases 1 and 2) showed evidence of the "staircase effect" where layering or layered marks were visible on 3D-printed parts, resulting in a rougher feel of the prototype. The "face" features of the designs were not distinguishable in remotely-printed prototypes from phases 1 and 2. The staircase effect was reduced in remotely-printed phase 2 to 5 designs with an increase in appearance, smoothness to touch, and overall improved quality. The feel of a solid dosage form greatly influences patient acceptability [19]. The theoretical surface area and volume were calculated using the formula for calculating a rectangular because the CAD was developed from a rectangular shape before further modifying into a gummy bear shape; therefore, the values were expected to be slightly greater. As a result of this, the values will be overestimated in the facial parts of the gummy bears as they were made up of irregular shapes.

3.4. Design 4—Different Infill Densities

Overall, the focus of the work detailed in this study was to explore the remote printability of simple and complex pharmaceutically relevant designs. Considerations of 3D printing in pharmaceutical sciences include varying the percentage infill density (also referred to as the infill percentage) as a strategy to generate chewable and more flexible solid dosage forms. Such formulations are ideal for patients with swallowing difficulties. To push the potential of remote 3D printing of solid dosage forms (prototypes) in this study using the DEFEND3D platform, the infill densities of design 4, as well as the phase 3 prototypes, were remotely 3D-printed at 0, 15, 50, and 100% infill densities (Figure 4). The flexibility (from a patient perspective) was explored by bending each resultant remotely-printed product by hand, with flexibility increasing with decreased infill densities, as shown in Figure 4. The infill density influenced the overall weight of the remotely-printed prototype (as expected), where 100% infill density had the greatest weight (i.e., 1.16 g) compared to the tablet with 0% infill density (0.58 g) (Table 5). This is because the greater the infill percentage, the more polymer is deposited inside the object, resulting in a lesser deformation [28,29]

4. Discussion

The proof-of-concept study detailed here addressed the potential of secure (using the SSTP, VICI-patented DEFEND3D platform) remote 3D (FDM) printing of simple and complex pharmaceutically relevant designs as it related to patient experiences when taking and accepting their medications, CAD, and printing optimisation. Solid dosage form prototypes were generated using model polymers, TPU and PLA. All simple and complex designs were successfully remotely and securely 3D-printed (FDM) using the DEFEND3D platform. For all designs, phase 5 models through the DEFEND3D profile (which involved modifications to optimise resolution and quality) were found to have the best quality, smoothest surfaces, good filament colour distributions, and improved resolutions compared to phases 1–4 of all designs. Physical properties (i.e., diameter, length, thickness, weight, surface area, and volume (both theoretical and experimental)) increased with increased prototype dimensions, as expected. Further work was explored with design 4 with remote 3D printing of prototypes with varied infill densities. Varying the infill density in the development of 3D-printed solid dosage forms expands the application of the resultant products as chewable and more flexible dosage forms. Design 4–phase 3 prototypes at 0, 15, 50, and 100% infill densities were successfully remotely 3D-printed. Flexibility (from a patient perspective) was greatest at the lowest infill density (i.e., 0% infill density %).

This work highlights the potential of secure remote 3D (FDM) printing of prototype solid dosage forms resulting in products with good reproducibility, resolution, and quality towards advancement in telemedicine and digital pharmacies. The ability to provide a healthcare service that would start with a consultation, diagnosis, a prescription, and ideally dispensing of the appropriate medicinal product remotely [2], will advance the potential of telemedicine to wider populations and regions globally. This has the potential to reduce global medicine access issues. The uptake of this emerging healthcare process requires barriers to be addressed to facilitate its advancement.

Medication manufacturing and dispensing as it relates to telemedicine and digital pharmacies can be supported by the implementation of 3D printing in the telemedicine care cycle. However, barriers to uptake need to be addressed. The cybersecurity risk associated with the remote digital transfer of a CAD file (acting as the electronic prescription to the printer) has been explored in this study with the use of the DEFEND3D platform, a patented SSTP, VICI designed to enhance the cybersecurity of remote 3D-printed products. The DEFEND3D pre-defines each printer's profile by selecting the appropriate print speed at various points, layer height, and infill percentage to ensure the optimised quality of prints to be produced [12]. DEFEND3D's commercial application allows the functionality to drag and drop CAD files into an application within a trusted environment without any knowledge of slicing software and with no 3D printing experience. These files are then sliced for use in several integrated FDM-type desktop machines that have been pre-defined by a DEFEND3D CAD engineer to allow an optimised print performance. This could be advantageous in digital pharmacies to ensure consistency across all prints, making sure that accurate doses are present in each formulation, as well as reducing the labour burden. Various regulatory concerns are circulating regarding the introduction of 3D printing into pharmacies. Copyright issues are often encountered in 3D printing. The CAD designed using dedicated 3D software by pharmacists undoubtedly involves human intellect, which is considered an intellectual property that needs to be protected against proliferation use [30]. DEFEND3D allows the secure transmission of virtual inventory to be delivered instantly without revealing intellectual property. The 3D file will always remain on the source computer, meaning the file cannot be stolen or manipulated by someone else.

5. Conclusions

Our work has confirmed the ability of the platform to successfully remotely 3D-print simple and complex pharmaceutically relevant designs at various infill densities. The limitation of the work presented here involves the use of model polymers and not pharmaceutically relevant polymers. This study focused on remote printability as it related to the shape complexity of pharmaceutical relevance and not the materials used. TPU and PLA were chosen due to their flexibility, ease of printing via FDM 3D printing, and to prevent breakage printing. This study has confirmed the possibility of secure remote printing of pharmaceutically relevant-shaped solid dosage forms.

Further work could be conducted using the same designs chosen in this study but with pharmaceutically relevant polymers used in hot-melt extrusion (HME) with demonstrated suitability for FDM 3D printing [31], such as poly(vinyl alcohol) [32]. However, it should be noted that any challenges that may occur with pharmaceutically relevant polymers are likely to be related to the polymer's printability and printer choice as opposed to the ability of the CAD file to be transferred to the printer remotely.

Author Contributions: Conceptualization, B.T.R.-A.; methodology, X.W.K., A.S., B.T.R.-A.; software, A.S., B.T.R.-A.; validation, X.W.K., A.S. and B.T.R.-A.; formal analysis, X.W.K.; investigation, X.W.K.; resources, B.T.R.-A. and A.S.; data curation, X.W.K.; writing—original draft preparation, X.W.K.; writing—review and editing, A.S. and B.T.R.-A.; visualization, B.T.R.-A. and A.S.; supervision, A.S. and B.T.R.-A.; project administration, B.T.R.-A.; funding acquisition, B.T.R.-A. All authors have read and agreed to the published version of the manuscript.

Funding: This research received no external funding.

Institutional Review Board Statement: Not applicable.

Informed Consent Statement: Not applicable.

Data Availability Statement: Data available on request.

Conflicts of Interest: Anisha Patel was employed by Wippit and now DEFEND3D.

References

1. Tan, D.K.; Maniruzzaman, M.; Nokhodchi, A. Advanced Pharmaceutical Applications of Hot-Melt Extrusion Coupled with Fused Deposition Modelling (FDM) 3D Printing for Personalised Drug Delivery. *Pharmaceutics* **2018**, *10*, 203. [CrossRef]
2. Araújo, M.R.P.; Sa-Barreto, L.L.; Gratieri, T.; Gelfuso, G.M.; Cunha-Filho, M. The Digital Pharmacies Era: How 3D Printing Technology Using Fused Deposition Modeling Can Become a Reality. *Pharmaceutics* **2019**, *11*, 128. [CrossRef]
3. Long, J.; Gholizadeh, H.; Lu, J.; Bunt, C.; Seyfoddin, A. Application of Fused Deposition Modelling (FDM) Method of 3D Printing in Drug Delivery. *Curr. Pharm. Des.* **2017**, *23*, 433–439. [CrossRef]
4. Lim, S.H.; Kathuria, H.; Tan, J.J.Y.; Kang, L. 3D printed drug delivery and testing systems—A passing fad or the future? *Adv. Drug Deliv. Rev.* **2018**, *132*, 139–168. [CrossRef]
5. Madla, C.M.; Trenfield, S.J.; Goyanes, A.; Gaisford, S.; Basit, A.W. 3D Printing technologies, implementation and regulation: An overview. In *3D Printing of Pharmaceuticals*, 1st ed.; Basit, A., Gaisford, S., Eds.; Springer: London, UK, 2018; Volume 31, pp. 21–40.
6. U.S. Department of Health and Human Services; Food and Drug Administration; Center for Devices and Radiological Health; Center for Biologics Evaluation and Research. *Technical Considerations for Additive Manufactured Medical Devices: Guidance for Industry and Food and Drug Administration Staff*; Center for Biologics Evaluation and Research: Silver Spring, MD, USA, 2017.
7. Mirza, M.A.; Iqbal, Z. 3D Printing in Pharmaceuticals: Regulatory Perspective. *Curr. Pharm. Des.* **2018**, *24*, 5081–5083. [CrossRef]
8. Doarn, C.R.; Merrell, R.C. Accessibility and Vulnerabilty: Ensuring Security of Data in Telemedicine. *Telemed. e-Health* **2015**, *21*, 143–144. [CrossRef]
9. Ahmed, S.; Sanghvi, K.; Yeo, D. Telemedicine takes centre stage during COVID-19 pandemic. *BMJ Innov.* **2020**, *6*, 252–254. [CrossRef]
10. Jalali, M.S.; Landman, A.; Gordon, W.J. Telemedicine, privacy, and information security in the age of COVID-19. *J. Am. Med. Inform. Assoc.* **2021**, *28*, 671–672. [CrossRef]
11. Montelongo, A.; Becker, J.L.; Roman, R.; de Oliveira, E.B.; Umpierre, R.N.; Gonçalves, M.R.; Silva, R.; Doniec, K.; Yetisen, A.K. The management of COVID-19 cases through telemedicine in Brazil. *PLoS ONE* **2021**, *16*, e02543399. [CrossRef]
12. DEFEND3D Official Website. Available online: https://www.defend3d.com/#about (accessed on 1 December 2021).

13. Trenfield, S.J.; Madla, C.M.; Basit, A.W.; Gaisford, S. The shape of things to come: Emerging applications of 3D printing in healthcare. In *3D Printing of Pharmaceuticals*, 1st ed.; Basit, A., Gaisford, S., Eds.; Springer: London, UK, 2018; Volume 31, pp. 1–19.
14. Fastø, M.M.; Genina, N.; Kaae, S.; Kälvemark Sporrong, S. Perceptions, preferences and acceptability of patient designed 3D printed medicine by polypharmacy patients: A pilot study. *Int. J. Clin. Pharm.* **2019**, *41*, 1290–1298. [CrossRef]
15. Ranmal, S.R.; Cram, A.; Tuleu, C. Age-appropriate and acceptable paediatric dosage forms: Insights from end-user perceptions, preferences and practices from the Children's Acceptability of Oral Formulations (CALF) Study. *Int. J. Pharm.* **2016**, *514*, 296–307. [CrossRef] [PubMed]
16. Jain, A.; Bansal, K.K.; Tiwari, A.; Rosling, A.; Rosenholm, J.M. Role of Polymers in 3D Printing Technology for Drug Delivery—An Overview. *Curr. Pharm. Des.* **2018**, *24*, 4979–4990. [CrossRef] [PubMed]
17. Baran, E.H.; Erbil, H.Y. Surface Modification of 3D Printed PLA Objects by Fused Deposition Modeling: A Review. *Colloids Interfaces* **2019**, *3*, 43. [CrossRef]
18. Van den Eynde, M.; van Puyvelde, P. *3D Printing of Poly(lactic acid), in Industrial Applications of Poly(lactic acid)*; di Lorenzo, M.L., Androsch, R., Eds.; Springer International Publishing: Cham, Switzerland, 2018; pp. 139–158.
19. Mazzanti, V.; Malagutti, L.; Mollica, F. FDM 3D Printing of Polymers Containing Natural Fillers: A Review of their Mechanical Properties. *Polymers* **2019**, *11*, 1094. [CrossRef] [PubMed]
20. Goyanes, A.; Scarpa, M.; Kamlow, M.; Gaisford, S.; Basit, A.W.; Orlu, M. Patient acceptability of 3D printed medicines. *Int. J. Pharm.* **2017**, *530*, 71–78. [CrossRef]
21. Guideline on Clinical Development of Fixed Combination Medicinal Products. 2017. Available online: https://www.ema.europa.eu/en/clinical-development-fixed-combination-medicinal-products (accessed on 14 December 2021).
22. Chew, S.L.; de Mohac, L.M.; Raimi-Abraham, B.T. 3D-Printed Solid Dispersion Drug Products. *Pharmaceutics* **2019**, *11*, 672. [CrossRef]
23. Gerrard, S.E.; Walsh, J.; Bowers, N.; Salunke, S.; Hershenson, S. Innovations in Pediatric Drug Formulations and Administration Technologies for Low Resource Settings. *Pharmaceutics* **2019**, *11*, 518. [CrossRef]
24. Pravin, S.; Sudhir, A. Integration of 3D printing with dosage forms: A new perspective for modern healthcare. *Biomed. Pharmacother.* **2018**, *107*, 146–154. [CrossRef]
25. Chung, M.; Radacsi, N.; Robert, C.; McCarthy, E.D.; Callanan, A.; Conlisk, N.; Hoskins, P.R.; Koutsos, V. On the optimization of low-cost FDM 3D printers for accurate replication of patient-specific abdominal aortic aneurysm geometry. *3D Print. Med.* **2018**, *4*, 2. [CrossRef]
26. Arnold, C.; Monsees, D.; Hey, J.; Schweyen, R. Surface Quality of 3D-Printed Models as a Function of Various Printing Parameters. *Materials* **2019**, *12*, 1970. [CrossRef]
27. Liu, F.; Ranmal, S.; Batchelor, H.K.; Orlu-Gul, M.; Ernest, T.B.; Thomas, I.W.; Flanagan, T.; Tuleu, C. Patient-centred pharmaceutical design to improve acceptability of medicines: Similarities and differences in paediatric and geriatric populations. *Drugs* **2014**, *74*, 1871–1889. [CrossRef] [PubMed]
28. Kuznetsov, V.E.; Solonin, A.N.; Urzhumtsev, O.D.; Schilling, R.; Tavitov, A.G. Strength of PLA Components Fabricated with Fused Deposition Technology Using a Desktop 3D Printer as a Function of Geometrical Parameters of the Process. *Polymers* **2018**, *10*, 313. [CrossRef] [PubMed]
29. Mogan, Y.P. Thermoplastic Elastomer Infill Pattern Impact on Mechanical Properties 3D Printed Customized Orthotic Insole. 2015. Available online: https://www.semanticscholar.org/paper/THERMOPLASTIC-ELASTOMER-INFILL-PATTERN-IMPACT-ON-3D-mogan/09914aeb177ebeebe9c1d13aa990f394d2b3bccc (accessed on 14 December 2021).
30. 3D Printing and Intellectual Property Futures. I.P. Office. Available online: https://assets.publishing.service.gov.uk/government/uploads/system/uploads/attachment_data/file/757767/3D-printing.pdf (accessed on 14 December 2021).
31. Cunha-Filho, M.; Araújo, M.R.; Gelfuso, G.M.; Gratieri, T. FDM 3D printing of modified drug-delivery systems using hot melt extrusion: A new approach for individualized therapy. *Ther. Deliv.* **2017**, *8*, 957–966. [CrossRef] [PubMed]
32. Azad, M.A.; Olawuni, D.; Kimbell, G.; Badruddoza, A.; Hossain, M.S.; Sultana, T. Polymers for Extrusion-Based 3D Printing of Pharmaceuticals: A Holistic Materials-Process Perspective. *Pharmaceutics* **2020**, *12*, 124. [CrossRef]

MDPI
St. Alban-Anlage 66
4052 Basel
Switzerland
Tel. +41 61 683 77 34
Fax +41 61 302 89 18
www.mdpi.com

Healthcare Editorial Office
E-mail: healthcare@mdpi.com
www.mdpi.com/journal/healthcare

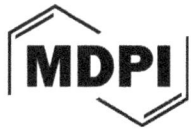

www.ingramcontent.com/pod-product-compliance
Lightning Source LLC
LaVergne TN
LVHW070452100526
838202LV00014B/1711